Springer Series in Cognitive Development

Series Editor
Charles J. Brainerd

Springer Series in Cognitive Development

Series Editor: Charles J. Brainerd

Recent Advances in Cognitive-Developmental Theory
Progress in Cognitive Development Research

Edited by
Charles J. Brainerd

Springer-Verlag
New York   Heidelberg   Berlin

Charles J. Brainerd
Department of Psychology
University of Western Ontario
London, Ontario
Canada N6A 5C2

...... ɔ5 Figures

Library of Congress Cataloging in Publication Data
Main entry under title:
Recent advances in cognitive-developmental theory.
   (Springer series in cognitive development)
   Contents: Social learning theory: a contextualist
account of cognitive functioning/Barry J. Zimmerman—
The development of two concepts/Robert S. Siegler and
D. Dean Richards—Gene-culture linkages and the
developing mind/Charles J. Lumsden—[etc.]
   1. Cognition in children—Addresses, essays, lec-
tures. I. Brainerd, Charles J. II. Series. [DNLM:
1. Child development.   2. Cognition—In infancy and
childhood.   WS 105.5.C7 R295]
BF723.C5R43   1983   155.4′13   82–19466

Typeset by Publishers' Service, Bozeman, Montana.
Printed and bound by R.R. Donnelley and Sons, Harrisonburg, Virginia.
Printed in the United States of America.
9 8 7 6 5 4 3 2 1

ISBN 0-387-90767-X   Springer-Verlag   New York   Heidelberg   Berlin
ISBN 3-540-90767-X   Springer-Verlag   Berlin   Heidelberg   New York

Series Preface

For some time now, the study of cognitive development has been far and away the most active discipline within developmental psychology. Although there would be much disagreement as to the exact proportion of papers published in developmental journals that could be considered cognitive, 50% seems like a conservative estimate. Hence, a series of scholarly books devoted to work in cognitive development is especially appropriate at this time.

The *Springer Series in Cognitive Development* contains two basic types of books, namely, edited collections of original chapters by several authors, and original volumes written by one author or a small group of authors. The flagship for the Springer Series is a serial publication of the "advances" type, carrying the subtitle *Progress in Cognitive Development Research*. Each volume in the *Progress* sequence is strongly thematic, in that it is limited to some well-defined domain of cognitive-developmental research (e.g., logical and mathematical development, development of learning). All *Progress* volumes will be edited collections. Editors of such collections, upon consultation with the Series Editor, may elect to have their books published either as contributions to the *Progress* sequence or as separate volumes. All books written by one author or a small group of authors are being published as separate volumes within the series.

A fairly broad definition of cognitive development is being used in the selection of books for this series. The classic topics of concept development, children's thinking and reasoning, the development of learning, language development, and memory development will, of course, be included. So, however, will newer areas such as social-cognitive development, educational applications, formal modeling, and philosophical implications of cognitive-developmental theory. Although it is anticipated that most books in the series will be empirical in orientation, theoretical and philosophical works are also welcome. With books of the latter sort, heterogeneity of theoretical perspective is encouraged, and no attempt will be made to foster some specific theoretical perspective at the expense of others (e.g., Piagetian versus behavioral or behavioral versus information processing).

C. J. Brainerd

Preface

This is the third contribution to the *Progress in Cognitive Development* sequence. Whereas the previous volumes were concerned with mathematical cognition and verbal processes, this one deals with current events in the area of cognitive-developmental theory.

The motivation for selecting such a theme arises from the present situation in cognitive-developmental theory. The situation can reasonably be described as one of extreme theoretical pluralism, coupled with much uncertainty about where we are going. This state of affairs has been brought about by a rapid decline in the influence of orthodox Piagetian theory, a fact that is now acknowledged by Piagetians and nonPiagetians alike. Until the mid-1970's, Piaget's ideas dominated the landscape the way Freudian thinking once ruled abnormal psychology. Since then, however, the picture has changed dramatically. Empirical and conceptual objections to the theory have become so numerous that it can no longer be regarded as a positive force in main stream cognitive-developmental research, though its influence remains profound in cognate fields such as education and sociology.

On the empirical side, the criticisms have tended to be of two sorts, namely, that the theory's predictions are not borne out by data and that its key predictions are untestable. Perhaps the best-known illustrations in the first category are predictions about learning. The theory says that children should not be able to learn concepts that are clearly above their current stage of cognitive development. It also says that children's susceptibility to training will increase as their current stage approaches the one at which the to-be-learned concept "spontaneously" appears. In Piaget's familiar words, children's learning will "vary very significantly as a function of the initial cognitive levels of the children," and "teaching children concepts that they have not acquired in their spontaneous development . . . is completely useless." These predictions have frequently been studied with concepts from the concrete-operational stage, especially conservation concepts, and the results have been consistently disconfirmatory. It has been found that children who are classified as preoperational can learn concrete-operational concepts, and it also has been found that children's susceptibility to learning does not covary to any marked degree with their pretraining stage classifications.

Turning to the other category of empirical objections, the most prominent example concerns invariant sequences in the developmental ordering of concepts. As everyone knows, children are supposed to pass through Piagetian stages in a universal order. This leads to what is undoubtedly the theory's most famous prediction: Children shall acquire certain concepts, those belonging to different stages, in an immutable sequence. Twenty years ago, putting this prediction to the test appeared to be a simple matter; all one had to do was administer tests for different-stage concepts to samples of children and see whether or not the tests were passed in the prescribed sequence. Although many studies of this sort were reported, it turns out that their data are completely uninterpretable for conceptual reasons. The main difficulties are the problem of measurement sequences and the problem of measurement errors. Regarding the former, most of the sequences featured in the theory have the peculiarity of being concerned with concepts that are linked via inclusion relationships. The prototype sequence is one where (*a*) there are two concepts, A and B, (*b*) the theory predicts "A before B," but (*c*) Concept A is a component of Concept B (i.e., Concept B = Concept A + other things) and not conversely. (An illustration that is commonly cited in the literature involves classification concepts. When a set of objects varies along more than one physical dimension, the theory anticipates that children will be able to classify the objects using one dimension before they will be able to classify them using two dimensions. But, logically, the ability to effect two-dimensional classifications presupposes one-dimensional classification.) If an inclusion relationship obtains, it is impossible to measure Concept B validly without also measuring Concept A and, for this reason, such relationships have come to be called measurement sequences. The difficulty with measurement sequences is that the opposite of the predicted ordering ("B before A") is a logical impossibility. Consequently, such sequences are not "predictions" at all; they are tautologies.

The measurement error problem is simply that there is more than one way for children to pass or fail any test for a target concept and we do not know how to distinguish these events in data. When children pass a concept test, it may be that they have the concept or it may be that they do not have it but a false positive error was committed. When children fail a concept test, it may be that they do not have the concept or it may be that they do have it but a false negative error was committed. Thus, if the data show that children pass an A test before they pass a B test, we cannot tell whether it is because there is a true A $\rightarrow$ B sequence or whether the false positive rate is higher on the A test or whether the false negative rate is higher on the B test.

Although these empirical criticisms are worrisome enough, there is a still deeper set of objections as to the theoretical utility of Piaget's conceptual machinery. Here, two of the most troublesome points are obscurity and seeming lack of explanatory power. The obscurity problem refers to the fact that no one is confident about the proper meanings of such fundamental notions as "stage," "cognitive structure," "equilibration," and so forth. Consequently, conflicting interpretations abound and, more important, we do not know how to set about measuring the relevant variables. For some years, it was fashionable to suppose that Piagetian constructs, like the ideas of quantum physicists, were merely difficult for the average mind to comprehend and that careful study of the theory would dispel the conceptual fog. As this has not happened, a more plausible hypothesis is that the theory is intrinsically opaque. Insofar as explanatory power is concerned, the litmus test for any theory in science is its capacity to explain the facts; to tell us why our data are as they are. It has become increasingly evident that whatever the ultimate definitions of "stage," "equilibration," etc. may be, they are at most descriptive generalizations from behavior. Hence, the chances are that any systematic attempt to use such concepts to explain data (e.g., as in "children do *x* because they are at Stage S" or "children do *x* because they have cognitive structure C") is doomed to circularity.

In the face of such perplexities, it is natural that students of cognitive development would turn to other lines of theoretical attack. But this new work presents an important difficulty of its own. As Piagetian writers have often remarked, the purview of post-Piaget theorizing has been quite narrow. The trend has been to develop theories that account for the fine-grain details of children's acquisition of single concepts (e.g., transitivity, object permanence), not to develop theories that account for the acquisition of several concepts. A case in point is that of the uncounted microtheories of conservation acquisition. Of course, microtheories have the advantage of usually being susceptible to test because, unlike Piagetian theory, their boundary conditions are well defined. But they leave us in the dark about cognitive development as a whole. It may be that our desire for an integrative account of cognitive development is intemperate, but it is nevertheless a desire that most researchers share.

Although post-Piaget theorizing has been narrow in scope, microtheories are not an inevitable consequence of the demise of Piagetian theory. In fact, several frameworks have been emerging lately that promise generality. Whether or not they deliver it is, naturally, another matter. The aim of this volume is to present some frameworks of this sort, each in a separate chapter, and thereby dispel the impression that microtheorizing has captured the field. The specific theories that are covered are contextualism (Zimmerman's chapter), the rule-oriented approach (Siegler and Richard's chapter), sociobiology (Lumsden's chapter), working-memory analysis (Brainerd's chapter), and ethology (Charlesworth's chapter). As a group, an interesting feature of these theories is that they have evolved from rather different traditions within the behavioral sciences. Contextualism is firmly rooted in social learning theory, sociobiological and ethological analyses of cognitive development have grown out of evolutionary biology, and the rule-oriented and working-memory approaches rely on modern information-processing concepts. Despite the fact that all the theories aspire to some level of generality, the phenomena with which they are most at home are not necessarily identical. For example, nomothetic aspects of concept development serve as the empirical background for the contextualist, rule-oriented, and working-memory chapters, whereas sociobiology and ethology hit their stride with individual differences.

In planning this volume, a tactical decision had to be taken about whether to cover as many emerging theories as possible, each in a brief chapter, or to cover fewer theories in longer chapters. At the time, it seemed that chapters of sufficient length to permit authors to present a thorough exegesis of their views would be of greater scholarly value than short, highlight chapters. However, this decision meant that certain theories had to be excluded to conform to the volume's overall space constraints. In the event, the inclusion or exclusion of specific theories was dictated almost entirely by the ability of authors to meet the production schedule. Thus, if a reader finds that some approach that he or she thinks is particularly promising is not treated, it was probably a passive omission due to unavailability of a relevant author.

C. J. Brainerd

Contents

Contributors

Charles J. Brainerd Department of Psychology, University of Western
Ontario, London, Ontario, Canada N6A 5C2.

William R. Charlesworth Institute of Child Development, University of
Minnesota, 51 East River Road, Minneapolis, Minnesota 55455,
U.S.A.

Charles J. Lumsden Department of Medicine, University of Toronto,
Toronto, Ontario, Canada M5S 1A8.

D. Dean Richards Department of Psychology, University of California,
Los Angeles, California 90024, U.S.A.

Robert S. Siegler Department of Psychology, Carnegie-Mellon University,
Pittsburgh, Pennsylvania 15213, U.S.A.

Barry J. Zimmerman Ph.D. Program in Education, Graduate Center,
City University of New York, 33 West 42nd Street, New York,
New York 10036, U.S.A.

1. Social Learning Theory: A Contextualist Account of Cognitive Functioning

Barry J. Zimmerman

Social learning theory grew out of the efforts of Bandura and Walters (1959, 1963) to explain how children acquired information and behavior by observing people in natural settings. Initially they investigated youngsters' simple imitation of common responses, such as aggression, by a model. Favorable results of this research prompted study of more complex classes of social learning, such as the development of emotional reactions (attraction and avoidance), cognitive and linguistic rules, self-regulating responses, personal standards, expectations, and self-efficacy judgments. This social interactionist approach to development revealed a distinctive but widely underestimated feature of children's knowledge: At all levels of complexity, it remained highly dependent on the social environmental context from which it sprang. This property of thought also became evident to other theorists as they began to study cognitive functioning in naturalistic settings. Several of these theorists have discussed the implications of their research on the basis of a general epistemology termed "contextualism."

This chapter is divided into two major sections. The first section provides a description of a growing consensus about the need for a contextual account of cognitive functioning, the metatheoretical form that contextualist formulations have adopted, and some implications of these formulations for cognitive-developmental research. In the second section, social learning theory is described and contextual features of this approach are delineated. Research revealing the contextual dependency of children's cognitive, mnemonic, and linguistic functioning is summarized and considered from a social learning viewpoint.

An Emerging Metatheoretical Consensus

The Need for a Contextual Account of Cognitive Functioning

During the last two decades there has been an increasing effort to study human concept formation, language acquisition, and mnemonic functioning outside the laboratory in naturalistic environmental settings. Researchers from practically every major theoretical tradition have undertaken naturalistic studies. Originally, most theorists were optimistic about the ability of classical cognitive theories derived from laboratory-based research to accommodate outcomes observed in the natural environment. However, conflicting results have led a number of theorists to question the suitability of classical cognitive theories. The label "classical cognitive theories" (Sampson, 1981) is meant to refer

> to that broad and diverse range of psychological approaches which emphasize the structures and processes within the individual's mind that are said to play the major role in behavior; a psychology of the subject rather than that of the object. (p. 730)

In particular, support for the use of mediational, cybernetic, and Piagetian models has eroded, and a major reassessment is currently under way (Jenkins, 1974; Neisser, 1976; Labouvie-Vief & Chandler, 1978; Sampson, 1981). These classical cognitive approaches are being challenged by increasing evidence that human thought and behavior are highly dependent on *context* (e.g., Jenkins, 1974; Nelson, 1974; Goodnow, 1976). Classical theorists' constructs such as associative word meaning, cognitive-developmental stages, and human information processing "programs" have been found to be of limited value in predicting human performance across situations or contexts (Rosenthal & Zimmerman, 1978). The need for theories that deal directly with knowledge and the context from which it is assumed to arise is now being widely discussed throughout the field of psychology, spanning such disparate areas as personality (e.g., Mischel, 1968), perception (e.g., Neisser, 1976), concept formation (e.g., Zimmerman, 1979), mnemonics (e.g., Jenkins, 1974), language acquisition (e.g., Nelson, 1974), and moral thought and behavior (e.g., Liebert, 1979). This recognition often came after years of experimentation, and in several cases it led prominent theorists to discard "classic" cognitive models that they had previously advocated. For example, Jenkins (1974) spent much of his early career attempting to define word meaning in terms of frequencies of association before the contextual implications of his research became evident.

> In place of the traditional [associative] analysis, I suggest a *contextualist* approach. This means not only that the analysis of memory must deal with contextual variables but also . . . that *what memory is depends on context.* (p. 786)

Jenkins discussed how major bodies of research that he had initially interpreted in support of a mediational associationist formulation of semantics was in fact qualified by contextual factors. For example, subjects' "subjective" clustering (Tulving, 1962) of words during free recall was originally explained on the basis of frequencies of word association. Hyde and Jenkins (1969) examined the context effects of an experimenter's verbal instructions on college students' associative clustering during free recall of word lists. One group of subjects was given a comprehension set that instructed them to rate the pleasantness of each word. The second group was given a form set that instructed them to look for certain letters in words. A substantially greater number of words were recalled by subjects who were given the comprehension instructions. These subjects also showed much greater associative clustering. Hyde and Jenkins suggested that their results indicated that recall is affected by the general context of the task (the socially implied purpose) rather than by the specific stimulus words to which the subjects were exposed.

Jenkins's conclusions about the deficiencies of associationist theories of mnemonic functioning are very similar to conclusions that have been drawn about many other currently popular cognitive theories of functioning (Sampson, 1981), particularly cybernetic information processing models and cognitive stage formulations. Perhaps the most dramatic acknowledgment of the need to consider the environmental context seriously in cognitive theories was that of Neisser (1976). Neisser's 1967 book, *Cognitive Psychology*, was a widely read, generally sympathetic description of the cybernetic version of information processing. However, in his 1976 text, significantly entitled *Cognition and Reality*, Neisser renounced the utility of cybernetic models of human thought because of their limited capacity to describe the complex reciprocal relationship between people and their proximal environment.

> If cognitive psychology commits itself too thoroughly to this model [the computer model], there may be trouble ahead. Lacking in ecological validity, indifferent to culture, even missing some of the main features of perception and memory as they occur in ordinary life, such a psychology could become a narrow and uninteresting specialized field. (p. 7)

He discussed the need for more ecologically valid studies, in which psychologists study cognition as it occurs in the ordinary environment in the context of natural, purposeful activity. Such a commitment, he argued, requires the researcher to pay greater attention to the details of the world in which people live and the structure of information that the world makes available to them. Neisser cited many examples from his research on human perception that indicate a need for a more reciprocally interactive, contextually sensitive psychological theory. For example, he suggested that cybernetic models are hard pressed to explain his common perceptual experiences such as seeing an approaching stranger. Neisser pointed out that unlike people, computers do not behave physically; they are active only "mentally" (i.e., they can manipulate information). However, existing research (Gibson, 1979) indicates that the act of perception involves eye, head, and body movements by the perceiver that continuously enhance the quality of information. From this rich and relationally complex stream of visual, auditory, and haptic information, as well from previously stored information about the context and approaching person, Neisser argued that one "constructs" the percept of a stranger approaching at a certain pace. Such perceptual experiences, which involve among other skills size constancy, are common to even very young children (Bower, 1966). Neisser concluded that in order to account for such common perceptual phenomena adequately, he needed to devise a new type of cognitive theory that was structurally different from existing cybernetic models. In his latest model, Neisser (1976) treats the perceiver as physically active as well as mentally active, and the environment is regarded as a richly detailed, dynamic entity. Such theories have been labeled either transactional (e.g., Gibb, 1979) or interactional (Labouvie-Vief & Chandler, 1978; Sampson, 1981).

There has been agreement among many contemporary theorists that evidence of the importance of context effects demands psychological theories that are explicitly interactive in nature (e.g., Bowers, 1973; Mischel, 1973; Sampson, 1981). Most contemporary cognitive theories have some features that can be described as interactional. However, they also have features that significantly limit the role that environmental stimuli can play in mental functioning. For example, Piaget's cognitive stage theory has been criticized for being insufficiently interactional to account for much evidence of contextualism in children's thought. Riegel (1976) has argued that although the child in Piaget's account is regarded as active, the environment is treated as universal and unchanging. Social events were not viewed by Piaget as having a dynamic of their own; they were not seen as capable of altering physical reality for the child. Piaget gave little attention to the effect of the social dimensions of the environment—the individual and collective behavior of other people—on children's reasoning. The concepts that he studied were generally nonsocial in nature (e.g., space, number, time, conservation, and mathematics) and thus were less likely to be contextually dynamic. One social concept (i.e., pertaining to man and his relations with other people) that Piaget (1948) studied extensively was morality.[1] Interestingly, his research indicated that children's judgments and reasoning failed to measure up to his criteria for a stage designation (pp. 194-195). Clearly his stage theory was limited in its allowance for interaction: Reality had to be accommodated *mentally*, it could not be created *physically*.

There are other features of Piaget's theory, and of stage theories in general, that limit their utility in dealing with evidence of contextualism in functioning. Perhaps the major limitation is that stage theories are based on idealist philosophic premises (Pepper, 1970). Cognitive stages are seen as imperfect approximations of an ideal adult standard of mental functioning. Labouvie-Vief and Chandler (1978) have described some of the consequences of these idealist premises:

> Change in such an account is construed as inherently directional, growth is understood as progress, and adulthood is regarded as success. Developmental research, in this tradition, becomes a kind of ontological ballistics, tracking growth along a unilinear trajectory toward its idealized apogee in maturity. The laws or principles of development generated in this context become prescriptive rather than descriptive and adulthood comes to play the role of a kind platonic absolute. (p. 184)

This idealistic model treats cognitive development as a universal process that exists apart from an experimenter's theorizing and experimentation. Given these philosophic assumptions, cultural factors as well as other situational differences are treated as noise variables that obscure but do not substantially alter the genotypic course of development (Pepper, 1970). The discrepancy between behavioral reality

---

[1]This social distinction excludes Piaget's work on animism, artificialism, and finalism. Although children did ascribe humanlike qualities to stimuli in these types of studies, the referents were not human.

and the idealistic model is "explained" by using a performance-competence distinction. However, both Chandler (1977) and Riegel (1975) have pointed out that a competence-performance distinction represents a concession by cognitive stage theorists that behavior variations are not well explained by their idealized stage model.

Another feature of cognitive stage theories that greatly detracts from their ability to account for environmental context effects is their reliance on internal balance or equilibration notions to explain human motivation. In Piaget's theory as well as in social psychological balance formulations, motivation is ascribed to people if they experience "cognitive conflict." Such conflicts are assumed to be noxious, and the individual is described as compelled to alleviate this state by forming a more mature concept (Piaget, 1952). The importance of the environment is minimal, since motivation is seen as residing internally, not externally, and the person is seen as acting *mentally* to resolve or accommodate these conflicts. Children's physical actions are viewed merely as exploratory probes of an unchanging world of objects (Riegel, 1976). Individual differences in response are thus attributed to structurally different constructions of a constant reality, a practice termed "subjective reductionism." Sampson (1981) discussed the drawback of subjective reductionism.

> In substituting thought for action, mental transformation for real-world transformation, cognitivism veils the objective sources and bases of social life and relegates individual potency to the inner world of gymnastics. (p. 735)

In the case of age-related differences in performance, the adult is often seen by consistency theorists as more adroit in denying or overcoming contextual cues. Piaget's (1950) discussion of preoperational children's failure to conserve is a case in point. Adults are believed to conserve because they can ignore spatial cues and rely instead on logical rules when making quantitative judgments. In these accounts, adults are viewed as more insensitive to environmental context than children (see Piaget, 1970). However, Piaget (1972) eventually recognized extensive evidence that (a) cognitive functioning during the formal operations period (adolescence and adulthood) varied extensively based on the content of a task (one contextual variable); (b) task effects on cognitive functioning became increasingly pronounced during this developmental period; and (c) cognitive proficiency was highly related to task-relevant experiences by the individual.

A final point should be made concerning cognitive consistency theories of human development. To date, there has been little progress by consistency theorists in devising operational measures of cognitive conflict that are *independent* of the behaviors that conflict constructs have been used to explain (Zimmerman & Blom, 1983). Typically, a "conflict" situation is experimentally created and then behavioral, cognitive, or attitudinal change is measured (e.g., Murray, 1972). Actual cognitive conflict is seldom (if ever) measured. Thus, the assumption that conflict is noxious and that people try to avoid confronting discrepant sources of information is not directly demonstrated by data. In fact, Riegel (1975) has argued that mature adults often *seek out* (rather than avoid) contradictions as a basis for innovation and creative work.

> The confirmation of contradictions, in contrast to their denial by cognitive and mentalistic psychologists, enables us to propose an alternative interpretation of crisis and catastrophes. For the individual, contradictions, doubts, questions, and

inner dialogues represent the very basis of his actions and thoughts. His social development likewise is founded upon and finds expression in conflicts, disagreements, debates, and dialogues. Both these inner and outer interactions are functional and beneficial for both the individual's development and that of the social group. (p. 101)

Although many people might also question Riegel's dialectical view of man as seeking out contradictions and crisis, it is certainly true that a researcher's ability to formulate conflicting alternative hypotheses has been the basis of much scientific discovery.

A third, middle-of-the-road, viewpoint on the motivational role of conflict has been proposed by *optimum stimulation* theorists (e.g., Hebb, 1949; Dember & Earl, 1957). These researchers assume that people seek an intermediate level of conflict where people stimulate themselves enough to avoid boredom but avoid excessive stimulation, which is assumed to be noxious. Berlyne's (1960, 1970) work on human curiosity and McClelland, Atkinson, Clark, and Lowell's (1953) theory of achievement motivation are examples of optimum stimulation models.

In short, a case can be made that people seek out conflict as much as they seek to avoid it. Each outcome is probably situationally dependent. As a result, contextually oriented scholars tend to avoid cognitive conflict assumptions altogether (Sampson, 1981; Zimmerman & Blom, 1983). Such assumptions have the net effect of focusing undue attention on an internal (unmeasured) cognitive state and ignoring effects of environmental context.

The term *reification* has been increasingly used by contextually oriented scholars for descriptions of human performance and outcomes that are abstracted from their social context and treated as independent cognitive entities (Lukacs, 1971). Because reified accounts of thought and functioning are not qualified by contextual considerations, they are alluring—appearing to be timeless and highly objective (see Adorno, 1967, 1976). But the inherent weakness of reified theories (Gergen, 1973, 1978; Sampson, 1977, 1978) is that although they explain the phenomena from which they were derived, they fare poorly when predicting behavior in other contexts. Piaget's notions of egocentrism and operativity are good examples. Their convergent validity across contexts has been found to be low (Berzonsky, 1971; Ford, 1979; Zimmerman, 1978, 1980).

Another particularly distressing side effect of reified cognitive theories has been discussed by Sampson (1981).

Psychological reifications clothe existing social arrangements in terms of basic and inevitable characteristics of individual psychological functioning; this inadvertently authenticates the status quo but now in a disguised psychological costume. What has been mediated by a sociohistorical process—the forms and contents of human consciousness and of individual psychological experience—is treated as though it were an "in-self," a reality independent of these very origins. (p. 738)

Many researchers have sought to test this immutability assumption with Piaget's theory by undertaking conservation training studies. Originally, Piagetian scholars (Smedslund, 1961a, 1961b; Wohlwill, 1959; Wohlwill & Lowe, 1962) were unable to teach preoperational children to conserve. They (Flavell, 1963) interpreted this outcome as due to inherent limitations of children's preoperational stage of reasoning. Subsequently, a vast number of training studies were conducted by critics as well as disciples of Piaget, and researchers generally found that even preschool children could be taught rather easily to conserve (for a review, see Brainerd, 1977). Thus the pessimistic prognosis of Piagetians for teaching young children to conserve was wrong. Brainerd (1978a) has noted that early unsuccessful training studies by Piagetians were all conducted by using complicated mechanical devices (e.g., balance scales). Subsequent research studies involving many of the same training variables (e.g., reinforcement, rule provision, and perceptual set induction) but without these devices generally proved successful. Brainerd's point underscores the concern expressed earlier that laboratory procedures which depart markedly from learning in naturalistic contexts can (but do not necessarily) produce unrepresentative results.

Contextualist Formulations

A number of philosophers of science (Berger & Luckman, 1966; Habermas, 1971; Kuhn, 1970; Sampson, 1981) have considered evidence of the contextual dependency of knowledge and the adequacy of classical cognitive theories in accounting for these outcomes, and they have called for the development of a new class of theories that are more explicitly interactional. This metatheoretical position has been widely termed *contextualism* (Pepper, 1970; Jenkins, 1974; Labouvie-Vief & Chandler, 1978), and it is associated with the pragmatic philosophical tradition of James (1890) and the functionalist tradition in American psychology (see Zimmerman & Whitehurst, 1979; Beilin, 1981). This viewpoint emphasizes the social contextual origins of knowledge and the adaptive quality of human cognition. The major tenets of contextualism are the following:

1. *Person-Environment Interaction.* The meaning of an event is the result of the interaction of a person and his or her proximal and distal environment (Jenkins, 1974). Each person's psychological functioning depends to a substantial degree on environmental events; and conversely, environmental events are determined to a substantial degree by a person's thoughts and actions. Yet both the subject and the environment are treated as separately dynamic. That is, a person cannot fully determine environmental events, nor are environmental events totally causative of a person's actions. This complex relationship is depicted in Figure 1-1. It should be noted that the environment term in this analysis includes the actions and speech of *other people* as well as changes in the physical environment. Contextualists generally regard the actions of other people as the most dynamic of environmental stimuli, and hence most contextualists give much attention to social-group and cultural forces in their theorizing (Sampson, 1981).

A contextualist views people as both physically and mentally active. People's behavioral skills enable them to manipulate their environment in such a way that certain outcomes become more probable or more evident, or both (Coates & Thoresen, 1979). Contextualists reject static, reified (person- and actionless) descriptions of children's environment with the same vigor with which they reject reified descriptions of children's thought. Environments are assumed to be just as sensitive to people as the reverse; both are constantly changing, in part as a result of the influ-

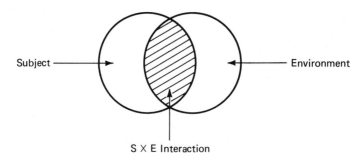

S X E Interaction

Figure 1-1. An interactionist view of subject and environmental contributions to causation of events.

ence of the other and in part because of other forces. The comprehensiveness and complexity of this interactive approach is revealed in Jenkins's (1974) description of a contextualist analysis of recall.

> What is remembered in a given situation depends on the physical and psycholog-ical context in which the event was experienced, the knowledge and skills that the subject brings to the context, the situation in which we ask for evidence for remembering, and the relation of what the subject remembers to what the experimenter demands. (p. 793)

Thus, cognition is inextricably linked to the context from which it emerges, and reified analyses of all types are inherently misleading.

2. *Events as Holistic Phenomena.* "Contextualism holds that experience consists of *events*. Events have a quality as a whole. By *quality* is meant the total meaning of the event" (Jenkins, 1974, p. 786). To the contextualist, events are more than the sum of discrete environmental stimuli. An event is experienced by the subject as a cognitively unified phenomenon, and it is not reducible to a more elemental or externally "objective" form. This tenet distinguishes the contextual account of cog-nition from reified *associationist* views of mental functioning. This holism-of-experi-ence assumption can be traced back to the very beginnings of American functional-ism. William James (1890) argued that the mind had to be studied as a dynamic whole, not as a composite of discrete elements, as had been suggested by his con-temporary Wundt (Watson, 1963). James viewed consciousness as a continuous stream of thoughts, each inextricably linked to preceding thoughts and embedded in the context of overt experience. He used the phrase "specious present" to sug-gest that people cognitively join sequential events into atemporal wholes.

Figure 1-2 is a diagrammatic effort to relate the contextualist psychology of Jenkins (1974) and Nelson (1974) to the philosophy of Pepper (1970). In Figure 1-2, the learner is assumed to respond interactively (denoted by a bidirectional arrow) to a particular environmental context. This event involves both motoric-perceptual acts (e.g., information gathering or enhancing) and phenomenal experi-ence (i.e., an expectancy or belief). Prior beliefs, which are depicted as previous events, determine which part of the current environmental context will be initially

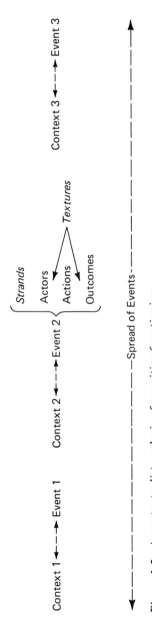

Figure 1-2. A contextualist analysis of cognitive functioning.

scrutinized and how the resulting information will be initially interpreted. However, current experiential outcomes also contribute significantly to how the event will be ultimately interpreted. An event (2) can be decomposed into elements, termed *strands*, and relationships among strands, called *textures*. The definition of a strand is considered arbitrary, and is left up to theorists to designate, depending on the purpose of their analysis. Words in a sentence can be conceptualized as strands and the relationship of words as textures. Pepper (1970) has identified a variety of basic textures that he has labeled "references." Most contextual psychologists are mainly interested in what Pepper termed an *instrumental reference*, which deals with a functional relationship among strands. A common instrumental reference (e.g., Nelson, 1974) focuses on the strands of *actors* or things that act (the subject of a sentence), *actions* or transformations (e.g., the predicate of a sentence), and *outcomes* of actions or transformations (e.g., the direct object or predicate nominative of a sentence). Textures are assumed to be deduced from the nature of the strands as they lie in a particular context. Although a person's conceptual decomposition of an event into such strands as actor, actions, and outcomes puts some constraint on the construction of textures, ultimately contextual information provides the "conceptual glue" for fusing the precise meaning of an event.

A contextualist account assumes that the beginning point in a psychological description of people's functioning is a current event (2). Contextualists are confident about current events and the implications they provide about neighboring events, but are less certain about the wider structure of the world. The meaning of an event is assumed to *spread* both backward and forward in time. It is related backward to preceding events (event 1) that share common contextual features (i.e., have interpenetrating strands and textures). For example, a man's interpretation of a woman's reasons for declining an invitation for a date on a given day are synthesized within the larger context of the reasons she offered for also refusing a previous day's invitation. The man may decide that *he* (and not the woman's expressed reasons) is the reason for the refusal! The meaning of an event can also be projected to future events (3) based on common strands and textures. This is particularly true of instrumental references. Such functional knowledge enables prediction and control of future events to some degree on the basis of common critical contextual features.

Jenkins (1974) used the example of sentence comprehension in this connection. He suggested that listeners construct the meaning of a sentence by relating words on the basis of such contextual cues as sentences previously heard, referents in the speaking situation, nonverbal cues in the face of the speaker, and perhaps common anticipated future events. For example, when asked "When will it come?" by a man, a woman may infer the meaning of the sentence from such contextual cues as the physical setting (bus stop), the facial expression of the man (agitated), and prior discussion (the man's questions about the neighborhood). The listener in this case deduces that (a) "it" refers to the bus, (b) the man is new to the neighborhood, and (c) the man is late for an appointment. These inferences extend considerably beyond the present context but are nevertheless directly dependent on contextual cues: Inference (b) extends immediately back in time, whereas inference (c) extends forward into the near future. In this sense, the meaning of an utterance spreads beyond the physical stimuli immediately present. Thus to a contextualist (Pepper, 1970), concepts are embedded within the contextual "layers" of successively larger units of experience (or events). Notice also in this contextualist account that the woman's concept about this event or experience is highly dependent on its *content* (the particular man encountered) as well as on other features of the physical environmental setting. Therefore, task content or attributes are viewed as a subvariety of a larger group of contextual cues that people use to construct concepts. Contextualist scholars have accordingly devoted considerable attention to the defining role that content features of children's experience play in their cognitive functioning (e.g., Zimmerman, 1978).

3. *Contextualism Is Comprehensive and Dynamic*. The assumption of the unity of cognitive experience and its adaptability to contextual features of the environment led James (1890) to rule out the possibility that the human mind could be usefully dissected by introspection or described in any static, elemental fashion. Instead, he suggested that the human mind should be studied "in motion" as a person adapted to changing environmental contexts. This functional approach for defining concept meaning is the hallmark of contemporary contextualists as well (Pepper, 1970; Jenkins, 1974). To James, "truths" were those concepts (and related actions) that led a person to make successful adaptations. Since adaptation was viewed as context dependent and since experiential contexts were seen as highly varied across individuals, groups, and societies, and as varying over time, truth was assumed to be culturally relative. Therefore, contextualists reject the suggestion that there can be a "complete" or "final" analysis that reveals the elemental structure of human knowledge. The belief in a reified, elemental structure derives from an idealist view of epistomology (Pepper, 1970). Reductionist theories as theoretically diverse as mediational associationism, cybernetic processing, and structuralism are rejected because they all assume that psychological events can be reduced to a set of basic associations, human computer programs, or logic structures (Jenkins, 1974; Neisser, 1976; Labouvie-Vief & Chandler, 1978). Contextualists, like all theorists, want to reduce the complexity of psychological phenomena in order to achieve parsimony and greater control over human thought and behavior. However, they differ from idealists in that they see reductive analyses as sheering away specific contextual meaning from a particular experience in order to relate it to a larger, more diverse context.

For example, after observing a series of conflicts between a boy and his teacher, a contextualist may notice that teacher criticism was correlated with increases in disruptive behavior by the student. A reinforcement (reductive) hypothesis would imply that teacher criticism (perhaps because it attracted peer attention) served as a reinforcer for the boy. Such an analysis might lead to testing the hypothesis that changing the teacher's attending practices from deviant to appropriate behavior would improve the boy's classroom deportment. A contextualist would, however, deny that this is *the* true psychological account of what occurred. Even if the reinforcement analysis proved valid (i.e., predictive) in these circumstances, it would not explain why all children were not disruptive in order to elicit teacher attention, nor would it suggest how the boy would respond to teacher criticism in a different context, such as his home (with his parents present). Many contextual details were excluded from this account that might provide answers to these questions. Thus, there is no *single* criterion of truth, no single elemental form of knowledge. Contextualists believe that the validity of psychological theories, as of all concepts, is never absolute but is relevant to specific purposes and particular contexts.

Contextualists argue that researchers must be acutely aware of the relative nature of their criteria for "truth." Pluralistic conceptions of truth are accepted, and the utility of each set of criteria must be carefully considered relative to specific scientific objectives (Jenkins, 1974). In contrast, idealist cognitive theories argue not only that a true reductionist account is possible, but also that there is great value in knowing the basic form of psychological phenomena (Pepper, 1970). Idealists assume that the use of an elemental structure allows them to make predictions across contexts, such as Piaget's claims that preoperational egocentrism limits children's performance in diverse social and physical situations.

Contextualists believe that failures by idealist theorists to recognize the social relativity of their analytic framework create problems in interpreting cross-cultural as well as developmental research. For example, Sampson (1981) has criticized Piaget for describing all children's cognitive development on the basis of the technological view of knowledge of industrialized societies. According to Piaget's formulation, abstract criteria for making judgments are assumed to be more cognitively mature than concrete-functional criteria. But people from at least one preindustrial society disagree with Piaget about the priority of such criteria. In a study of object grouping, Cole, Gay, Glick, and Sharp (1971) found that African tribesman, the Kpelle, tended to cluster stimuli in concrete-functional categories, such as putting a knife and orange together "because a knife is used to cut oranges." Glick (1975) noted that the tribesmen often supported their groupings by saying, "A wise man would do things in the way it was done." Once, in exasperation, the experimenter retorted, "How would a fool do it?" The tribesmen responded by grouping the objects on the basis of Piaget's preferred abstract criteria (foods in one pile, tools in another, etc.). Although both criteria were known to these tribesmen, the concrete-functional criterion was valued more highly than the abstract one. There are analogous difficulties with Kohlberg's stage theory of moral reasoning (Dannhauser, 1981). Kohlberg (e.g., 1968) argues that the highest level of moral reasoning involves adherence to "universal" rules of conduct such as the golden rule. His research in third world countries indicated that few people achieved this level of moral reasoning. Yet Liebert (1979) has pointed out that many non-Christian cultures do not accept the golden rule as self-evident truth. It will be recalled that this rule was derived from the parable of the Good Samaritan, who risked his life to help a foreigner who had been mugged along the road. Liebert points out that in China it is considered irresponsible to risk one's life to save a stranger, since a person's foremost moral obligation is to his or her family. In traditional societies, the loss of a productive family member is seen as bringing hardship to the rest.

4. *Development Is Ongoing and Diverse.* Contextualists challenge universalist concepts of human development (Rosenthal & Zimmerman, 1978; Sampson, 1981).

They believe that claims of developmental universality are made at considerable hidden expense. Variations in performance by children of a particular age, by children across tasks and settings, and by children of different cultural groups are treated as a form of measurement error (Kohlberg, 1971; Wohlwill, 1973). In contrast, the contextualist argues for multiformity in developmental adaptation. No single stage is seen as ending the process of development. Such teleological assumptions are seen as another form of idealist bias by theorists who regard early adulthood as the epitome of human behavior. Young children's and senior citizens' thinking invariably are described pejoratively relative to the young adult age standard (Labouvie-Vief & Chandler, 1978). Contextualists argue that maturity cannot be captured by a universal epigenetic formula; mature thought and behavior are neither universal nor static but shift to suit cultural demands (Campbell, 1975). According to this view, a lack of formalized thinking should not be interpreted as deficient socialization of the young or old; rather, it reflects a common relationship between age-group context variables and behavior (Berger & Luckman, 1966; Buck-Morss, 1975; Campbell, 1975; Garbarino & Bronfenbrenner, 1976; Kohn, 1969).

The arbitrariness of the assumption that young adult reasoning is the ideal standard has been revealed in several studies. For example, Weir (1964) ingeniously reversed the usual age-group context bias in a study of problem solving by subjects who ranged in age from 3 to 20 years. The task involved finding and pulling the correct lever in a mechanical game. Correct lever pulling was reinforced according to a 33% or 66% variable ratio (VR) schedule. Young children consistently outperformed older subjects even after 80 trials under the 33% VR schedule. Older subjects finally caught up with the 3- and 5-year-olds after 50 trials under the 66% VR schedule. Weir concluded that adults fared poorly relative to children because they expected that it was possible to be reinforced on all trials. Thus, adult expectations about the form of a correct answer, which normally give them an edge over children, worked to their disadvantage in this instance. A similar finding was reported by Russell (1976). He administered a conservation of area task to adults and preoperational stage children. Conservation of area differs from Piagetian conservation concepts in that transformations in shape alter the amount of exposed surface area. As contextualists would predict, the preoperational children (who are believed to rely on spatial configuration cues) correctly solved the problem. In contrast, the college students tended to rely on a "perimeter" compensation rule and came to erroneous conclusions. Thus, the validity of supposedly "logical" rules or strategies is, in fact, ultimately context dependent. But this relative property of rules is obscured in research studies in which task or other context parameters are not varied.

Many contextualists agree with stage theorists, however, that age-related changes in behavior are often discontinuous or qualitative (Labouvie-Vief & Chandler, 1978). Nevertheless, they assume that such shifts reflect efforts by people to adapt to often quite abrupt, age-related changes in social context (Flavell, 1970; Datan & Ginsberg, 1975). Some changes may depend on physiological maturation, such as an infant's development of articulatory facility, an adolescent's undergoing puberty, or an elderly person's loss of motoric control. Other age-related changes are due to such historic events as children's entrance into school, adults' selection of mates, or the elderly's retirement from active work or loss of a spouse. Thus, what appears to be maturationally "normal" in cognition and performance reflects, upon closer examination, a culturally imposed system of "prods and brakes" (Neugarton & Datan, 1973). That the approximate ages 2, 7, and 12 are chosen to herald developmental shifts by such diverse stage theorists as Piaget (1954), Erikson (1963), Kohlberg (1968), and Freud (1938) is not surprising to the contextualist, nor is it regarded as evidence of the universality of cognitive development. Such shifts are viewed as caused by age-related social contextual events. In fact, Erikson's (1963) life span theory of development implicitly links stage functioning to important age-related, social contextual events such as entrance into school, puberty, marriage, and retirement. Contextualists believe that such social variables will ultimately predict performance shifts more accurately than age (Baltes & Labouvie, 1973; Bengtson, 1973; Bruner, Olver, & Greenfield, 1966; Lindsley, 1964; Seligman, 1975; Zimmerman & Lanaro, 1974). Support for this prediction is evident in cross-cultural studies of development wherein social events often occur at somewhat different ages (Cole & Bruner, 1971; Cole & Scribner, 1974; Buck-Morss, 1975). In a sense, however, stage theorists (e.g., Kohlberg, 1968) have already conceded ground on this point, since they have followed Piaget's lead (1954) in dissociating age from stage.

5. *Research Methods and Goals Must Be Revised.* The contextualist perspective requires that developmental psychologists reconsider their research methods and goals. The validity of traditional cross-sectional and longitudinal designs is questioned by contextualist scholars, since with them little attention is given to the confounding effects of historical and social context variables on age. Some researchers have recommended cohort-group designs as more valid. However, the control afforded by nonexperimental[2] versions of this design for social historical events is quite limited. Consider, for example, carrying out a study of three cohort groups (4-, 5-, and 6-year-olds) designed to produce normative data for a 3-year period of children's cognitive development. Consider further the possibility of an effective educational television program as a confounding event. If the television program begins after the first year of the study, its impact would be indicated by the superior performance by the last two cohort groups. The researcher still needs to attribute the enhanced performance of the second and third cohort groups to the television program from the other experiences occurring during the second year. If the program began before the outset of the study and continued throughout the 3-year period, its impact would not be detected. Obtained age-group norms would be erroneously accepted as valid, since they were replicated across all three cohort groups. Thus nonexperimental cohort-group designs provide little control for social or historical events that extend in duration throughout the developmental period of study. These are perhaps the most important of all such events because their influence continues over a span of time, perhaps even as long as a generation.

The possibility of such confounding has led some life span developmental psy-

---

[2]In experimental cohort-group designs, the effects of a treatment are examined over time on successive cohort groups (e.g., the evaluation of the national Follow Through Program). Such designs can assess the impact of social historical events if they can be specified a priori and can be experimentally controlled.

chologists to question whether "developmental decrement" descriptions of the reasoning by the elderly may be due to different social history influences on successive generation groups (Nesselroade, Schaie, & Baltes, 1972; Schaie & Labouvie-Vief, 1974; Schaie, Labouvie, & Buech, 1973; Schaie & Strother, 1968a, 1968b). Schaie and Labouvie-Vief (1974) describe how the social context can lead to decrement interpretations of the capacity of the elderly:

> Most of the adult life span is characterized by an absence of decisive intellectual decrements. In times of rapid cultural and technological change, it is primarily in relation to younger populations that the aged can be described as deficient, and it is erroneous to interpret such cross-sectional age differences as indicating ontogenetic change patterns. (p. 319).

This explanation is particularly appealing since it also explains why the elderly are viewed as wise in tradition-bound, illiterate cultures such as tribal groups. For these groups, knowledge of such matters as hunting, herding, food gathering, or crop raising remains functional for successive generations. Such information must be acquired from social sources or by more hazardous and less efficient trial and error. For such cultural groups, the wisdom of the elderly is a valued resource, and the elderly hold a revered status.

Mounting evidence of context influences on human thought and behavior has prompted many developmental psychologists to concede that changes must be made in research methodology. These discussions have led to a consensus that the ecological validity of research needs to be improved. The most comprehensive statement of the principles by which ecological validity can be achieved was offered by Bronfenbrenner (1979). He cautioned researchers to consider carefully the influence of diverse contextual stimuli, such as social-group effects and the role of historical events, when they conduct studies and interpret their results. Brofenbrenner questioned the ecological validity of much laboratory research where phenomena are studied without regard to context and where context clues are typically eliminated through experimental control. He grants that although results may be replicable, it is unlikely they are generalizable to real-world situations.

Many readers of Bronfenbrenner's treatise have concluded erroneously that he argued that ecological validity was determined by the location for conducting research and that laboratory studies were therefore invalid. Careful scrutiny of his work reveals the inaccuracy of this interpretation.

> Ecological validity refers to the extent to which the environment experienced by the subjects in a scientific investigation has the properties it is supposed or assumed to have by the investigators. . . . This definition does not designate any particular kind of research locale as valid or invalid on a priori grounds. Thus depending on the problem, the laboratory may be an altogether appropriate setting for an investigation, and certain real-life environments may be highly inappropriate. . . . At a more general level, the comparison of results obtained in laboratory and real-life settings provides an illustration of the basic strategy through which ecological validity can be demonstrated or found wanting. . . . It is therefore not sufficient to show only that a certain variation in the environment has produced an alteration in behavior; it is also necessary to demonstrate that this change exhibits some invariance across time, place, or both. (pp. 29-34).

Thus Bronfenbrenner's definition of ecological validity does not require that research be judged according to a criterion of "contextual naturalness" but rather according to the generality of results across settings that vary in contextual correspondence.

Misinterpretations of Bronfenbrenner's position undoubtedly stem from the great emphasis he placed on conducting experimental studies in naturalistic settings. However, he readily admitted the paucity of such research and the difficulties involved in drawing causal inferences in available studies. Researchers from the operant tradition (e.g., Bijou & Baer, 1978) have probably devoted much effort to establishing functional relationships between contextual events and responding in natural settings through the use of time series designs. However, behavioral ecologists (e.g., Willems, 1974) have criticized them for being narrow in their selection of contextual variables and classes of response for study.

Many contextualist scholars (e.g., Botwinick, 1973; Jenkins, 1974; Bandura, 1978a) are less optimistic than Bronfenbrenner about researchers' ability to determine the importance of contextual stimuli from studies conducted in unstructured natural settings and have opted instead to recreate learning events in a laboratory where context factors can be controlled more precisely. These researchers have been particularly interested in descriptive data indicating context-related variations in children's functioning in the natural environment, and from these data they have identified specific stimuli (e.g., setting cues, task content, models, reinforcement) for laboratory testing. Their subsequent laboratory studies were distinguished from those conducted by classical cognitive theorists by the inclusion of contextual events that were present during functioning in natural, unstructured settings. In traditional laboratory studies, primary consideration was given to internal cognitive states or processes, and perhaps as a result, relatively few contextual features of the natural environment were studied.

Contextualists engaging in laboratory research historically have attempted to establish the generality of their results through the use of systematic tests of transfer wherein key contextual elements remain present but irrelevant elements are systematically altered (e.g., Zimmerman & Rosenthal, 1974b). This practice is in accordance with Brofenbrenner's criterion of ecological validity. Once causal relationships have been established across transfer tasks, they are used to explain correlation between children's performance and natural context features, as well as guide intervention studies designed to demonstrate the predictive validity of laboratory conclusions with regard to performance in naturalistic contexts (e.g., Bandura, Blanchard, & Ritter, 1969; Zimmerman & Pike, 1972; Henderson, Swanson, & Zimmerman, 1975; Bandura & Schunk, 1981).

In view of the extensive evidence of the usefulness of contextualist descriptions of children's cognitive functioning, McClelland (1973) has argued that *situational sensitivity* of measures should be the highest criterion of validity in psychological testing. The more sensitive a measure is to change due to experience or to changes in context, the more confidence researchers should place in their results. This contextual sensitivity criterion stands in contrast to the consistency criterion advocated by psychometric theories and structural theories of cognitive development (Kohlberg, 1971; Wohlwill, 1973). The latter approaches require stability across situations in the validation of cognitive measures. Variation in response to specific items is viewed as inconsistency, not contextual sensitivity, and it is treated statistically as a form of error (Mischel, 1968). Proshansky (1976) cautioned, however, that these practices may lead to "phenomenon legitimacy" wherein ecological scope and relevance are sacrificed in favor of internal consistency and theoretical purity.

Conclusions

During the last two decades, a steadily increasing body of research indicating the importance of environmental context in children's functioning has led to a gradual change in theorizing about the nature of cognition. This evolution in theory began in diverse areas of psychological research when investigators undertook studies bearing on children's functioning in naturalistic settings. This change in research focus and often in setting was precipitated by two notable historical events of the 1960s: (a) the massive federal support given for research and development designed to improve the functioning of disadvantaged youngsters in naturalistic contexts such as the day-care center, the home, and the school; and (b) the development of the portable television camera and videotape system for recording children's behavior in naturalistic settings and the electronic computer for storing and analyzing vast amounts of data (Mussen, 1982). Subtle conceptual dimensions of human performance and its interdependency with environmental context emerged under the focus of these "behavioral microscopes." In addition to a recording function, videotapes could be programmed to present naturalistic cognitive and social experiences to children in laboratory settings.

The evolution of psychological theories to accommodate evidence of contextualism has reached the point where several researchers have concluded that a fundamental shift in epistemology is required. They have adopted a contextualist epistemology (Pepper, 1970) to guide their theorizing. This approach is interactional or transactional in essential form: Both developing children and their surrounding environmental events are assumed to be separately dynamic yet complexly related. Contextualists question assumptions about the existence of a single, elemental structure of either the world or the human mind. Instead, contextualists assume that reality is dynamic and continuous in flow and that knowledge is the ever-changing cumulative product of one's personal transactions with the proximal and distal environment.

Several conclusions emerge from this contextualist account concerning psychological descriptions of developing children: (a) A contextualist description and analysis of an event in the life of a child includes cognitive-phenomenological factors as well as environmental and behavioral factors. (b) Contextualist descriptions of children's functioning enable prediction and explanation across personal events on the basis of common contextual elements. (c) Universalist psychological descriptions of children's functioning are believed to be imprecise at best and to be often misleading because they ignore personal differences in experience and the resulting contextual properties of an individual child's thought. (d) Developmental psychologists need to give much greater attention to context-related variations in children's performance instead of regarding them as error variance or assuming that contextual experiences are controlled in developmental designs. (e) The validity of contextual descriptions of children's functioning is never assumed to be absolute but instead is judged relative to specific objectives. (f) The validity of psychological descriptions of children's functioning must ultimately be judged by their effectiveness in facilitating performance in naturalistic contexts. (g) Although performance in naturalistic contexts must be the ultimate focus of psychological analysis, this setting is not necessarily optimal for conducting all research.

Social Learning Theory

Perhaps the first fully interactionist contextualist theory to emerge in modern psychology was Bandura's social learning formulation (Bandura & Walters, 1959, 1963). Like other contextualists, Bandura and his colleagues were particularly interested in explaining children's performance in naturalistic contexts such as the home or school. Bandura was concerned with the influences of social experience, particularly the influence of social models, on children's development and functioning. Prior to Bandura, behaviorists (e.g., Thorndike, 1913; Miller & Dollard, 1941; Skinner, 1953) had relegated vicarious learning phenomena to the category of instrumental conditioning of an imitative response (Rosenthal & Zimmerman, 1978). Bandura's research (see Bandura, 1965) revealed many features of children's vicarious learning that conflicted with noncognitive accounts: (a) Children could learn by observation alone without imitating immediately (which Bandura termed "no trial learning"); (b) children learned vicariously without ostensible rewards; (c) children would imitate models who were unfamiliar with them; (d) children's learning often was not manifested in their performance for extended periods of time; and (e) children's learning was readily transferable to novel tasks (e.g., Bandura & McDonald, 1963). Bandura (1962, 1965) concluded that vicarious learning was fundamentally a cognitive process: Children appeared to be forming naturalistic concepts from the actions of the models they observed. These concepts were then used to guide observers' performance during a postmodeling observation phase in Bandura's methodology. This cognitive interpretation of vicarious learning led Bandura (1965) to distinguish between concept formation, or *acquisition*, and *performance*. This theoretical distinction enabled him to explain not only response imitation by observers but also many other outcomes of social experiences, such as counterimitation, inhibition-disinhibition, generalized response facilitation, and rule learning (Zimmerman & Rosenthal, 1974b).

A particularly attractive feature of Bandura's approach was his modeling research paradigm; it enabled researchers to present social experiences presumed to be important in influencing children's development in simulated naturalistic settings. Bandura and Walters (1963) described the goals of this approach as

to reproduce as closely as possible the social stimuli and responses that occur in real life situations concerning which the experimenter wishes to make causal statements. However, this does not imply that laboratory experiments should be designed to reproduce real-life in toto; if they were, the experimenter would necessarily relinquish the crucial scientific strategy of manipulating one variable while holding others constant, and thereby forfeiting the possibility of establishing precise cause-effect relationships. (p. 46)

Modeling experiences could be recorded in naturalistic settings on film or videotape or could be directly enacted by live models in laboratory settings designed to simulate the environment of the home, school, or playground. Because this methodology permitted a high degree of experimental control, researchers could unambiguously determine the relationship between concept acquisition and performance. For example, social learning researchers have been able to develop explicit descriptions of how children's concepts affect their motivation and self-regulation. This account will be discussed later.

Social Learning Subprocesses

Bandura's theory (1971) distinguishes four fundamental interdependent subprocesses in human behavior. Two processes are primarily cognitive (attention and retention) and two are primarily noncognitive (motivation and motoric processes). Attention refers to processes by which children orient themselves to certain features of their environment. For children to learn from models, they must perceive and attend to such models. In support of this distinction, Yussen (1974) found children's attentional responses to be highly correlated with acquisition. Conversely, conditions that obstruct observation or divert attention have been found to impede learning (Bandura & Rosenthal, 1966; Clark & Brownell, 1975; Gerst, 1971; Rosenbaum & Schultz, 1967).

In addition to attending, Bandura suggested that the learner or observer must contribute cognitively before acquisition can occur. Comprehension and retention are viewed as personally activated processes. Failure by a learner to encode events symbolically into vivid images or into verbal meanings was predicted to impair vicarious acquisition. There is extensive evidence to support this hypothesis (Bandura & Jeffery, 1973; Bandura, Jeffery, & Bachicha, 1974). Bandura referred to this second cognitive subprocess as retention. Retention also includes the intentions and beliefs held by a person and the role these processes play in the creation and interpretation of experience. For example, Bandura has cited numerous studies (e.g., Kaufman, Baron, & Kopp, 1966; Chatterjee & Ericson, 1962) indicating that people's performance is determined by their beliefs about the nature of reinforcement contingencies rather than by the actual contingencies themselves. Social learning scholars assume that a person's contemporary experience is seldom, if ever, so informationally complete that prior experience can be ignored. Rather, contemporary experience is seen as creating a situational or contextual framework that is cognitively "embellished" by using information gained from prior experiences (Zimmerman & Jaffe, 1977). Thus the meaning of a "no-feedback" consequence (see Dulaney, 1968) can be reinforcing (if contrasted with a negative feedback), punishing (if contrasted with a positive feedback), or ambiguous (if contrasted with positive and negative feedback). The contextual origins of the "meaning" of reinforcement are clearly evident in this social learning analysis.

The final two subprocesses in Bandura's theory are motoric skill and motivation. Motoric processes are overt response executions. Learning is more than knowing *what* to do. It also involves knowing *how* to do it. Frequently, the terminal behaviors in laboratory studies of concept formation have been relatively trivial—pushing a button, pointing to a picture, or answering yes or no. However, concept learning in naturalistic contexts often requires sophisticated motoric capabilities. Consider the motoric elements needed by a child in order to solve a division problem in mathematics. Numerals must be clearly written and properly placed, and "carry" marks must be duly noted. These motoric components, as elementary school teachers will attest, are not trivial but central to successful solution. Social learning theory assumes that an observer can attend to a social model and can extract appropriate meaning from the modeling sequence, but may still not perform if he or she lacks the requisite motoric capability. The phrase *capability training* is often used by social learning therapists to describe procedures designed to improve motoric functioning (Bandura, 1980).

Motivation describes the processes by which competence becomes activated as behavior. In terms of vicarious learning, a child observer can attend to a model, can extract meaning from a modeling array, and can be behaviorally competent, but performance may remain unchanged if the child is not motivated to perform. For example, Bandura (1965) found that children who witnessed a punished model display novel acts acquired the behavior but did not imitate the model unless informed that they, unlike the model, would be rewarded for performing the act. Nearly all cognitive theories accept the premise that prediction of actual performance requires consideration of motivational processes. In social learning theory, however, motivation and information acquisition are given equal status. In fact, motivation is assumed to reciprocally affect the cognitive subprocesses of attention and retention as well as terminal motoric performance. Both external events (such as reinforcement contingencies) and internal events (the interpretation of contingencies) combine to determine motivation (Bandura, 1977b).

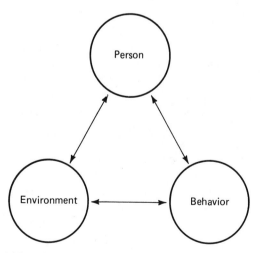

Figure 1-3. A social learning view of reciprocal determinism.

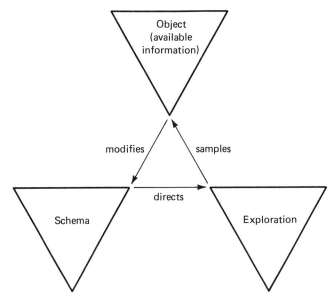

Figure 1-4. Neisser's perceptual cycle. (From *Cognition and Reality* by Ulrich Neisser. Copyright 1976 by W. H. Freeman and Company. Adapted by permission.)

Reciprocal Determinism

These four subprocesses are said to interact reciprocally with environmental stimuli. The two cognitive and two behavioral processes are combined in a tripartite depiction (see Figure 1-3). The person element refers to internal cognitive and affective events, and the environment element refers to social (actions of others) as well as physical stimuli. Changes in any one element are assumed to have an impact on the other elements. A change in environmental contingency is expected to change a person's beliefs as well as his or her behavioral functioning. For example, a teacher can decrease the incidence of much student misbehavior by withdrawing his or her attention from these responses and by purposely attending to positive responses when they occur (e.g., Allen, Henke, Harris, Baer, & Reynolds, 1967). This type of teaching style often affects students' beliefs about themselves (e.g., Davidson & Lang, 1950; Flanders, 1965). Conversely, a change in belief can lead a person to behaviorally restructure his or her environment (Thoresen & Mahoney, 1974; Bandura, 1982b). For example, if college students decide that the quality of their study environment is related to their grades, they may decide to leave a noisy fraternity or sorority house to study in the quiet of the library.

It is interesting to note that Neisser's (1976) interactionist description of perceptual functioning is based on a similar triadic model (see Figure 1-4). In comparing these two accounts we note that the object in Neisser's perceptual cycle is similar to the social learning notion of environment; schema is similar to person; and exploration is similar to behavior. Like social learning theorists' (e.g., Zimmerman, 1981) conclusions regarding general psychological functioning, Neisser sees perception as a constructive process both physically (i.e., exploration) and mentally (i.e., one's scheme). He (Neisser, 1976) describes the interactive perceptual process as follows:

> At each moment the perceiver is constructing anticipations of certain kinds of information, that enable him to accept it as it becomes available. Often he must explore the optic array to make it available, by moving his eyes or his hand or his body. These explorations are directed by the anticipating schema, which are plans for perceptual action as well as readinesses for particular kinds of optical structure. The outcome of the explorations—the information picked up—modifies the original schema. Thus modified, it directs further exploration and becomes ready for more information. (pp. 20-21)

The covergence of these two models is not accidental. It reflects metatheoretical consensus by two contextualists, each interested in quite different phenomena, about the fundamental interactive nature of psychological functioning.

Bandura's (1982a) reciprocal model of interaction differs fundamentally from nonmediational accounts of functioning and unidirectional cognitive accounts in the proposed direction of causality. In theories of the latter sort, the environment is treated as the beginning point in the explanatory process rather than as an interactive entity. Bandura's triadic model also differs from dyadic models of interaction, in which $B = f(P \leftrightarrow E)$, which are in vogue even among some contextualist researchers. The latter approaches do not treat a person's behavior as separately interactive in determining intrapersonal and environmental events. Instead, behavior is regarded as a one-directional outcome of a behaviorless person in an environmental setting. Bandura argues that a person's behavior is an interactive determinant of an event, not a detached by-product. This triadic formulation assumes that people behave in ways that simultaneously change their environment and their concepts, beliefs, emotions, and expectations. This reciprocal dependency model has some notable advantages. It allowed Bandura to explain the longevity of irrational phobias (Bandura, Grusec, & Menlove, 1967b; Bandura, Blanchard, & Ritter, 1969) as well as self-fulfilling prophecies (e.g., R. Rosenthal, 1966). Phobias were interpreted as sustained by avoidance behavior that protected the individual from discrepant outcomes; self-fulfilling prophecies were seen as triggering approach actions by persons that improved the quality of their experiences in a particular area. For example, a person told of an aptitude for music might undertake special voice training. These actions by both phobics and aspiring musicians were conceptualized by Bandura (Bandura & Walters, 1963) as self-regulating in the sense that they determined, in part, long-term outcomes for that individual.

This social learning description of self-regulation has been supported in numerous studies. Not only can self-regulation skills be taught to learners (e.g., Bandura & Kupers, 1964; Bandura, Grusec, & Menlove, 1967a), but the impact of self-produced changes in a person's environment has been found to correspond to that of changes directly created by other people (e.g., Bandura & Perloff, 1967; Glynn, 1970). Research on self-regulation has led to extensive use of these procedures in the clinic, the home, and the school to improve human functioning (e.g., Bandura, 1969; Mahoney, 1974; Thoresen & Mahoney, 1974; Bandura, 1982a).

This self-regulation feature of social learning theory has explicit utility for describing the interface between conceptual functioning and human performance, that is, people's motivation. Social learning scholars view motivation as determined most directly by cognitive factors (Bandura, 1977a; Zimmerman & Ringle, 1981). While the role of internal emotional responses in functioning is acknowledged (e.g., Bandura & Rosenthal, 1966; Bandura, 1982a), available evidence (Bandura, 1969) indicates that people's emotions derive primarily from their beliefs rather than the reverse. The value of somatic indicators of affect in predicting behavior is poor, whether measured physiologically (Rachman & Hodgson, 1974) or through self-report (Liebert & Morris, 1967). Bandura (1969, 1977b) has cited evidence that learning occurs in subjects whose somatic feedback has been blocked by surgery or drugs (Black, 1958; Taub, Bacon, & Berman, 1965). Social learning scholars have concluded from this body of evidence that people's impulse to act ultimately has a cognitive source (e.g., Bandura, 1978b).

Self-Efficacy and Related Expectations

Social learning theorists see people as acting in purposeful ways in order to obtain what are viewed as positive outcomes and to avoid what are viewed as negative ones. This cognitive approach to motivation differs from simplistic reinforcement approaches in the emphasis placed on a person's beliefs about stimuli rather than on the inherent qualities of those stimuli. In support of this position, there is evidence that social influences such as the actions of a model greatly affect children's judgments about the value of stimuli (e.g., Zimmerman & Koussa, 1975, 1979) or about the propriety of certain classes of behavior (e.g., Bandura, Ross, & Ross, 1963; Zimmerman & Kinsler, 1979). This cognitive view of outcomes can explain why people might endure considerable punishment rather than accede to what they regard as unjust or immoral (Bandura, 1977b).

Bandura (1977a, 1982a) has provided a detailed account of the cognitive processes that determine when an attractive goal will motivate requisite responses. He has used the construct of "self-efficacy" to describe the directive role of people's knowledge on their overt performance. He distinguishes between two types of expectancies: an outcome expectation and an efficacy expectation (see Figure 1-5). "An *outcome expectancy* is defined as a person's estimate that a given behavior will lead to certain outcomes" (Bandura, 1977a, p. 193, italics added). According to Bandura, outcome expectancies are not sufficiently context specific to enable us to predict an individual's behavior. Bandura suggests that people's self-perception of behavioral competence is a critical contextual factor in determining whether they will act. He terms this an *efficacy expectation*, which he defines as "the conviction that one can successfully execute the behavior required to produce the outcomes" (Bandura, 1977a, p. 193). Bandura suggested that seeing a model execute a sequence of responses leading to a particular environmental outcome will induce observers to form an outcome expectation but not necessarily an efficacy expectation. However, if that model is viewed as similar in competence to oneself, the same experience will also affect personal efficacy expectations. Behavior enactment is expected in the latter case, and there is research that supports Bandura's hypothesis (Brown &

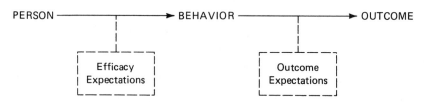

Figure 1-5. A diagrammatic representation of the difference between efficacy expectations and outcome expectations. (From "Toward a Unifying Theory of Behavioral Change," by A. Bandura, *Psychological Review,* 1977, *84,* 191-215. Copyright by the American Psychological Association. Reprinted by permission.)

Inouye, 1978). There is also a growing body of evidence (Bandura & Schunk, 1981; Schunk, 1981; Salomon, in press) that children's self-efficacy judgments are highly predictive of their behavioral functioning.

Thus social learning scholars assume that people's knowledge determines their performance; it enables them to regulate their environment to produce desired outcomes. It is implicit in the self-regulation notion that this knowledge of action-environment outcomes is not limited to short-term immediate relationships. The self-regulation notion posits that immediate action-outcome relationships are embedded in sequences leading to long-term outcomes in classic contextualist fashion (see contextualism point 3). One implication of this formulation is that deficiencies in children's self-regulation (e.g., poor study habits, lack of persistence in problem solving, poor test performance) can be corrected by making them aware of long-term outcomes of contemporaneous actions (outcome expectations) as well as by providing these people with competence-building experiences that transform outcome expectations into personal efficacy judgments. This view of self-regulation has been translated by Bandura (1976) into a training technique, termed *participant modeling*, in which outcome expectations and self-percepts of coping efficacy are enhanced when observers witness proficient models deal effectively with problems and are induced to imitate. There is growing evidence of the effectiveness of this procedure (Bandura, 1982a). For example, Schunk (1981) found that participant modeling experiences greatly improved self-efficacy judgments and mathematics proficiency of children who initially showed gross deficits and disinterest in this subject matter. Thus, Bandura's description of self-regulation and self-efficacy has not only emerged as an explicit account of the role of children's beliefs on their actions; it has also been found socially useful in remedying deficiencies in children's functioning on real-world tasks.

Cognitive Rule Learning

An important question is to consider at this point involves the fundamental unit of human knowledge that underlies people's expectancies. Three levels of knowledge have been suggested by social learning theorists: (a) At the most generic level, *plans* or conceptions have been proposed for sequencing behaviors to attain goals (Mischel, 1968). (b) At an intermediate level, *rules* have been proposed for organizing, judging, and producing instances (Bandura, 1969; Zimmerman & Rosenthal, 1974b). (c) At the most specific level, subskills and self-instructions have been proposed (Mahoney, 1974; Zimmerman, 1977) for orchestrating effective enactments. These distinctions can be illustrated by using the example of a child who is presented with several rods to seriate on the basis of length (see Zimmerman, 1977). One subskill would involve judging the relative length of each rod. A rule would provide the basis for judging whether the rods were properly aligned from long to short (e.g., "Do the rods descend like stairs?"). A plan would enable a child to align or realign the rods properly according to length. (An example of such a plan is "Select the largest rod from the array and start a new array; continue the practice, placing subsequently selected rods to the right of previously selected ones.") A common feature of all three levels of knowledge is a functional quality. A functional or conditional relationship takes the generic form "If (necessary conditions), then (outcome expectations)." Perhaps the most widely used description of knowledge in the social learning literature is the rule. In applying this term to children's learning, it is recognized that higher order rules can be used to organize basic rules and that an unlimited number of embeddings of rules within superordinate rules is possible. Bandura (1969) described vicarious rule learning in the following way:

> Observers must abstract common attributes exemplified in diverse modeled responses and formulate a principle for generating similar patterns of behavior. Responses performed by subjects that embody the observationally derived rule are likely to resemble the behavior that the model would be inclined to exhibit under similar circumstances, even though the subjects never witnessed the model's behavior in these particular situations. (p. 149)

This learning account suggests that children, as well as adults, form rules by watching models recurrently act upon their environment and by discriminating or abstracting common features of those interactions. Social learning scholars also recognize that rules can be induced personally without social support or guidance, but such learning is believed to be usually inefficient because it depends on prior rule learning and naturalistic reinforcement. Whether experience is vicarious or direct, social learning theorists assumed that the diversity involved in a learning sequence (i.e., the degree of variation in context that is dealt with) determines the generality or degree of transfer (Rosenthal, Zimmerman, & Durning, 1970). In support of this hypothesis, there is evidence that the greater the variability in modeling, context interactions, the greater the degree of transfer (Zimmerman, 1974).

Social learning theorists have argued that the rule as a contextually defined construct is sufficiently flexible to explain such "cognitively generative" performance as the use of grammar in speech, problem solving, and even creative responses. In fact, the rule learning paradigm has been used to specifically teach or induce these generative performances (Zimmerman & Rosenthal, 1974b). A particularly compelling, unexpected finding that emerged during these studies was over- and undergeneralization errors that were previously reported in naturalistic investigations, such as children's use of regular verb endings (e.g., -ed) on irregular verbs (e.g., eat; Schumaker & Sherman, 1970). These generative errors had been emphasized by organismic theorists as conflicting with experiential accounts of concept formation (e.g., McNeill, 1970).

Rules are believed by social learning theorists to be inherently functional constructs. Modeling actions that do not produce discernible environmental outcomes are not assumed to be abstracted (Bandura, 1969, p. 149). This contingency has been termed the *informative* function of reinforcement (Rosenthal & Zimmerman, 1978). Further, if outcomes that are associated with a model's actions are not desired by the observer, the rule is not expected to be implemented in performance (Bandura, 1965). This contingency has been termed the *incentive* function of reinforcement (Rosenthal & Zimmerman, 1978). These formulations are supported by experiments showing increases in rule acquisition on the basis of informative outcomes when they are separated from incentive contingencies (Rosenthal & Whitebook, 1970; Rosenthal & Carroll, 1972).

Social learning theorists suggest that drawing information from environmental outcomes in naturalistic settings is usually a complex cognitive process, unlike the impression often conveyed in laboratory studies of concept learning from reinforcement. In naturalistic settings, the meaning of consequences, the promptness of their delivery, and even their likelihood of occurrence are usually far from certain. Considerable prior rule acquisition often must occur before reinforcement effects can happen under these informationally degraded conditions. Bandura (1978b) has used the term *self-reinforcement* to describe learning under such conditions. He theorized that self-reinforcement involves people's relating outcomes to personally held goals and standards.

This self-reinforcement interpretation of children's learning was recently tested by Bandura and Schunk (1981). A group of children with substantial deficits in mathematics and low levels of self-efficacy were engaged in a program of self-directed learning to subtract. In this study, children's goal setting was manipulated by encouraging one group to set proximal goals (e.g., accomplishing a certain number of pages of problems on a certain day) and another group to set distal goals (e.g., number of pages accomplished by the end of the study). From a social learning position, the setting of proximal goals is considered optimal, since they serve as a concrete standard by which children can immediately evaluate their performance. Children who were encouraged to set proximal goals displayed substantially higher levels of subtraction performance than youngsters encouraged to set distal goals or youngsters not encouraged to set goals. Children in the proximal goal group showed significantly greater increases in self-efficacy and in intrinsic interest in the task than youngsters in the other two group. This study provided clear evidence of the substantial role that self-evaluative processes play in children's self-directed learning. In this study, goal setting was influenced by an experimenter's instructions. Researchers have also reported that self-reinforcement standards are formed during observation of the behavior of models (e.g., Bandura & Kupers, 1964; Mischel & Liebert, 1966; Bandura, Grusec, & Menlove, 1967a).

This self-reinforcement construct also implies the possibility that reinforcement effects can occur in situations when experimenters are not actively controlling consequences. For example, in a study by Rosenthal, Zimmerman, and Durning (1970), children displayed vicarious acquisition of a question-asking rule even though no feedback was provided. However, the experimenter asked the model to compose questions to pictorial stimuli and then passively accepted the model's interrogative responses. The model was an adult (and could be assumed to know what to do), and the experimenter's tacit acceptance could be construed to indicate some degree of approval. Such outcomes are subsumable as forms of self-reinforcement, and in fact rule learning occurred in this study.

In summary, social learning theorists have stressed rules as the basic units of cognition. Rules are believed to be abstracted from specific, contextually delimited events. Rules are functional, dynamic entities. They fuse context-action conditions that produce particular environmental outcomes. Rules vary in their inclusiveness. *Plans, strategies,* and *conceptions* are terms used to describe broader or higher order rules. Although all rules are believed to enable people to control their environment, higher order rules enable people to exert greater control over future outcomes. If the relationship between successive action-outcome rules is understood through the formation of higher order rules, plans, or strategies, then people can act in the present context in ways that are instrumental to their attainment of long-term goals. Self-regulating actions (such as self-reinforcing, weakly externally reinforced actions; choosing settings or social groups that are consonant with long-term goals; or restructuring one's personal environment in ways that remove counterproductive stimuli) will assist the individual to achieve future goals. In this sense, social learning theory explains not only the formation and alteration of people's knowledge, but also how such knowledge directs people's behavior in naturalistic settings.

The Development of Cognitive Functioning

Social learning theorists assume that children's level of knowledge is a critical factor in explaining age differences in cognitive functioning. But social learning scholars avoid reified, macromentalistic descriptions of knowledge states of particular age groups of children, and instead favor contextually specific analyses (Zimmerman & Whitehurst, 1979). They assume that children's knowledge is organized around specific features of their prior experience, particularly social experiences with parents, siblings, and peers. Physical maturation is, however, believed to play an important indirect role in mental development. In other words, since concepts are assumed to arise from children's interactive experiences and since experience is dependent to some degree on children's physical capabilities (e.g., motoric dexterity, articulatory facility) and socially valued physical attributes (e.g., size and apparent maturity), and then children's knowledge levels will to that degree be correlated with their physical development and with their age.

This formulation yields several testable hypotheses about cognitive development. One hypothesis is that socializing agents such as parents and peers will respond variably to children according to their age. There is some support for this hypothesis. Research on language acquisition indicates that parents (Snow, 1972; Phillips, 1973) and older children (Shatz & Gelman, 1973) modify the linguistic complexity of their speech based on the age of a child.

A second testable hypothesis is that in cases where experience is unrelated to a person's age, experience as a variable will predict learning outcomes, whereas age will not. One contextually specific way to define experience is *familiarity* with a task or object. Familiarity with a task has been manipulated by selecting people

with known experiential backgrounds in a particular area and has been operationally defined by the results of specific content area tests of knowledge (e.g., Tobias,
1976). Such content-related descriptions of knowledge stand in contrast to content-
free constructs, such as information processing capacity, generic mnemonic strategies, or operations, used by classical cognitive theorists.

The relative importance of children's age versus their level of prior knowledge
was tested in a study by Chi (1978). She studied not only recall but also the predictive skills of adults and 10-year-old children on digit span and chess tasks. The
twist in the experiment involved the 10-year-olds. They were chess experts, whereas
the adults were only novices. The recall task of interest involved examining an
organized arrangement of chess pieces on a board for 10 seconds and then recon-
structing the display from memory on another chess board. The subjects were asked
to predict the number of trials that they would require in order to obtain the correct answer. Such metamemory measures are believed to reflect adult-level awareness
of the utility of mnemonic strategies (Flavell & Wellman, 1977). Children were not
only better than adults in their recall on chess piece positions, they were also more
accurate in predicting the number of required trials. As expected, adults showed
their usual age-group superiority in recall of digits. Chi concluded that differences
in specific task-related knowledge outweighed all other factors (including information processing capacity measures) in explaining age differences in recall.

There is other evidence that the content of people's prior knowledge determines
the quality of generic memorization strategies. Myers and Perlmutter (1978) studied
word recall by 2-year-olds and 4-year-olds and found that age-related improvements
in recall were uncorrelated with the use of such general strategies as rehearsal, elaboration, or organization. They concluded that age differences in recall were due to
the older children's superior content knowledge.

Cross-cultural data also indicate that contextually specific experience is more
influential on learning and memory than extensive training in the use of mnemonic
strategies. Wagner (1978) studied recognition of oriental rugs by Koranic scholars
and by rug merchants. As a result of extensive formal training, the Koranic scholars
had great skill in memorizing textual passages, whereas the rug merchants had more
specific knowledge about rugs. The rug merchants proved to be much better than
the scholars at recognizing previously seen rugs. Wagner concluded that the rug
sellers' greater knowledge of task stimuli (in terms of attributes and functions of
rugs) aided them in identifying distinctive features of particular rugs. Thus, it
appears that a person's organizational skills, long known to be a critical process in
long-term memory (Tulving, 1962; Mandler, 1967; Atkinson & Shiffrin, 1968), are
more dependent on the *content* of one's knowledge than one one's possession of
contextually free mnemonic strategies.

In general, social learning researchers have attempted to establish the relation of
sociocontextual experience to children's level of cognitive functioning through training studies (see Zimmerman & Rosenthal, 1974b). The first step in such experiments
is to identify groups of children who have not yet "naturally" attained a particular
level of cognitive functioning. The children are then provided with contextually
rich social modeling experiences in which a developmentally advanced rule is exem-

plified. If the children show rule acquisition and retention, the importance of social contextual experience in cognitive development is demonstrated. To the degree that such rules are transferred to new tasks, a "constructive" or "generative" or "productive" level of cognitive functioning has been attained (Zimmerman & Whitehurst, 1979). In contextualist terms, such data indicate that rules can be used interactively by the child.

These training studies spanned a wide range of cognitive phenomena of interest to developmental psychologists, such as question-asking styles (Rosenthal, Zimmerman, & Durning, 1970; Rosenthal & Zimmerman, 1972a; Zimmerman & Pike, 1972), concept formation (Zimmerman & Rosenthal, 1972a; Rosenthal, Alford, & Rasp, 1972), conservation (Rosenthal & Zimmerman, 1972b; Zimmerman & Lanaro, 1974; Zimmerman & Rosenthal, 1974a), language rules (e.g., Bandura & Harris, 1966; Odom, Liebert, & Hill, 1968; Carroll, Rosenthal, & Brysh, 1972; Vasta & Liebert, 1973; Harris & Hassemer, 1972), problem solving (Laughlin, Moss, & Miller, 1969; Lamal, 1971; Zimmerman & Rosenthal, 1972b), cognitive tempo (Debus, 1970; Ridberg, Parke, & Hetherington, 1971; Debus, 1976), categorization (Zimmerman, 1974; Zimmerman & Jaffe, 1977), Piagetian seriation (Henderson, Swanson, & Zimmerman, 1975; Zimmerman & Kleefeld, 1977), and creative production (Harris & Evans, 1973; Harris & Fisher, 1973; Zimmerman & Dialessi, 1973; Belcher, 1975; Arem & Zimmerman, 1976). This list is not exhaustive, but it illustrates the vast literature on modeling training studies. With few exceptions, the results of these training efforts were positive.

In addition to age-related differences in experience, social learning theorists suggest that rule interdependence is another source of correlation between children's level of cognitive functioning and their age. Zimmerman and Lanaro (1974) and Rosenthal and Zimmerman (1978) have noted that complex rules such as Piagetian conservation of number, seriation, and two-dimensional classification are dependent on a child's prior mastery of subordinate rules. In the case of conservation of number, subordinate rules such as counting or one-to-one matching are essential. Brainerd (1978b) has termed such interdependencies "measurement sequences" and has convincingly argued that a distinction should be drawn between learning sequences that are logically inevitable and those that are not. He reasoned that *logically* interdependent sequences do not require *psychological* constructs, such as a stage, to be explained. He surveyed Piaget's studies of children's cognitive development and concluded that many sequentially related skills are logically interdependent.

Social learning theorists (e.g., Zimmerman & Rosenthal, 1972b) assume that children who lack subordinate rules may require considerable exposure to complex modeling performances before a terminal rule can be induced. Many times, special efforts are necessary in order to restructure the task in ways that make subordinate rules evident before inexperienced children can learn from modeling (Zimmerman, 1977). Social learning theorists (Henderson, Swanson, & Zimmerman, 1975) have suggested that subordinate rules should be taught first, and once acquired (Zimmerman, 1981) will be utilized by the observer to induce superordinate rules from social experiences. This process of secondary (tertiary, etc.) rule learning is complex but lawful. It yields the prediction that children will show individual differences in learning from a common modeling experience based on prior rule learning. Unlike stage assumptions, secondary rule learning leads to the hypothesis that children can learn if they are taught subordinate rules first (see Gagne, 1968). Evidence in support of this hypothesis will be discussed later.

Rule interdependence assumptions can thus explain the sequential appearance of increasingly complex performances by children. Since children are constantly aging, their level of cognitive sophistication will, of course, be correlated with their age to some degree. This analysis is related to point 5 in the discussion of contextualism, which cautioned researchers that sociocultural experiences are typically confounded with age in developmental research.

Rule Interdependence and Learning

It has been suggested that constructing accurate rules from contextually rich social experiences is not a simple one-step process. Salient but irrelevant contextual features of modeling experiences often have to be eliminated before an observer will attend to other features. The behavior of a model can assist the observer in focusing on the relevant cues. But the interpretation of the model's actions usually requires a considerable amount of prior rule learning as well. Intentional cues such as a model's eye contact, body orientation, hand movements, and speech are behavioral events that children must learn to use to decode contextual experiences. Once such cues become meaningful, children are able to respond to social contextual experiences at new and more sophisticated levels (i.e., they can form more advanced rules).

Social learning researchers have devoted much attention to the contextual conditions that facilitate decoding. For example, the *degree* and *type of organization* in a modeling sequence have been found to affect the type and amount of observational learning that occurs. If the sequence of a model's actions is isomorphic with an underlying rule structure, learning is facilitated (Rosenthal & Zimmerman, 1973, 1976), retention is improved (Liebert & Swenson, 1971b), transfer is enhanced (e.g., Zimmerman & Bell, 1972), and the observer becomes more capable of accurately predicting future actions of the model (Liebert & Swenson, 1971a).

The completeness of modeling experiences has also been found to be a particularly important dimension affecting young children's rule learning. For example, Zimmerman (1974) instructed preschool children in a new method for grouping pictures that differed from the rule used spontaneously by these children. After training, the older children, who were 5 years of age, could use either the new rule or the old method for grouping pictures, but the 3- and 4-year-olds could not shift back to the old rule. The younger children were then exposed to a modeling sequence wherein the model flexibly used both rules, and the youngsters were subsequently able to group pictures by using either rule. Therefore, individual differences in cognitive rule learning occurred when only part of the desired terminal behavior was demonstrated. These differences were eliminated when the modeling episode depicted the shifting strategy as well as the new rule.

The possibility of an interaction between the completeness of modeling sequences and children's level of development was studied by Zimmerman and Jaffe (1977). They taught a rule for grouping pictures to children from Grades 1, 2, and

3. Three modeling sequences were studied: (a) a low-structure condition, in which the model's categorical groupings were presented after the fact; (b) an intermediate-structure condition, in which the model sorted the cards in front of the child; and (c) a high-structure condition, in which the model pointed to the relevant contextual feature on each card before assigning it to a group. No significant age differences were evident under either the high- or low-structure modeling conditions; however, significant differences among the three grade groups occurred at the intermediate level of structure. These results were interpreted as follows: Age differences occur with learning tasks that are informationally deficient in some way that older youngsters can fill in but younger children cannot. Unfortunately, the relevant pre-existing knowledge possessed by older children was not determined in this study.

Together, these studies on the effects of the completeness of a model's performance on children's rule learning imply that social learning in naturalistic circumstances is often far from optimal from the point of view of a naive child. Deficient contextual conditions can lead to age-related differences in learning. It was suggested earlier that older children generally have greater contextually relevant knowledge.

Language is another important age-related capacity that is assumed by social learning psychologists to affect children's cognitive rule learning. There is extensive evidence that providing adjunctive statements greatly facilitates learning by people at all age levels (e.g., Zimmerman & Rosenthal, 1972a, 1972b). Verbal codes have been found to enhance vicarious learning whether they were provided by a model (Rosenthal & Zimmerman, 1972b), by an experimenter (Zimmerman & Rosenthal, 1972a), or by the observers themselves (Gerst, 1971). Verbal cues such as descriptions or rationales for a model's performance appear to play a particularly important but complex role in young children's rule learning. It is well known (Bloom, 1975) that a young child's competence in language is far from complete, and hence it can be expected that language cues will assist children to acquire information more effectively as they grow older. As imperfect as a young child's language system is, however, it can reduce the contextual complexity of social experiences. For example, telling a preoperational child a conservation rule outside the context of relevant modeling actions has been found to be ineffective (Rosenthal & Zimmerman, 1972b, Experiment 3), but rule statements that correspond to nonverbal model enactments facilitate learning (Rosenthal & Zimmerman, 1972b, Experiment 1). Therefore, young children's rule learning depends on their ability to map words onto contextual referents and to map sentences onto event sequences. The complex interactive process by which language, as a second rule system, is acquired is discussed below.

Some researchers have assisted young children who had difficulty vicariously acquiring complex rules by breaking the modeling sequence into shorter, subordinate rule episodes and by linking simplified verbal descriptions to contextual events. For example, Rosenthal and Zimmerman (1972b, Experiment 4) found that middle-class 4-year-old children had difficulty abstracting a conservation rule from six sequentially connected modeling demonstrations of various conservation concepts. When the task was divided into separate task episodes, however, vicarious learning occurred, and subsequently generalization was evident. Zimmerman and Lanaro (1974) reported that further subdivisions had to be made in order to teach disadvantaged 4-year-olds to conserve. In each of these studies, young children had difficulty mapping verbal rationales onto complex modeling sequences but could do so when contextual complexity was reduced.

These outcomes led Henderson, Zimmerman, Swanson, and Bergan (1974) to use task analysis procedures to teach complex rules to preschool-aged native American children. These children were disadvantaged in practically every sense of the word. They were poor and lived in isolated homes in a rural desert region of Arizona. The skills selected for training were numeration, conservation, seriation, and question asking. Each skill was decomposed into a hierarchy of subordinate rules. The rules were taught by culturally appropriate puppets and by adult and child characters using a series of videotapes. Rule instruction proceeded sequentially, with subordinate rules being presented and mastered before more complex rules were presented. The results were positive despite the difficulty of the rules, the age of these children, and their level of disadvantage (e.g., Henderson, Swanson, & Zimmerman, 1974, 1975).

The importance of decomposing tasks into simple units, sequencing the units from simple to complex, and mapping simplified rule statements onto modeling sequences was further studied by Zimmerman and Kleefeld (1977). They compared the instructional effectiveness of a group of teachers trained in the use of social learning techniques with a control group of elementary school teachers. Both groups were given the task of teaching a 4-year-old preoperational child to seriate during a single instructional session. The length of the session was left to the teacher's discretion. Children who were taught by social learning teachers displayed significantly more seriation on posttest than children taught by uninstructed teachers and children in a no-teaching control group. The latter two groups did not differ. In addition, social learning teachers used approximately half the instructional time required by untrained teachers.

Together, these studies reveal some of the difficulties encountered by young children as they attempt to form rules from unstructured, naturalistic modeling experiences. However, they also indicate that systematic efforts by adults to reduce the contextual complexity of social experiences and explicitly map rule statements on the simplified modeling sequences were quite successful in overcoming age disadvantages of younger children. The relationship between children's linguistic and cognitive development is, however, a complex issue. Fortunately, a fair amount of research has been devoted to this topic.

Language Acquisition

Social learning theorists (e.g., Bandura & Harris, 1966; Bandura, 1969, 1977b) view language acquisition as a process of second-order rule learning. Rules of language are assumed to be abstracted during naturalistic encounters that a child witnesses between speakers and listeners. Such linguistic rules cannot be abstracted, it is assumed, unless the child first understands contextual relationships among nonlinguistic referential stimuli. Bandura (1977b) has described language acquisition in the following manner.

> The process of acquiring language involves not only learning grammatical relations between words, but also correlating linguistic forms with the events to

which they apply. Language learning therefore depends upon semantic aids and nonlinguistic understanding of the events to which the utterances refer. . . . Verbal expressions that convey grammatical relations are usually matched to meaningful ongoing activities about which children already have some knowledge. (pp. 176-177)

A similar contextualist view of language acquisition has been advocated by several psycholinguists as well. For example, Bloom (1974) said, "In a naturalistic situation, a child might respond to [a grammatical form] when he hears it, but what he understands of the form might be heavily dependent on the situation in which he hears it or on the state of affairs to which it refers" (p. 298). MacNamara (1972) reviewed an extensive series of psycholinguistic studies of language acquisition by infants and young children and came to a similar conclusion. He described how children infer the meaning of a sentence from the nonlinguistic context:

Children initially take the main lexical items in the sentences they hear, determine referents for these items, and then use their knowledge of the referents to decide what the semantic structures intended by the speaker must be. . . . Their final task is to note the syntactic devices, such as word order, prepositions, number of affixes etc. which correlate with the semantic structures. (p. 9)

In support of contextualist views of language acquisition there is extensive evidence (e.g., Bloom, 1970; Snow, 1972) that when parents talk in the presence of young children, they typically converse about objects, people, and action sequences that are readily observable.

In early studies, social learning theorists examined the effects of an adult model's speech patterns on elementary-school-aged children's use of language. In these studies, the children had opportunities to observe an adult make statements about selected stimuli (e.g., pictures, words, or dolls). At some point during the experiment, the children were asked to generate statements about new (transfer) stimuli, and the correspondence between the structure of their utterances and that of the model's statements was determined. The model's statements were organized according to such linguistic rules as verb tense and prepositional phrases (Bandura & Harris, 1966; Odom, Liebert, & Hill, 1968; Carroll, Rosenthal, & Brysh, 1972), sentence length and complexity (Harris & Hassemer, 1972), conditional phrases (Harris & Siebel, 1976), and interrogative forms (Zimmerman & Pike, 1972). With few exceptions, children altered the structure of their generated sentences to accord with that of the model whether they were instructed to imitate (e.g., Bandura & Harris, 1966) or not (e.g., Harris & Hassemer, 1972). Because their language performance was altered on transfer tasks, it was clear that the children had adopted a rule. There was typically little imitation of the exact semantic content of the model's speech on these transfer tasks, just emulation of the syntactic rule form (e.g., Rosenthal, Zimmerman, & Durning, 1970).

In recent descriptive research on verbal interactions between mothers and their 2- to 3-year-old child, Hood and Bloom (1979) also found modeling effects. They reported essentially perfect agreement in mother-child phrase ordering of causal language. For example, children of mothers who reasoned from effect to cause (e.g., "Get another pen, it's dirty") showed a predominance of the same type of reasoning in their own speech. Particularly impressive about these agreements in reasoning pattern *within* mother-child dyads was evidence of tremendous differences in reasoning *across* the eight mother-child dyads. Thus, evidence of modeling effects on children's language patterns is not limited to laboratory studies but has been found in research conducted in naturalistic settings as well.

These initial experimental modeling studies were not directed at *de novo* syntactic rule learning. Most of the children were already of age where the modeled syntactic forms had been acquired. However, operant psychologists (e.g., Guess, Sailor, Rutherford, & Baer, 1968; Schumaker & Sherman, 1970; Clark & Sherman, 1975) have undertaken numerous studies that used modeling to teach novel language rules to atypical children, such as retarded youngsters. In these studies (see Rosenthal & Zimmerman, 1978), children were presented with a stimulus (pictures, words, objects, etc.) and were asked to describe it. The stimulus was designed to elicit a particular linguistic structure, such as a prepositional phrase. If the children produced this structure, they were reinforced with praise and/or tangible rewards. If they did not, the experimenter modeled the correct statement and then asked the children to imitate. Correct imitations were similarly reinforced. Training was discontinued after the children displayed correct answers to a specified series of new items without modeling assistance.

Although operant studies demonstrated *de novo* language rule learning, they say little about how linguistic rules are acquired by normal populations of children in natural settings. Psycholinguistics such as McNeill (1970) and Brown (1973) have discounted the relevance of operant findings, arguing that no systematic use of reinforcement is evident in observations of parent-child interactions in natural settings such as the home. McNeill and Brown's conclusion, however, rests on how reinforcement is defined and studied in such settings. Obviously, parents do not praise or provide tangible rewards to their children each time they utter a certain statement. However, reinforcement is not defined so narrowly by social learning psychologists. A wide variety of parental responses (e.g., appropriate verbal or nonverbal responses, tacit acceptance of self-evident statements, eye contact) is considered reinforcing if the responses are contingently related to children's statements.

With this point in mind, other studies (e.g., Moerk, 1976; Mann & Van Wagenen, 1975) have revealed that, contrary to conclusions by McNeill (1970) and Brown (1973), parents respond contingently during verbal exchanges with their children in naturalistic contexts. They frequently provide phonetic, semantic, and grammatical corrections after incomplete or incorrect utterances by their offspring. Thus, parents do appear to reinforce their children systematically for appropriate language, and they were also observed to reduce such support as the youngsters acquired linguistic competence.

Despite the extensive use of reinforcement by parents during linguistic interaction with their children, the usefulness of modeling alone in teaching language rules is a theoretically interesting question. Whitehurst and Novak (1973) and Whitehurst, Ironsmith, and Goldfein (1974) studied the effects of modeling alone and modeling with reinforcement on several syntactic rules in 4- and 5-year-old children. They found that modeling by itself was ineffective, and they concluded that children could not imitate a model's use of a syntactic structure that was not already comprehended. (Comprehension was assessed by asking the youngsters to point to the correct referent after hearing an utterance of a particular form.) This conclusion led Whitehurst and colleagues to hypothesize a three-step sequence in which comprehension precedes imitative rule learning, which in turn precedes productive use of the rule.

Morgulas and Zimmerman (1979) have reported evidence that provided some support for the comprehension-imitation-production (CIP) hypothesis. Groups of 4- and 5-year-olds were tested for comprehension of sentences with passive verbs, a linguistic structure that is not typically acquired until children are approximately 6 years old. Half of the subjects were exposed to a model who consistently used the passive form (e.g., "The ball was hit by the boy") to describe pictures. The children alternated with the model in composing descriptions of different pictures. The children's degree of rule usage in their speech was found to be directly related to their initial level of rule comprehension. However, a small but significant degree of learning was found with even the lowest comprehenders.

It is important to point out that the modeling procedures used in studies by Whitehurst and colleagues and by Morgulas and Zimmerman (1979) were not optimal according to social learning theory. All of these modeling studies used line drawings as linguistic referents with which to test and to train the children. Such referents are contextually very sparse compared to naturalistic interaction experience. In particular, the model's sentences were not accompanied by appropriate nonverbal action in contextually relevant settings.

A direct test of Bandura's account of language acquisition was reported by Brown (1976). This researcher compared linguistic modeling in which a picture was used as the referent with linguistic modeling in which doll enactments were used as the referential context. The targeted language rule was the passive-voice sentence form. The children ranged in age from 3½ to 5 years. Children in the enactive modeling condition achieved significantly higher posttest comprehension scores than children in the pictorial referent modeling condition and significantly higher scores than youngsters who were exposed to verbal modeling without any referents present. As in prior research, modeling with picture referents failed to produce significant acquisition (relative to the control group). This study demonstrated that dynamic physical activity is the critical contextual cue for abstracting linguistic meaning. Brown's data indicated that a social learning formulation can explain children's learning to comprehend linguistic rules as well as their learning to use them in their speech. Together these studies indicated that both comprehension and imitative performance were influenced by observational learning. Considering these and other results, Bandura (1977b, p. 179) has questioned CIP assumptions that comprehension and imitation are causally linked. He suggested that both linguistic outcomes be viewed as manifestations of a common observational rule learning process.

This social learning account of language acquisition as arising from specific dynamic experience has been supported by a growing body of research gathered by psycholinguistics scholars. Nelson (1974) has examined developmentally the meaning of young toddlers' first words and found that dynamic, functional qualities of referents were abstracted before concrete physical dimensions. Words such as *dog, cat, ball,* and *car* were among the 10 most common "thing" words that these children used (Nelson, 1973b). When examining clothing words of these youngsters, it was found that two-thirds referred to shoes and other footwear. Nelson argued that these were items that children typically acted on (i.e., used functionally). Perhaps most interesting was the absence from these children's vocabularies of any words that referred to stationary or functionally unresponsive stimuli (e.g., furniture), despite their presence in the environment of children. From these as well as other data (e.g., Nelson, 1973a) she concluded:

> It seems likely from these considerations that the relations at the functional core of the child's first concepts will be actions and the results of actions, whether these are caused by the child himself or by others, animate or inanimate. This fundamental functional center may emerge from the perceptual salience of movement or variation, from the importance of the child's active involvement with objects, or possibly from some inherent cognitive processing disposition. (pp. 279-280)

Nelson's conclusion is in essential agreement with the contextualist argument that meaning arises from physical as well as mental interaction with stimuli and with the conclusions by social learning scholars that human knowledge is functional in its essential form.

Nelson (1974) has suggested that children's meaning for words changes developmentally and that concrete, physical dimensions of referents are eventually discriminated and mapped onto functional core meanings. But the functional nature of human knowledge remains fundamental to older verbal children, as it is to preverbal youngsters. In more recent research, Nelson (1978) asked a group of 4-year-olds to describe eating situations at home, at a day-care center they attended, and at a McDonalds' fast food restaurant. The children's "scripts" revealed a predominant concern for utilitarian types of information. For example, the order of the children's recall of events corresponded to the correct sequence. Actions that were functionally related to eating, such as traveling to McDonald's, were mentioned by virtually every child. Events likely to occur on such trips but irrelevant to the act of eating (e.g., seeing other people entering and leaving the restaurant) were seldom mentioned. Finally, the few inaccurate statements that were made (e.g., paying for the meal at McDonald's after eating instead of before) were consistent with the sequential patterns followed in restaurants as a class of events. Although such data were collected under naturalistic conditions without much experimental control, they do suggest that older children organized their recall on the basis of functional relationships or rules. Such outcomes are concordant with a social learning utilitarian view of knowledge.

In addition to emphasizing the importance of dynamic contextual events in children's construction of meaning from spoken language, Bandura's (1977b) reciprocal-interactionist description of language acquisition assumes the importance of previously acquired knowledge. The impact of preexisting knowledge, both linguistic and nonlinguistic in form, has emerged in several social learning studies. Such outcomes were often age related. For example, Liebert, Odom, Hill, and Huff (1969) studied 5-, 8-, and 14-year-old children's exact imitation (mimicry) of a model's grammatical and ungrammatical phrases (e.g., *the door at*). They found no age differences in imitation of grammatical sentences but did find differences with ungrammatical phrases. Older children displayed more accurate mimicry of ungrammatical phrases than younger children. The authors concluded that older children were more sensitive to the contextual constraints of the experimental situation and more expecting of improbable statements than younger children (see also Vasta & Liebert, 1973). The younger children were observed to reformulate ungrammatical phrases into grammatically correct ones. Similar age-related differences in accuracy have been found with children's comprehension of language as well. Strohner and Nelson (1974, Experiment 1) studied 4- to 6-year-old children's comprehension of probable ("The cat chases the mouse") or improbable sentences ("The mouse chases the cat"). All age groups of children were comparable in correctly decoding probable sentences; however, age differences in comprehension occurred with improbable sentences. The data revealed that with age the children became increasingly adept at understanding anomalous sentences.

The foregoing research indicates that there are quantitative differences in errors in language comprehension and mimicry associated with a child's age. There is also evidence that there are qualitative differences in errors associated with a child's age. Brown, Smiley, Day, Townsend, and Lawton (1977) presented a brief story to second, fourth, and sixth graders and then asked the youngsters to recall it. These researchers found qualitative differences in the intrusion errors among the three age groups. Older children's intrusions were more often relevant to the theme of the story. Brown and colleagues attributed these differences to greater preexisting knowledge about the topic by the older children. Interestingly, there were no age differences in the quantity of intrusions in this study. It is important to note that very stringent criteria were used to score accuracy in this study. In many studies, thematically relevant intrusions would not be considered errors, but would be regarded as evidence of generalization or comprehension. The absence of age-related differences in the quantity of errors under these demanding criteria implies that they were not due to age differences in mental capacity but appeared more attributable to age-related differences in the quality of children's knowledge. Such an interpretation coheres with previously discussed evidence reported by Chi (1978), Myers and Perlmutter (1978), and Wagner (1978) about the importance of contextually specific knowledge.

A social learning explanation for age differences in linguistic accuracy focuses on the availability of contextually relevant knowledge to children as they encounter new experience. That such knowledge may be age associated is interesting but inessential to this account. To date, few efforts have been undertaken within the social learning tradition to experimentally manipulate prior knowledge and examine its interactive relationship to language acquisition. One such study has recently been completed. Morgulas (1982) studied young children's acquisition of a passive-voice sentence comprehension rule with 4- and 5-year-olds. A very demanding screening procedure was followed in order to eliminate children displaying any evidence of comprehension of passive-voice sentences. The youngsters were randomly assigned to modeling conditions that used either puppet models as dynamic referents, or pictorial referents, or no referents at all. Half of the youngsters in each condition were given contextually relevant information about the personality (i.e., the likely behavior patterns) of the protagonists in the story. Then the story was presented according to one of the three modeling formats. All sentences in the story were reversible passive-voice constructions, that is, sentences in which either character could plausibly be the actor or the recipient of the action specified by the verb. Such a story is a stringent test of passive-voice learning, since all non-passive-voice syntactic cues (e.g., interspersed active-voice sentences and nonreversible passive-voice sentences, wherein only one meaning is plausible) have been eliminated. Three separate posttests of comprehension of passive-voice rules were conducted; they varied in degree of stringency of transfer (i.e., contextual overlap with the training story). Significant acquisition of the passive-voice rule was evident for only those children who had been familiarized with the characters and were exposed to enactive modeling. Passive-voice rule learning was evident on the most stringent posttest as well as on the least stringent posttest. Such findings provide clear-cut support for Bandura's account of language acquisition: Only those children who were provided with information about the meanings of contextual referents for words and saw the words behaviorally enacted were able to abstract the linguistic rule.

Conclusion

The claim that human knowledge emerges from specific person-environment encounters and is organized on the basis of specific features of such experiences was made by social learning theorists before contemporary psychological interest in contextualism surfaced with the republication of Pepper's book in 1970. In 1968, Mischel published *Personality and Assessment*, a book-length treatment of the contextual nature of people's personality and social functioning. He argued for the need for a fully interactionist psychological theory to explain such outcomes and recommended Bandura's social learning theory. At the time, he used the phrase "situational specificity" to describe the fundamental contextual character of human knowledge.

> The phenomena of discrimination and generalization lead to the view that behavior patterns are remarkably situation specific, on the one hand, while also evokable by diverse and often seemingly heterogeneous stimuli on the basis of generalization effects. The person's prior experiences with related conditions and the exact details of the particular evoking situation determine the meaning of the stimuli—that is, their effects on all aspects of his life. Usually generalization effects involve relatively idiosyncratic *contextual* and semantic generalization dimensions. (p. 189, italics added)

Mischel (1968) comprehensively reviewed the available literature in personality and social functioning and found that reified constructs such as mental "traits" and "cognitive styles" were severely taxed by evidence of "situationism." His book raised a storm of controversy in the field of personality (e.g., Bowers, 1973) by critics who mistook Mischel's position to be noncognitive or noninteractionist. In his rebuttals, Mischel went to some length to clarify these misinterpretations of his position (Mischel, 1973, 1977, 1979).

In retrospect, it is now clear that evidence of contextualism in human functioning was even more pervasive than Mischel had claimed, extending to many other areas of research, such as developmental psychology, cognitive psychology, and educational psychology. The movement toward contextualist explanations was not limited to social learning theorists; it was in fact a metatheoretical implication of many research studies conducted in naturalistic settings. Because of their early concern with observational learning in naturalistic settings, social learning theorists (e.g., Bandura & Walters, 1959) were among the first to confront evidence of contextualism.

Although social learning theory has previously been identified with other contextual theories (Rosenthal & Bandura, 1978), the present account is the first systematic effort to specify in detail how it fits within the broad metatheoretical movement of contextualism and to point out its common features with other contextual theories concerned with such phenomena as concept formation, perception, language acquisition, and memory. Pepper's (1970) philosophic treatment of contextualism provides a broad framework for integration at this metatheoretical level. It is hoped that it will also make more explicit the fundamental interactionist, nonreductionist nature of social learning theory as well. Unfortunately, some critics of social learning theory have had difficulty understanding these features and have misclassified the approach as mechanistic and reductionist (e.g., Beilin, 1981) or as reified cognitivist (Smedslund, 1978; Sampson, 1981). Pepper's (1970) distinction between contextualism and universalist accounts such as mechanism and organicism should help clarify, at a metatheoretical level, the distinctiveness and cohesiveness of contextualist viewpoints.

The central concern of this chapter has been (a) to describe the emergence of contextualism as a broad-based metatheoretical movement dealing with children's development, (b) to note the intimate relationship between contextualist accounts and naturalistic research on children's cognitive functioning, (c) to indicate the contributions of social learning theorists to the contextualist movement, and (d) to provide a brief overview of a social learning account of children's development of cognitive functioning. These goals plus the constraint of page space necessarily limited the depth of the present review of research. The social learning literature on children's cognitive functioning is extensive, and readers who desire summaries of this evidence are referred to several recent reviews (e.g., Zimmerman & Rosenthal, 1974; Bandura, 1977b; Zimmerman, 1977; Rosenthal & Zimmerman, 1978).

Contextualist accounts of cognitive development, such as social learning theory, may not prove attractive to developmental psychologists who desire elegant simplicity at a theoretical level. Although it should now be clear how contextualist approaches deliver explanation and prediction beyond immediately observable events, such accounts are by nature contextually qualified. These theories require disciplined, cautious interpretations of children's behavior. Decision making in the absence of data about specific children in particular contexts is all but ruled out. Unlike universalist theories, however, contextual accounts such as social learning theory require few restrictive assumptions about children's ability to learn to understand the world around them and to adapt behaviorally to it. As evidence of the contextual dependency of children's knowledge continues to mount, universalist accounts of cognitive development will become less viable unless they too are qualified contextually. As they become more complex, their apparent advantage will concomitantly dissipate.

Acknowledgments. I would like to express my gratitude to Albert Bandura, Charles J. Brainerd, Ted L. Rosenthal, and Grover J. Whitehurst for their invaluable comments on initial drafts of this chapter. I would also like to thank my colleague Geoffrey Saxe for providing secretarial assistance with the preparation of this manuscript and for his helpful discussions of several of the issues treated in this paper. Finally, I would like to acknowledge the contribution of Betty Einerman; her patience and expert typing were greatly appreciated.

References

Adorno, T. W. Sociology and psychology. *New Left Review*, November-December 1967, 67-80.

Adorno, T. W. Introduction. In T. W. Adorno, H. Albert, R. Dahrendorf, J. Habermas, H. Pilot, & K. R. Popper (Eds.), *The positivist dispute in German sociology.* New York: Harper & Row, 1976.

Allen, K. E., Henke, L. B., Harris, F. R., Baer, D. M., & Reynolds, N. J. Control of hyperactivity by social reinforcement of attending behavior. *Journal of Educational Psychology*, 1967, *58*, 231-237.

Arem, C. A., & Zimmerman, B. J. Vicarious effects on the creative behavior on retarded and nonretarded children. *American Journal of Mental Deficiency*, 1976, *81*, 289-296.

Atkinson, R. C., & Shiffrin, R. M. Human memory: A proposed system and its control processes. In K. W. Spence & J. T. Spence (Eds.), *The psychology of learning and motivation* (Vol. 2). New York: Academic Press, 1968.

Baltes, P. B., & Labouvie, G. V. Adult development of intellectual performance: Description, explanation, and modification. In D. Eisdorfer & M. P. Lawton (Eds.), *The psychology of adult development and aging.* Washington, D.C.: American Psychological Association, 1973.

Bandura, A. Social learning through imitation. In M. R. Jones (Ed.), *Nebraska Symposium on Motivation* (Vol. 10). Lincoln: University of Nebraska Press, 1962.

Bandura, A. Influence of a model's reinforcement contingencies on the acquisition of imitative responses. *Journal of Personality and Social Psychology*, 1965, *11*, 587-595.

Bandura, A. *Principles of behavior modification.* New York: Holt, Rinehart & Winston, 1969.

Bandura, A. *Psychological modeling—Conflicting theories.* Chicago: Atherton/Aldine, 1971.

Bandura, A. Effecting change through participant modeling. In J. D. Krumboltz & C. E. Thoresen (Eds.), *Counseling method.* New York: Holt, Rinehart & Winston, 1976.

Bandura, A. Self efficacy: Toward a unifying theory of behavioral change. *Psychological Review*, 1977, *84*, 191-215. (a)

Bandura, A. *Social learning theory.* Englewood Cliffs, N.J.: Prentice-Hall, 1977. (b)

Bandura, A. On paradigms and recycled ideologies. *Cognitive Therapy and Research,* 1978, *2*, 79-103. (a)

Bandura, A. The self system in reciprocal determinism. *American Psychologist,* 1978, *33*, 344-358. (b)

Bandura, A. The self and mechanisms of agency. In J. Suls (Ed.), *Social psychologi-*

cal perspectives on the self. Hillsdale, N.J.: Erlbaum, 1980.

Bandura, A. Self-efficacy mechanism in human agency. *American Psychologist, 1982, 37*, 122-147. (a)

Bandura, A. The psychology of chance encounters and life paths. *American Psychologist, 1982, 37*, 747-755. (b)

Bandura, A., Blanchard, E. B., & Ritter, B. The relative efficacy of desensitization and modeling approaches for inducing behavioral, affective, and attitudinal changes. *Journal of Personality and Social Psychology, 1969, 13*, 173-199.

Bandura, A., Grusec, J. E., & Menlove, F. L. Some social determinants of self-monitoring reinforcement systems. *Journal of Personality and Social Psychology, 1967, 5*, 449-455. (a)

Bandura, A., Grusec, J. E., & Menlove, F. L. Vicarious extinction of avoidance behavior. *Journal of Personality and Social Psychology*, 1967, *5*, 16-23. (b)

Bandura, A., & Harris, M. B. Modification of syntactic style. *Journal of Experimental Child Psychology*, 1966, *4*, 341-352.

Bandura, A., & Jeffery, R. W. Role of symbolic coding and rehearsal processes in observational learning. *Journal of Personality and Social Psychology, 1973, 26*, 122-130.

Bandura, A., Jeffery, R. W., & Bachicha, D. L. Analysis of memory codes and cumulative rehearsal in observational learning. *Journal of Research in Personality, 1974, 7*, 295-305.

Bandura, A., & Kupers, C. J. The transmission of patterns of self reinforcement through modeling. *Journal of Abnormal and Social Psychology, 1964, 69*, 1-9.

Bandura, A., & McDonald, F. J. Influences of social reinforcement and the behavior of models in shaping children's moral judgments. *Journal of Abnormal and Social Psychology*, 1963, *67*, 274-281.

Bandura, A., & Perloff, B. Relative efficacy of self-monitored and externally imposed reinforcement systems. *Journal of Personality and Social Psychology, 1967, 7*, 111-116.

Bandura, A., & Rosenthal, T. L. Vicarious classical conditioning as a function of arousal level. *Journal of Personality and Social Psychology, 1966, 3*, 54-62.

Bandura, A., Ross, D., & Ross, S. A. Imitation of film mediated aggressive models. *Journal of Abnormal and Social Psychology, 1963, 66*, 3-11.

Bandura, A., & Schunk, D. Cultivating competence, self efficacy, and intrinsic interest through proximal self motivation. *Journal of Personality and Social Psychology, 1981, 41*, 586-598.

Bandura, A., & Walters, R. H. *Adolescent aggression*. New York: Ronald Press, 1959.

Bandura, A., & Walters, R. *Social learning and personality development*. New York: Holt, 1963.

Beilin, H. *Piaget and the new functionalism*. Paper presented at the 11th symposium of the Jean Piaget Society, Philadelphia, May 1981.

Belcher, T. L. Modeling original divergent responses: An initial investigation. *Journal of Educational Psychology, 1975, 67*, 351-358.

Bengtson, V. L. *The social psychology of aging*. New York: Bobbs-Merrill, 1973.

Berger, P. L., & Luckman, T. *The social construction of reality*. Garden City, N.Y.: Doubleday, 1966.

Berlyne, D. E. *Conflict, arousal, and curiosity*. New York: McGraw-Hill, 1960.

Berlyne, D. E. Children's reasoning and thinking. In P. H. Mussen (Ed.), *Carmichael's manual of child psychology* (3d ed.). New York: Wiley, 1970.

Berzonsky, M. D. Interdependence of Inhelder and Piaget's model of logical thinking. *Developmental Psychology,* 1971, *4,* 469-476.

Bijou, S., & Baer, D. *Behavioral analysis of child development.* Englewood Cliffs, N.J.: Prentice-Hall, 1978.

Black, A. H. The extinction of avoidance responses under curare. *Journal of Comparative and Physiological Psychology,* 1958, *51,* 519-524.

Bloom, L. Language development: Form and function in emerging grammars. Cambridge, Mass.: M.I.T. Press, 1970.

Bloom, L. Talking, understanding, and thinking. In R. L. Schiefelbusch and L. L. Lloyd (Eds.), *Language perspectives—Acquisition, retardation, and intervention.* Baltimore: University Park Press, 1974.

Bloom, L. Language development review. In F. D. Horowitz (Ed.), *Review of child development research* (Vol. 4). Chicago: University of Chicago Press, 1975.

Botwinick, J. *Aging and behavior.* New York: Springer-Verlag, 1973.

Bower, T. G. R. The visual world of infants. *Scientific American,* 1966, *215,* 80-92.

Bowers, K. S. Situationism in psychology: An analysis and a critique. *Psychological Review,* 1973, *80,* 307-336.

Brainerd, C. J. Cognitive development and concept learning: An interpretive review. *Psychological Bulletin,* 1977, *84,* 919-939.

Brainerd, C. J. Learning, research, and Piagetian theory. In L. S. Siegel & C. J. Brainerd (Eds.), *Alternatives to Piaget.* New York: Academic Press, 1978. (a)

Brainerd, C. J. The stage question in cognitive-developmental theory. *The Behavioral and Brain Sciences,* 1978, *2,* 173-213. (b)

Brofenbrenner, U. *The ecology of human development.* Cambridge, Mass.: Harvard University Press, 1979.

Brown, A. L., Smiley, S. S., Days, J. D. Townsend, M. A., & Lawton, S. C. Intrusion of a thematic idea in children's comprehension and retention of stories. *Child Development,* 1977, *48,* 1454-1466.

Brown, I., Jr. Role of referent concreteness in the acquisition of passive sentence comprehension through abstract modeling. *Journal of Experimental Child Psychology,* 1976, *22,* 185-199.

Brown, I., Jr., & Inouye, D. K. Learned helplessness through modeling: The role of perceived similarity in competence. *Journal of Personality and Social Psychology,* 1978, *36,* 900-908.

Brown, R. Development of the first language in the human species. *American Psychologist,* 1973, *28,* 97-106.

Bruner, J. S., Olver, R. R., & Greenfield, P. B. *Studies in cognitive growth.* New York: Wiley, 1966.

Buck-Morss, S. Socio-economic bias in Piaget's theory and its implication for cross-culture studies. *Human Development,* 1975, *18,* 35-49.

Campbell, D. T. On conflicts between biological and social evolution and between psychology and moral tradition. *American Psychologist,* 1975, *30,* 1103-1126.

Carroll, W. R., Rosenthal, T. L., & Brysh, C. G. Social transmission of grammatical parameters. *Journal of Educational Psychology,* 1972, *63,* 589-596.

Chandler, M. Social cognition and life-span approaches to the study of cognitive development. In H. W. Reese (Ed.), *Advances in child development and behavior* (Vol. 11). New York: Academic Press, 1977.

Chatterjee, B. B., & Ericson, C. W. Cognitive factors in heart rate conditioning. *Journal of Experimental Psychology,* 1962, *64,* 272-279.

Chi, M. T. Knowledge structures and memory development. In R. S. Siegler (Ed.), *Children's thinking: What develops?* Hillsdale, N.J.: Erlbaum, 1978.

Clark, H. B., & Sherman, J. A. Teaching generative use of sentence answers to three forms of questions. *Journal of Applied Behavior Analysis,* 1975, *8,* 321-330.

Clark, H. H., & Brownell, H. H. Judging up and down. *Journal of Experimental Psychology: Human Perception and Performance,* 1975, *1,* 339-352.

Coates, T. J., & Thoresen, C. E. Behavioral self-control and educational practice or do we really need self control? In D. Berliner (Ed.), *Review of research in education.* Washington, D.C.: American Educational Research Association, 1979.

Cole, M., & Bruner, J. S. Cultural differences and inferences about psychological processes. *American Psychologist,* 1971, *26,* 867-876.

Cole, M., Gay, J., Glick, J., & Sharp, D. *The cultural context of learning and thinking.* New York: Basic Books, 1971.

Cole, M., & Scribner, S. *Culture and thought: A psychological introduction.* New York: Wiley, 1974.

Dannhauser, W. J. A review of the philosophy of moral development. (*Moral stages and the idea of justice,* Vol. 1: *Essays on moral development* by L. Kohlberg). *New York Times Book Review,* 1981, *8* (August 9), 11.

Datan, N., & Ginsberg, L. H. (Eds.). *Life span developmental psychology: Normative life crises.* New York: Academic Press, 1975.

Davidson, H. R., & Lang, G. Children's perceptions of their teachers' feelings toward them related to self-perception, school achievement, and behavior. *Journal of Experimental Education,* 1960, *29,* 107-188.

Debus, R. L. Effects of brief observation and model behavior on conceptual tempo of impulsive children. *Developmental Psychology,* 1970, *2,* 22-32.

Debus, R. L. *Observational learning of reflective strategies by impulsive children.* Paper presented at the Congrès International de Psychologie, Paris 1976.

Dember, W. N., & Earl, R. W. Analysis of exploratory, manipulatory, and curiosity behaviors. *Psychological Review,* 1957, *64,* 91-96.

Dulaney, D. E. Awareness, rules, and propositional control: A confrontation with S-R behavior theory. In T. R. Dixon and D. L. Horton (Eds.), *Verbal behavior and general behavior theory.* Englewood Cliffs, N.J.: Prentice-Hall, 1968.

Erikson, E. *Childhood and society* (2nd ed.). New York: Norton, 1963.

Flanders, N. A. Teacher influence, pupil attitudes, and achievement. *Cooperative Research Monograph,* 1965 (No. 12). U.S. Department of Health, Education and Welfare, Office of Education, Washington, D.C.

Flavell, J. H. *The developmental psychology of Jean Piaget.* Princeton, N.J.: Van Nostrand-Reinhold, 1963.

Flavell, J. H. Cognitive changes in adulthood. In P. B. Baltes & L. R. Goulet (Eds.), *Life span developmental psychology.* New York: Academic Press, 1970.

Flavell, J. H., & Wellman, H. M. Metamemory. In R. V. Vail & J. H. Hagen (Eds.), *Perspectives on the development of memory and cognition.* Hillsdale, N.J.: Erlbaum, 1977.

Ford, M. E. The construct validity of egocentrism. *Psychological Bulletin,* 1979, *86,* 1169-1188.

Freud, S. *The basic writings of Sigmund Freud* (F. A. Brill, Ed.). New York: Modern Library, 1938.

Gagne, R. M. Contributions of learning to human development. *Psychological Review,* 1968, *75,* 177-191.

Garbarino, J., & Brofenbrenner, U. The socialization of moral judgment and behavior in cross-cultural perspective. In T. Lickona (Ed.), *Moral development and behavior*. New York: Holt, Rinehart & Winston, 1976.

Gergen, K. J. Social psychology as history. *Journal of Personality and Social Psychology, 1973, 26*, 309-320.

Gergen, K. J. Toward generative theory. *Journal of Personality and Social Psychology, 1978, 36*, 1344-1360.

Gerst, M. S. Symbolic coding operations in observational learning. *Journal of Personality and Social Psychology, 1971, 19*, 7-17.

Gibb, J. C. The meaning of ecologically oriented inquiry in contemporary psychology. *American Psychologist, 1979, 34*, 127-140.

Gibson, J. J. *An ecological approach to visual perception*. Boston: Houghton-Mifflin, 1979.

Glick, J. Cognitive development in cross-cultural perspective. In F. D. Horowitz (Ed.), *Review of child development research* (Vol. 4). Chicago: University of Chicago Press, 1975.

Glynn, E. L. Classroom applications of self determined reinforcement. *Journal of Applied Behavior Analysis, 1970, 3*, 123-132.

Goodnow, J. J. The nature of intelligent behavior: Questions raised by cross-cultural studies. In L. Resnick (Ed.), *The nature of intelligence*. Hillsdale, N.J.: Erlbaum, 1976.

Guess, D., Sailor, W., Rutherford, G., & Baer, D. M. An experimental analysis of linguistic development: The productive use of the plural morpheme. *Journal of Applied Behavior Analysis, 1968, 1*, 297-306.

Habermas, J. *Knowledge and human interests*. Boston: Beacon Press, 1971.

Harris, M. B., & Evans, R. C. Models and creativity. *Psychological Reports, 1973, 33*, 763-769.

Harris, M. B., & Fisher, J. L. Modeling and flexibility in problem solving. *Psychological Reports, 1973, 33*, 19-23.

Harris, M. B., & Hassemer, W. G. Some factors affecting the complexity of children's sentences: The effects of modeling, age, sex, and bilingualism. *Journal of Experimental Child Psychology, 1972, 13*, 447-455.

Harris, M. B., & Siebel, C. E. Effects of sex, occupation, and confidence of model and sex and grade of subject on imitation of language behaviors. *Developmental Psychology, 1976, 12*, 89-90.

Hebb, D. O. *The organization of behavior*. New York: Wiley, 1949.

Henderson, R. W., Swanson, R., & Zimmerman, B. J. Inquiry response induction of preschool children through televised modeling. *Developmental Psychology, 1974, 11*, 523-524.

Henderson, R. W., Swanson, R., & Zimmerman, B. J. Training seriation responses in young children through televised modeling of hierarchically sequenced rule components. *American Educational Research Journal, 1975, 12*, 474-489.

Henderson, R. W., Zimmerman, B. J., Swanson, R., & Bergan, J. R. Televised cognitive skill instruction for Papago native American children. Tucson: Arizona Center for Education Research and Development, 1974.

Hood, L., & Bloom, L. What, when, and how about why: A longitudinal study of early expressions of causality. *Monographs of the Society for Research in Child Development, 1979, 44* (6, Serial No. 181).

Hyde, T. S., & Jenkins, J. J. Differential effects of incidental tasks on the organization of recall of a list of highly associated words. *Journal of Experimental Psychology*, 1969, *82*, 472-481.

James, W. *The principles of psychology*. New York: Holt, 1890.

Jenkins, J. J. Remember that old theory of memory? Well, forget it! *American Psychologist*, 1974, *29*, 785-795.

Kaufman, A., Baron, A., & Kopp, R. E. Some effects of instructions on human operant behavior. *Psychonomic Monograph Supplements*, 1966, *1*, 243-250.

Kohlberg, L. Stage and sequence: The cognitive-developmental approach to socialization. In D. H. Goslin (Ed.), *Handbook of socialization theory and research*. Chicago: Rand McNally, 1968.

Kohlberg, L. From is to ought: How to commit the naturalistic fallacy and get away with it in the study of moral development. In T. Mischel (Ed.), *Cognitive development and epistomology*. New York: Academic Press, 1971.

Kohn, M. *Class and conformity: A study in values*. Homewood, Ill.: Dorsey Press, 1969.

Kuhn, T. S. *The structure of scientific revolutions* (2nd ed.). Chicago: University of Chicago Press, 1970.

Labouvie-Vief, G., & Chandler, M. J. Cognitive development: Idealism vs. contextualism. In P. B. Baltes (Ed.), *Life span development and behavior*. New York: Academic Press, 1978.

Lamal, P. A. Imitative learning of information-processing. *Journal of Experimental Child Psychology*, 1971, *12*, 223-227.

Laughlin, P. R., Moss, I. L., & Miller, S. M. Information processing in children as a function of adult model, stimulus display, school grade, and sex. *Journal of Educational Psychology*, 1969, *60*, 188-193.

Liebert, R. M. Moral development: A theoretical and empirical analysis. In G. J. Whitehurst & B. J. Zimmerman (Eds.), *Functions of language and cognition*. New York: Academic Press, 1979.

Liebert, R. M., & Morris, L. W. Cognitive and emotional components of text anxiety: A distinction and some initial data. *Psychological Reports*, 1967, *20*, 975-978.

Liebert, R. M., Odom, R. D., Hill, J. H., & Huff, R. L. The effects of age and rule familiarity on the production of modeled language constructions. *Developmental Psychology*, 1969, *1*, 108-112.

Liebert, R. M., & Swenson, S. A. Abstraction, inferences, and the process of imitative learning. *Developmental Psychology*, 1971, *5*, 500-504. (a)

Liebert, R. M., & Swenson, S. A. Association and abstraction as mechanisms of imitative learning. *Developmental Psychology*, 1971, *4*, 289-294. (b)

Lindsley, O. R. Geriatric behavioral prosthetics. In R. Kastenbaum (Ed.), *New thoughts on old age*. New York: Springer-Verlag, 1964.

Lukacs, G. *History and class consciousness*. New York: Random House, 1971.

MacNamara, J. Cognitive basis of language learning in infants. *Psychological Review*, 1972, *7*, 195-203.

Mahoney, M. J. *Cognition and behavior modification*. Cambridge, Mass.: Ballinger, 1974.

Mandler, G. Organization and memory. In K. W. Spence & J. T. Spence (Eds.), *The psychology of learning and motivation: Advances in research and theory* (Vol. 1). New York: Academic Press, 1967.

Mann, M. E., & Van Wagenen, R. K. *Alteration of joint mother-child linguistic styles, involving procedures of extension, elaboration and reinforcement*. Paper presented at the biennial meeting of the Society for Research in Child Development, Denver, April 1975.

McClelland, D. C. Testing for competence rather than "intelligence." *American Psychologist*, 1973, *28*, 1-14.

McClelland, D. C., Atkinson, J. W., Clark, R. W., & Lowell, E. L. *The achievement motive*. New York: Appleton-Century-Crofts, 1953.

McNeill, D. *The acquisition of language: The study of developmental psycholinguistics*. New York: Harper & Row, 1970.

Miller, N. E., & Dollard, J. *Social learning and imitation*. New Haven: Institute of Human Relations, Yale University Press, 1941.

Mischel, W. *Personality and assessment*. New York: Wiley, 1968.

Mischel, W. Toward a cognitive social learning reconceptualization of personality. *Psychological Review*, 1973, *80*, 252-283.

Mischel, W. The interaction of person and situation. In D. Magnusson & N. S. Endler (Eds.), *Personality at the cross roads: Current issues in interactional psychology*. Hillsdale, N.J.: Erlbaum, 1977.

Mischel, W. On the interface of cognition and personality: Beyond the person-situation debate. *American Psychologist*, 1979, *34*, 740-754.

Mischel, W., & Liebert, R. M. Effects of discrepancies between observed and imposed reward criteria on their acquisition and transmission. *Journal of Personality and Social Psychology*, 1966, *3*, 45-53.

Moerk, E. L. Processes of language teaching and language learning in the interaction of mother-child dyads. *Child Development*, 1976, *47*, 1064-1078.

Morgulas, S. *The effect of information about sentence referents on children's observational learning of a syntactic rule*. Unpublished doctoral dissertation, Graduate School of the City University of New York, 1982.

Mogulas, S., & Zimmerman, B. J. The role of comprehension in children's observational learning of a syntactic rule. *Journal of Experimental Child Psychology*, 1979, *28*, 455-468.

Morris, L. W., & Liebert, R. M. Relationship of cognitive and emotional components of test anxiety to physiology arousal and academic performance. *Journal of Consulting and Clinical Psychology*, 1970, *35*, 332-337.

Murray, F. B. Acquisition of conservation through social interaction. *Developmental Pyschology*, 1972, *6*, 1-6.

Mussen, P. H. Foreward. In R. Vasta (Ed.), *Strategies and techniques of child study*. New York: Academic Press, 1982.

Myers, N. A., & Perlmutter, M. Memory in the years two to five. In P. H. Ornstein (Ed.), *Memory development in children*. Hillsdale, N.J.: Erlbaum, 1978.

Neisser, U. *Cognitive psychology*. New York: Appleton-Century-Crofts, 1967.

Neisser, U. *Cognition and reality*. San Francisco: W. H. Freeman, 1976.

Nelson, K. Some evidence for the cognitive primacy of categorization and its functional basis. *Merrill Palmer Quarterly*, 1973, *19*, 21-39. (a)

Nelson, K. Structure and strategy in learning to talk. *Monograph of the Society for Research in Child Development*, 1973, *38*(1-2, Serial No. 149). (b)

Nelson, K. Concept, word, and sentence: Interrelations in acquisition and development. *Psychological Review*, 1974, *81*, 267-285.

Nelson, K. How children represent knowledge of their world in and out of language: A preliminary report. In R. S. Siegler (Ed.), *Children's thinking: What develops?* Hillsdale, N.J.: Erlbaum, 1978.

Nesselroade, J. R., Schaie, K. W., & Baltes, P. B. Ontogenetic and generational components of structural and quantitative change in adult cognitive behavior. *Journal of Gerontology,* 1972, *27,* 222-228.

Neugarten, B. L., & Datan, N. Sociological perspectives on the life cycle. In P. B. Baltes & K. W. Schaie (Eds.), *Life span developmental psychology: Personality and socialization.* New York: Academic Press, 1973.

Odom, R. D., Liebert, R. M., & Hill, J. H. The effects of modeling cues, rewards, and attention set on the properties of grammatical and ungrammatical syntactic constructions. *Journal of Experimental Child Psychology,* 1968, *6,* 131-140.

Pepper, S. C. *World hypotheses.* Berkeley: University of California Press, 1970.

Phillips, J. R. Syntax and vocabulary of mother's speech to young children. *Child Development,* 1973, *44,* 182-185.

Piaget, J. *The moral judgment of the child.* Glencoe, Ill.: Free Press, 1948.

Piaget, J. *The psychology of intelligence.* New York: Harcourt and Brace, 1950.

Piaget, J. *The origins of intelligence in children.* New York: International Universities Press, 1952.

Piaget, J. *The construction of reality in the child* (M. Cook, trans.). New York: Basic Books, 1954.

Piaget, J. Piaget's theory. In P. H. Mussen (Ed.), *Carmichael's manual of child psychology.* New York: Wiley, 1970.

Piaget, J. Intellectual evolution from adolescence to adulthood. *Human Development,* 1972, *15,* 1-12.

Proshansky, H. M. Environmental psychology and the real world. *Psychologist,* 1976, *31,* 303-310.

Rachman, S. J., & Hodgson, R. I. Synchrony and desynchrony in fear and avoidance. *Behavior Research and Therapy,* 1974, *12,* 311-318.

Ridberg, E. H., Parke, R. D., & Hetherington, E. M. Modification of impulsive and reflective cognitive style through observation of film-mediated models. *Developmental Psychology,* 1971, *5,* 185-190.

Riegel, K. F. Adult life crises: A dialectical interpretation of development. In N. Datan and L. H. Ginsburg (Eds.), *Life span developmental psychology.* New York: Academic Press, 1975.

Riegel, K. F. From traits and equilibrium toward developmental dialectics. In W. J. Arnold (Ed.), *Nebraska Symposium on Motivation* (Vol. 23). Lincoln: University of Nebraska Press, 1976.

Rosenbaum, M. E., & Schultz, L. J. The effects of extraneous response requirements on learning by performers and observers. *Psychonomic Science,* 1967, *8,* 51-52.

Rosenthal, R. *Experimenter effects in behavioral research.* New York: Appleton-Century-Crofts, 1966.

Rosenthal, T. L., Alford, G. S., & Rasp, L. M. Concept attainment, generalization, and retention through observation and verbal coding. *Journal of Experimental Child Psychology,* 1972, *13,* 183-194. (a)

Rosenthal, T. L., & Bandura, A. Psychological modeling: Theory and practice. In S. L. Garfield & A. E. Bergan (Eds.), *Handbook of psychotherapy and behavior change* (2nd ed.). New York: Wiley, 1978.

Rosenthal, T. L., & Carroll, W. R. Factors in vicarious modification of complex grammatical parameters. *Journal of Educational Psychology,* 1972, *63,* 174-178.

Rosenthal, T. L., & Whitebook, J. S. Incentives versus instructions in transmitting grammatical parameters with experimenter as model. *Behavior Research and Therapy,* 1970, *8,* 187-196.

Rosenthal, T. L., Zimmerman, B. J., & Durning, K. Observationally-induced changes in children's interrogative classes. *Journal of Personality and Social Psychology,* 1970, *16*, 681-688.

Rosenthal, T. L., & Zimmerman, B. J. Instructional specificity and outcome expectation in observationally induced question formulation. *Journal of Educational Psychology,* 1972, *63*, 500-504. (a)

Rosenthal, T. L., & Zimmerman, B. J. Modeling by exemplification and instruction in training conservation. *Developmental Psychology,* 1972, *6*, 392-401. (b)

Rosenthal, T. L., & Zimmerman, B. J. Organization, observation and guided practice in concept attainment and generalization. *Child Development,* 1973, *44*, 606-613.

Rosenthal, T. L., & Zimmerman, B. J. Organization and stability of transfer in vicarious concept attainment. *Child Development,* 1976, *47*, 110-117.

Rosenthal, T. L., & Zimmerman, B. J. *Social learning and cognition.* New York: Academic Press, 1978.

Russell, J. Nonconservation of area: Do children succeed where adults fail? *Developmental Psychology,* 1976, *12*, 467-468.

Salomon, G. Television is "easy" and print is "tough": The differential investment of mental effort in learning as a function of perceptions and attributions. *Journal of Educational Psychology,* in press.

Sampson, E. E. Psychology and the American ideal. *Journal of Personality and Social Psychology,* 1977, *35*, 767-782.

Sampson, E. E. Scientific paradigms and social values: Wanted—A scientific revolution. *Journal of Personality and Social Personality,* 1978, *36*, 1332-1343.

Sampson, E. E. Cognitive psychology as ideology. *American Psychologist,* 1981, *36*, 730-743.

Schaie, K. W., Labouvie, G. V., & Buech, B. U. Generational and cohort-specific differences in adult cognitive functioning: A fourteen-year study of independent samples. *Developmental Psychology,* 1973, *9*, 151-166.

Schaie, K. W., & Labouvie-Vief, G. Generational versus ontogenetic components of change in adult cognitive behavior: A fourteen-year cross-sequential study. *Developmental Psychology,* 1974, *10*, 305-320.

Schaie, K. W., & Strother, C. R. A cross-sectional study of age changes in cognitive behavior. *Psychological Bulletin,* 1968, *70*, 671-680. (a)

Schaie, K. W., & Strother, C. R. The effects of time and cohort differences on the interpretation of age changes in cognitive behavior. *Multivariate Behavior Research,* 1968, *3*, 259-294. (b)

Schumaker, J., & Sherman, J. A. Training generative verb usage by imitation and reinforcement procedures. *Journal of Applied Behavior Analysis,* 1970, *3*, 273-287.

Schunk, D. H. Modeling and attribution effects on children's achievement: A self-efficacy analysis. *Journal of Educational Psychology,* 1981, *73*, 93-105.

Seligman, M. E. P. *Helplessness.* San Francisco: W. H. Freeman, 1975.

Shatz, M., & Gelman, R. The development of communication skill modification in the speech of young children as a function of listener. *Monograph of the Society for Research in Child Development,* 1973, *38* (5, Serial No. 152).

Skinner, B. F. *Science and human behavior.* New York: Macmillan, 1953.

Smedslund, J. The acquisition of conservation of substance and weight in children, II: External reinforcement of conservation of weight and operations of addition and subtraction. *Scandinavian Journal of Psychology,* 1961, *2*, 71-84. (a)

Smedslund, J. The acquisition of conservation of substance and weight in children. *Scandinavian Journal of Psychology,* 1961, *3*, 153-155. (b)

Smedslund, J. Bandura's theory of self-efficacy: A set of common sense theorems. *Scandinavian Journal of Psychology*, 1978, *19*, 1-14.

Snow, C. E. Mother's speech to children learning language. *Child Development*, 1972, *43*, 549-565.

Strohner, H., & Nelson, K. The young child's development of sentence comprehension: Influence of event probability, non-verbal context, syntactic form, and strategies. *Child Development*, 1974, *45*, 189-193.

Taub, E., Bacon, R. C., & Berman, A. J. Acquisition of a trace-conditioned avoidance response after deafferentation of the responding limb. *Journal of Comparative and Physiological Psychology*, 1965, *59*, 275-279.

Thoresen, C. E., & Mahoney, M. J. *Behavioral self-control.* New York: Holt, 1974.

Thorndike, E. L. *Educational psychology*, Vol. 1: *The original nature of man.* New York: Teachers College, Columbia University, 1913.

Tobias, S. Achievement treatment interactions. *Review of Educational Research*, 1976, *46*, 61-74.

Tulving, E. Subjective organization in free recall of related words. *Psychological Review*, 1962, *69*, 344-354.

Vasta, R., & Liebert, R. M. Auditory discrimination of novel prepositional constructions as a function of age and syntactic background. *Developmental Psychology*, 1973, *9*, 79-82.

Wagner, D. A. Memories of Morocco: The influence of age, schooling, and environment on memory. *Cognitive Psychology*, 1978, *10*, 1-28.

Watson, R. I. *The great psychologists.* Philadelphia: Lippincott, 1963.

Weir, M. W. Developmental changes in problem solving strategies. *Psychological Review*, 1964, *71*, 473-490.

Whitehurst, G. J., Ironsmith, M., & Goldfein, M. Selective imitation of the passive construction through modeling. *Journal of Experimental Child Psychology*, 1974, *17*, 288-302.

Whitehurst, G. J., & Novak, G. Modeling, imitation training, and the acquisition of sentence phrase. *Journal of Experimental Child Psychology*, 1973, *16*, 332-345.

Willems, E. P. Behavioral technology and behavioral ecology. *Journal of Applied Behavior Analysis*, 1974, *7*, 151-166.

Wohlwill, J. F. Un essai d'spprentissage dans le domaine de la conservation due nombre. *Études d'Epistémologie Génétique*, 1959, *9*, 125-135.

Wohlwill, J. F. *The study of behavioral development.* New York: Academic Press, 1973.

Wohlwill, J. F., & Lowe, R. C. An experimental analysis of the conservation of number. *Child Development*, 1962, *33*, 153-167.

Yussen, S. R. Determinants of visual attention and recall in observational learning by preschoolers and second graders. *Developmental Psychology*, 1974, *10*, 93-100.

Zimmerman, B. J. Modification of young children's grouping strategies: Effects of modeling, verbalization, incentive, and age. *Child Development*, 1974, *45*, 1032-1041.

Zimmerman, B. J. Modeling. In H. Hom & P. Robinson (Eds.), *Psychological processes in children's early education.* New York: Academic Press, 1977.

Zimmerman, B. J. A social learning explanation for age-related changes in children's conceptual behavior. *Contemporary Educational Psychology*, 1978, *3*, 11-19.

Zimmerman, B. J. Concepts and classification. In G. J. Whitehurst & B. J. Zimmerman (Eds.), *Functions of language and cognition.* New York: Academic Press, 1979.

Zimmerman, B. J. *Operativity: A critic's view of the construct and related research.* Paper presented at the sixth biennial meeting of the Southeastern Conference on Human Development, Alexandria, Va., April 1980.

Zimmerman, B. J. Social learning theory and cognitive constructivism. In I. E. Sigel, D. M. Brodzinsky, & R. M. Golinkoff (Eds.), *New directions in Piagetian theory and practice.* Hillsdale, N.J.: Erlbaum, 1981.

Zimmerman, B. J., & Bell, J. A. Observer verbalization and abstraction in vicarious rule learning, generalization, and retention. *Developmental Psychology,* 1972, *7,* 227-231.

Zimmerman, B. J., & Blom, D. E. *Cognitive conflict and learning: An empirical test of the construct. Development Review,* 1983, in press.

Zimmerman, B. J., & Dialessi, F. Modeling influences on children's creative behavior. *Journal of Educational Psychology,* 1973, *65,* 127-134.

Zimmerman, B. J., & Jaffe, A. Teaching through demonstration: The effects of structuring, imitation, and age. *Journal of Educational Psychology,* 1977, *69,* 773-778.

Zimmerman, B. J., & Kinsler, K. The effects of exposure to a punished model and verbal prohibitions in children's toy play. *Journal of Educational Psychology,* 1979, *71,* 388-395.

Zimmerman, B. J., & Kleefeld, C. F. Toward a theory of teaching: A social learning view. *Contemporary Educational Psychology,* 1977, *2,* 158-171.

Zimmerman, B. J., & Koussa, R. Sex factors in children's observational learning of value judgments of toys. *Sex Roles: A Journal of Research,* 1975, *1,* 121-133.

Zimmerman, B. J., & Koussa, R. Social influences on children's toy preferences: Effects of model rewardingness and affect. *Contemporary Educational Psychology,* 1979, *4,* 55-66.

Zimmerman, B. J., & Lanaro, P. Acquiring and retaining conservation of length through modeling and reversibility cues. *Merrill-Palmer Quarterly,* 1974, *20,* 145-161.

Zimmerman, B. J., & Pike, E. O. Effects of modeling and reinforcement on the acquisition and generalization of question asking behavior. *Child Development,* 1972, *43,* 892-907.

Zimmerman, B. J., & Ringle, J. Effects of model persistence and statements of confidence on children's self efficacy and problem solving. *Journal of Educational Psychology,* 1981, *73,* 485-493.

Zimmerman, B. J., & Rosenthal, T. L. Concept attainment, transfer, and retention through observation and rule provision. *Journal of Experimental Child Psychology,* 1972, *14,* 139-150. (a)

Zimmerman, B. J., & Rosenthal, T. L. Observation repetition and ethnic background in concept attainment and generalization. *Child Development,* 1972, *43,* 605-613. (b)

Zimmerman, B. J., & Rosenthal, T. L. Conserving and retaining equalities and inequalities through observation and correction. *Developmental Psychology,* 1974, *10,* 260-268. (a)

Zimmerman, B. J., & Rosenthal, T. L. Observational learning of rule governed behavior by children. *Psychological Bulletin,* 1974, *81,* 29-42. (b)

Zimmerman, B. J., & Whitehurst, G. J. Structure and function: A comparison of two views of the development of language and cognition. In G. J. Whitehurst and B. J. Zimmerman (Eds.), *The functions of language and cognition.* New York: Academic Press, 1979.

2. The Development of Two Concepts

Robert S. Siegler and D. Dean Richards

The purpose of this chapter is to explore ways in which we can characterize conceptual development. We will briefly examine existing approaches to studying the topic, point to their strengths and weaknesses, propose an alternative approach, and illustrate the alternative with examples involving children's concepts of numbers and of life. The recurring theme will be that conceptual understanding is multi-faceted, and that our approaches to studying it must be consistent with this fact.

Existing Approaches to Conceptual Development

At one time, not very long ago, there was a large degree of consensus as to how best to characterize children's knowledge of concepts. Piaget had identified tasks that came to be accepted as necessary and sufficient indices of conceptual under-standing. Children were said to understand the concept of classes when and only when they could succeed on the class inclusion task, to understand the concept of ordering when and only when they could succeed on the seriation task, to under-stand the concept of perspective when and only when they could succeed on the three-mountain task, and so on. Even though Piaget examined numerous tasks before reaching his conclusions, many investigators relied on just one of his tasks as their sole index of understanding of each concept.

Accompanying the view that understanding could be assessed by performance on a single task was the view that children possessed a single understanding to measure. This view was reflected in the multitude of studies in which researchers attempted to establish *the* age at which children master particular concepts. It was also reflected in the titles that investigators, both Piagetians and non-Piagetians, chose for their reports. Illustratively, two of the most influential monographs on children's understandings of numbers have been those of Piaget (1952) and Brainerd (1979). Piaget titled his book *The Child's Conception of Number*. Brainerd titled his book *The Origins of the Number Concept*. The use of the singular in the terms *conception* and *number* and of the definite article together with the singular in the phrase *the number concept* is striking. The implication is that there exists a single number concept to be understood and that children have a particular conception of it.

Mathematicians and philosophers have long debated whether there exists any core concept of number to be understood. However, the results of the past 20 years of empirical research render completely untenable the view that children possess a single understanding of number or of other complex concepts. Even within a single basic problem, wide variability in performance, depending on the details of the task, has been the rule. To cite one illustration, although most children do not succeed on Piaget's number conservation problem until age 6 or 7 (Beilin, 1968; Miller, 1976; Rothenberg & Courtney, 1969), most children can succeed on variants of it by age 2 or 3 (Bever, Mehler, & Epstein, 1968; Bryant, 1974; Gelman, 1972). There does not seem to be any simple, principled way to decide which form of this task is optimally suited to assessing understanding (Flavell, 1971; Siegler, 1981). The same point could be made about class inclusion, seriation, and other common cognitive-developmental tasks.

The situation becomes even more complicated when we consider not just variants of a single task but also the many possible tasks that might reasonably be said to correspond to any concept. Rather than assessing knowledge of numbers by the number conservation problem, we might assess it in terms of ability to count objects, to compare numerical magnitudes, to understand the relation between arithmetic and algebra, to understand number theory, and so on. Again, there is no apparent principled way to choose.

The issue can be considered at a very general level. Braine (1959) and Brown (1976) have advocated specific criteria for defining conceptual understanding. Braine argued for a criterion of initial competence, Brown for a criterion of stable usage. The dilemmas that each of these proposals lead to suggest that no single standard of conceptual understanding can be adequate. Consider Braine's (1959) statement:

> It is clear that if one seeks to state an age at which a particular type of response develops, the only age that is not completely arbitrary is the earliest age at which this type of response can be elicited using the simplest experimental procedure. (p. 16)

This statement is entirely reasonable, as far as it goes. When one considers the long time period separating initial and mature understanding of concepts, however, a paradox becomes evident. Adopting the initial competence criterion puts us in the position of saying that many concepts develop at relatively young ages, yet of also saying that children fail many reasonable indices of understanding for years thereafter. Stated another way, much—perhaps most—conceptual growth would be seen as occurring after the concept "develops."

Brown (1976) implicitly suggested an alternative criterion in her discussion of the development of seriation:

> Under optimal circumstances, they can indeed seriate a succession of pictures representing a time course. . . . Yet how robust is their concept of succession? Is it truly operative according to the defining features argument? The answer must be 'no,' for their concept of order appears to be extremely fragile and is disrupted by seemingly trivial changes in the optimal task. (p. 77)

The paradox that is implicit in Brown's observation is pointed out in Braine's comment. What exactly does a child understand when he can use a concept in some situations but fails to qualify as having an operative understanding of it? As Braine suggested, it does seem arbitrary to identify understanding with anything other than the earliest form of understanding; however, it seems misleading to identify understanding with the earliest form of understanding.

How then can we study conceptual development? The foregoing critique suggests a three-stage procedure. First, examine performance on a variety of tasks corresponding to different aspects of a concept. For the same reasons that psychometricians sample numerous content domains in order to infer intelligence, developmental psychologists might sample content within more narrowly specified domains in order to infer conceptual understanding. Second, characterize the representations and processes that people use to perform each task. The reasons for formulating models that distinguish between representations and processes have been discussed by Anderson (1976, 1978) and will be further discussed in a later section of this chapter. Third, integrate the findings from each task into a general characterization of knowledge about the concept. Such characterizations inevitably would be incomplete, but might capture the most important features of conceptual understanding at various ages. In the remainder of this chapter, we will apply this strategy to analyzing children's concepts of numbers and of life.

Children's Concepts of Numbers

The first domain that we will discuss is preschoolers' knowledge of numbers. This section focuses on four parts of numerical understanding: knowledge of number conservation, counting, numerical magnitudes, and addition. The number conservation research focuses on the development of understanding of transformations that increase, decrease, or do not affect quantity, and on the applications of this knowledge to different-sized sets. The counting research emphasizes children's knowledge of the structure of the number string and the effects of this knowledge on their stopping points, omissions, repetitions, and use of nonstandard numbers in counting. The research on magnitudes examines the preschoolers' subjective grouping of numbers into categories based on size, and the effects of the categorizations on their magnitude comparisons, labeling of numbers, and ability to learn more about magnitudes. The investigation of addition spotlights the way in which 4- and 5-yearolds regulate their use of visible and audible strategies so that they employ them in precisely those situations in which the strategies will do the most good. At the ends of each of the four sections on children's knowledge about a numerical domain, we present models of expertise in that domain that generate performance similar to the children's. Finally, after we have examined all four domains, we present comprehensive models of preschoolers' knowledge of numbers that integrate the models of understanding of number conservation, counting, magnitudes, and addition.

Number Conservation

A study of Piaget's number conservation problem (Siegler, 1981, Experiments 3 & 4) was instrumental in convincing us of the need to adhere to the above-described procedures in order to characterize children's knowledge. This study began with a consideration of the role of transformations in conservation problems. Analysis suggested that transformations play a crucial role in conservation. The one sure way to determine whether the value of a particular dimension will be preserved in a situation is to know the type of transformation that will be performed. Adding to that dimension necessarily results in more, subtracting from it results in less, and neither adding nor subtracting anything results in the same amount as before.

Piaget and subsequent researchers focused almost exclusively on transformations that do not affect quantity: pouring water, molding clay, moving objects apart, and so on. Transformations that do affect quantity—addition and subtraction—are of at least equal importance, however. A conserver might reasonably be expected to understand not only that spreading a row of objects leaves the number of objects unchanged, but also that spreading them and adding an object meant that the row now has more objects than before and that spreading them and taking away an object means that the row now has less.

In Siegler's (1981) study, 3- to 9-year-olds were presented number conservation problems in which the starting configuration always had two equally numerous and equally long rows of objects. Transformations varied in their effect on the rows' number and length. Some problems involved adding objects to a row, some involved subtracting objects from a row, and some involved neither adding nor subtracting objects. Some problems involved lengthening the transformed row of objects, some involved shortening the row, and some involved moving the objects but ultimately returning the row to its original length. Finally, on some problems the rows had few objects and on others they had many. The pattern of correct answers and errors on these problems was sufficient to allow us to induce children's rules for performing the task (see Siegler, 1976, 1978, 1981, for descriptions of the rule assessment approach that was used).

Most children used one of five rules on the conservation problems. As shown in Figure 2-1A, the youngest children, most of them 3-year-olds, chose the longer row as having more objects in almost all cases—whenever the problem involved a large number of objects, and even with small arrays when nothing was added or subtracted. When the number of items was small and something had been added or subtracted, however, they quantified the numbers of objects and chose the row with more as having more.[1]

---

[1] Children using Rules I, II, and III may have used set size and type of transformation cues as direct bases of judgment rather than as indices of when to quantify. Available evidence did not allow discrimination between these two interpretations.

(A)

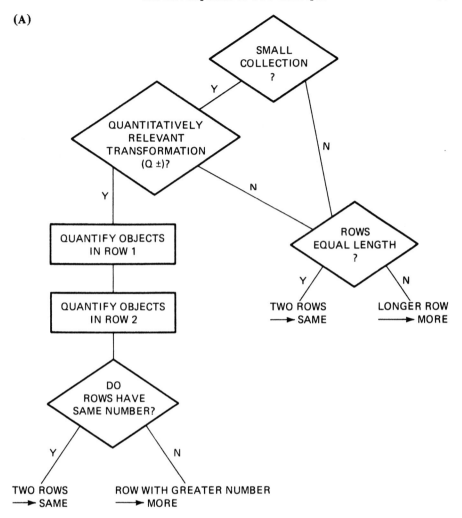

Figure 2-1. (A-E) Rules on number conservation task. (A) Rule I.

Somewhat older children used a simplified version of this approach (Figure 2-1B). When presented with only a few items, they always quantified and chose the more numerous row. However, when presented with many objects, the children chose the longer row as having more.

In Rule III (Figure 2-1C), if the rows had few items, regardless of the transformation, or if they had many and something had been added to or subtracted from one of them, relative quantities determined conservation judgments. If the rows had many items and nothing had been added or subtracted, however, children still chose the longer row as having more. Interestingly, this last holdout is precisely the traditional conservation of number problem.

Rule IV children answered all types of number conservation problems correctly. This achievement did not conclude the development of the concept, however.

(B)

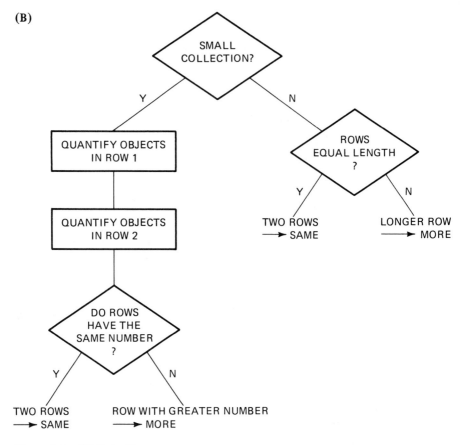

Figure 2-1. (B) Rule II.

Whereas Rule IV children solved number conservation problems by comparing quantities (Figure 2-1D), Rule V children realized even without quantifying that adding necessarily meant that that row had more, that subtracting necessarily meant that it had less, and that doing neither meant that it necessarily had the same number of objects as before (Figure 2-1E).

The same 3- to 9-year-olds whose understanding of number conservation was assessed were also tested on liquid and solid quantity conservation tasks. Two findings suggested that an understanding of number conservation was crucial to an understanding of the other two conservation problems. First, no children consistently solved liquid and solid quantity conservation problems who did not also consistently solve number conservation problems. Second, among children who consistently solved number conservation problems, those who justified their responses on those problems by citing the type of transformation were much more likely to solve the other two types of conservation problems than children who justified their responses by citing relative numbers.

These findings suggested an overall model of conservation acquisition. After

(C)

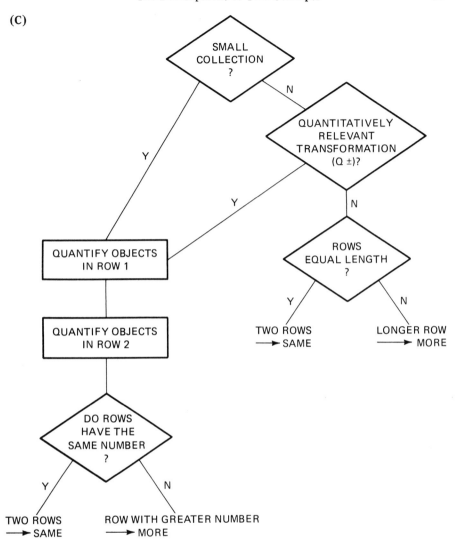

Figure 2-1. (C) Rule III.

using rules that consistently solve some but not all number conservation problems, children come to solve all problems by using the quantifiers of counting, subitizing, or comparing. Later, they note that these tests always indicate that when something has been added there are more objects than before, that when something has been subtracted there are fewer, and that when nothing has been added or subtracted there are the same number. Therefore, they rely on the type of transformation to solve the number conservation problems. Finally, the children apply what they have learned about transformations in the number context to other domains involving transformations but not allowing simple quantifiers, specifically conservation of liquid and solid quantity.

(D)

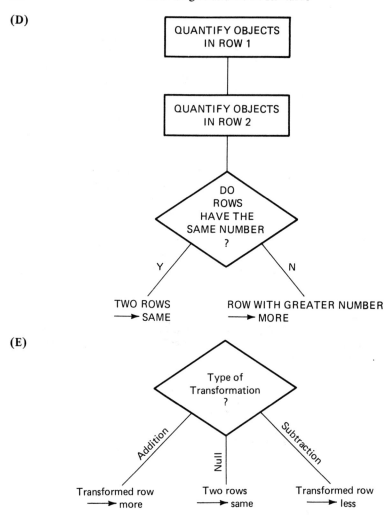

Figure 2-1. (D) Rule IV; (E) Rule V.

This investigation persuaded us of several points. First, it illustrated the difficulty of defining conceptual understanding. If understanding of number conservation were defined as "in at least some situations, answering on the basis of number despite opposing perceptual cues," then Rule I would be the point of understanding. If understanding were defined as "for the traditional number conservation
transformation, in at least some situations answering correctly despite opposing
perceptual cues," then Rule II would be chosen. If it were defined as an "ability to
consistently solve number conservation problems," then Rule IV would be chosen.
If it were defined as "an abstract understanding of the quantitative effects of transformations that does not depend upon requantification and that can be transferred

to other types of conservation problems," then Rule V would be chosen. Each one of these definitions seems sensible within particular theoretical contexts; no one of them seems absolutely more sensible than the others.

A second lesson was the desirability of separating children's representations of information from the processes that they apply to their representations. This distinction is related to the storing-processing distinction in working-memory systems (see Chapter 4 in this volume). The rule models specified the processes that children used to solve the conservation problems but only implicitly addressed the content on which the processes operated. Children's knowledge about liquids, solids, and countable objects may have influenced their choice of selection rules. However, it is unclear how such information could have been included within the rule format.

Anderson's (1976) suggestion that representations and processes be separately described held out the promise of more precise yet also more economical characterizations. Specifying the representation would force us to consider the structure of the relevant knowledge domains as well as the interrelations among knowledge domains that children draw upon. Specifying the processes would force us to consider the ways in which children manipulate this information to meet task demands. In addition, characterizing knowledge in terms of representations and processes seemed congruent with the present emphasis on people possessing multiple understandings of concepts. Different processes can operate on the same content and similar processes can operate on diverse content to produce varied understandings of a single domain.

A third lesson was that even on a single problem, a variety of skills may be crucial to success. Consider the skills that were likely to be involved in using Rules IV and V on the number conservation problem. Children using Rule IV judged the results of transformations by counting each row of objects. After counting, the children compared the magnitudes of the numbers in order to determine which row, if either, had more. Similarly, children using Rule V needed to know about the directional effects of addition and subtraction in order to decide, without enumerating, which row had more.

The likely involvement of counting, comparing, and adding in the mastery of number conservation was one incentive to study these operations. Other motivations were even more compelling, though. Counting, comparing, and adding are basic mathematical skills. They are activities in which very young children are interested, in which they frequently engage, and at which they possess considerable skill. The skills have numerous possible interrelationships, in addition to the common involvement in number conservation. For example, Groen and Parkman (1972) postulated that when people add two integers, they compare the numbers in order to determine the larger one and then count up the number of times indicated by the smaller. Finally, the three skills are sufficiently diverse that data on them, together with the already collected data on number conservation, should allow reasonably broad-based inferences about children's knowledge of numbers. In the next three sections of this chapter, we describe experiments intended to reveal how knowledge of counting, numerical magnitudes, and addition develops in the preschool period.

Counting

Existing Research. It seems likely that children first encounter many numbers in the context of counting. Although words denoting small numbers have many semantic referents (e.g., two ears, three people in our family, four legs on a table), words denoting larger numbers do not. Learning about numbers in the counting context may help children learn about them in other contexts as well. Pollio and Whitacre (1970) reported that the length of preschoolers' counting strings is an excellent predictor of their ability to establish one-to-one correspondence, to divide objects into equally numerous sets, to insert the missing number into a series, and to count-on from an arbitrarily chosen point within the number string. The first goal of the present series of experiments, therefore, was to establish the representation and process that children apply in abstract counting (i.e., use of the number string in the absence of objects).

Three models of children's organization of the counting string seemed plausible. Ginsburg (1977) postulated a great deal of structure, beginning in the teens.

> The beginning of the sequence—the first 12 numbers or so—is completely arbitrary. There is no rational basis for predicting what comes after a certain number. Therefore, children have to memorize the smaller numbers in rote fashion. After a period of time, they discover that the numbers after about 13 contain an underlying pattern. Using it, children develop a few simple rules by which to generate the numbers up to about 100 (p. 9).

At the other extreme, Greeno, Riley, and Gelman (Note 1) postulated a representation with no explicit organization, that is, one in which numbers are connected only by the "next" relation between successive items. The third possibility suggested an intermediate amount of organization. Children might detect the relatively transparent structure that appears beyond the number 20 but not the less obvious structure that is present in the teens.

These three models predicted counts that differed in many respects. Consider just one: stopping points. If, as in Greeno et al.'s model, only "next" connections bind the numbers, children should be equally likely to stop at all points. Alternatively, if, as in Ginsburg's model, children treat the teens as the first decade with a repetitive structure, they should stop most often at points where the structure does not indicate the name of the next number: 19, 29, 39, and so on. Finally, if, as in the third possibility, children abstract the number string's structure only beyond the number 20, then they would be expected to stop relatively often at 29, 39, and 49, but not at 19.

Counting from One. Neither Ginsburg nor Greeno et al. presented data that supported their model or failed to support other models. At the time we wrote this section, no other detailed description of young children's abstract counting was available, although one such description has since been published (Fuson, Richards, & Briars, 1982). Therefore, in our first experiment, we asked 3-, 4-, and 5-year-olds from an upper-middle-class preschool to count as high as they could, in order to obtain a data base from which to generate models of preschoolers' abstract counting.

Examination of the data revealed three distinct patterns: one for children who stopped counting at or before 19, one for children who stopped between 20 and 99, and one for children who proceeded beyond 100. As shown in Table 2-1 and Figure 2-2, children in the three stopping-point-defined groups differed in the distribution of digit place values of their stopping points, in their omissions and repetitions, and in their use of nonstandard numbers.

First consider the distribution of stopping points. Children who stopped before 20 did not display any obvious regularities in the points at which they stopped (Figure 2-2). In contrast, an absolute majority of the counts of children who stopped between 20 and 99 terminated with a number that ended in 9. Children who counted beyond 100 often ended their counts at a 9 number but even more often at a 0.

The three groups also differed in their omissions. None of the children in the least expert group skipped 10 or more consecutive numbers, but roughly half of those in the two more expert groups did. All but 3 of the 43 decade omissions involved jumps from a number ending in 9 to the beginning of another decade (e.g., 27, 28, 29, 50).

The quality of repetitions also varied with expertise. Only 3% of the repetitions of children in the 1-19 group and 0% of the repetitions of children in the 100+ group involved more than three numbers. In contrast, 22% of the repetitions of those who stopped counting between 20 and 99 involved at least nine numbers. On all but two of the extended repetitions, children reached a 9 number and then regressed to a number ending in 0 or 1 in an already completed decade.

A sizable minority of children in the two more expert groups used at least one nonstandard number (Table 2-1). The nonstandard numbers invariably involved concatenations of standard numbers. The nonstandard numbers of children who stopped counting between 20 and 99 generally came immediately after a number ending in 9 and themselves began with the same decade name followed by a 10 (e.g., 29, 20-10). The nonstandard strings ended soon after they began; all but one ended by the time the child reached the decade name followed by a 12. Children who counted beyond 100 never produced this type of nonstandard number, but fairly often produced a variant in which they reached 100 and then concatenated hundreds names (e.g., 100-100, 100-200). Children who stopped below 20 never produced either type of nonstandard number.

Counting-On from a Point Beyond One. The counting of children who did not reach the number 20 differed in a large number of respects from the counting of children who proceeded beyond that point. Two explanations for these differences seemed plausible. Children who did not count as far as 20 may not have been aware of the generative rule that applies in the 20s and succeeding decades. Alternatively, these children might have known the rule but had no occasion to use it, because their counts ended before the point at which it becomes applicable.

Asking children to count-on from various points within and beyond their counting range was one way to probe the possibility of such unrevealed knowledge. If a child who stopped counting at 12 knew the generative rule for counting in the

Table 2-1 Data on Counting

Measure	Group		
	1-19 (N=10)	29-99 (N=26)	100+ (N=6)
Stopping Point			
Percentage of counts that stop at 9	14	69	38
Percentage of counts that stop at 0	10	4	50
Percentage of children who finish at least one count with 9	40	96	83
Percentage of children who finish at least one count with 0	20	14	100
Omissions			
Percentage of counts including any omission	70	75	67
Percentage of counts with omission of entire decade	0	32	41
Percentage of children omitting at least one number	100	96	83
Percentage of children omitting at least one entire decade	0	46	67
Repetitions			
Percentage of counts including any repetitions	92	52	54
Percentage of counts with repetitions of entire decades	0	11	0
Percentage of children repeating one or more numbers	100	85	100
Percentage of children repeating one or more decades	0	15	0
Nonstandard Numbers			
Percentage of counts including nonstandard numbers	0	29	12
Percentage of children who used nonstandard numbers at least once	0	54	33
Percentage of nonstandard numbers concatenating decade name with 10, 11, or 12 (e.g., 20-10)	—	83	0
Percentage of nonstandard numbers concatenating hundreds name to another number (e.g., 100-200)	—	0	100

Note: These percentages reflect 4 counts/child.

Note: From "The Development of Numerical Understandings," in H. Reese & L. P. Lipsitt (Eds.), *Advances in Child Development and Behavior Vol. 16.* Copyright 1982 by Academic Press. Reprinted by permission.

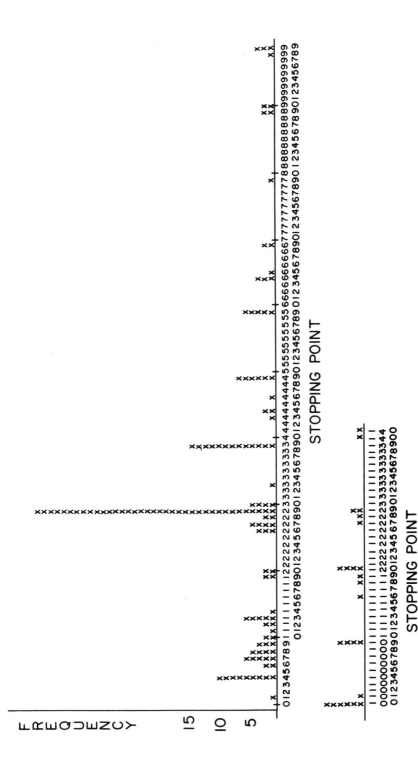

Figure 2-2. Distribution of stopping points in counting. From "The Development of Numerical Understandings," in H. Reese & L. P. Lipsitt (Eds.), *Advances in Child Development and Behavior Vol. 16.* Copyright 1982 by Academic Press. Reprinted by permission.

Table 2-2 Data on Counting-On

Criterion	Group		
	1-19 (*N*=6)	20-99 (*N*=25)	100+ (*N*=8)
Criterion Digit Within Child's Demonstrated Counting Competence[a]			
Percentage of counts on which child reached next 9 after starting point	0	75	100
Percentage of counts on which child reached next 0 after starting point	0	17	75
Criterion Digit Beyond Child's Demonstrated Counting Competence			
Percentage of counts on which child reached next 9 after starting point	0	90	100
Percentage of counts on which child reached next 0 after starting point	0	6	31

[a] Within child's counting competence means that the child has previously counted from 1 to at least the point of the criterion digit.

Note: From "The Development of Numerical Understandings," in H. Reese & L. P. Lipsitt (Eds.), *Advances in Child Development and Behavior Vol. 16*. Copyright 1982 by Academic Press. Reprinted by permission.

20s then starting him by saying "21, 22, 23" and asking him to continue seemed likely to reveal the additional knowledge. Similarly, the beyond-counting-range trials seemed likely to reveal whether the counting of children who continued beyond 20 was based on rote learning or on knowledge of an abstract rule. Only mastery of the abstract rule would allow children. to reach the ends of decades at points beyond those at which they previously stopped.

Therefore, the children who participated in the earlier counting experiment were again examined. The starting points for the counting-on procedure were varied for the three expertise groups so as to give each child the opportunity to count-on both from within and from beyond his or her previously demonstrated counting range.

As shown in Table 2-2, children who had not previously counted beyond 19 almost never were able to continue much beyond the experimenter's initial prompt. By contrast, children who stoppped between 20 and 99 almost always reached the following 9. They did so as often when the following 9 number was beyond as when it was within their previously demonstrated counting range. However, they rarely proceeded beyond that 9 number. Children who had counted beyond 100 showed yet a third pattern. They almost always completed the initial decade, sometimes went on to the next decade when it was within their counting range, and occasionally went on to the next decade even when it was beyond any of their previous counts.

Models of Three Levels of Counting Expertise. Three models, one corresponding to each level of counting expertise, are shown in Figure 2-3. Model I depicts the knowledge hypothesized to underlie counts that ended before 20 (Figure 2-3A).

(A)

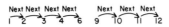

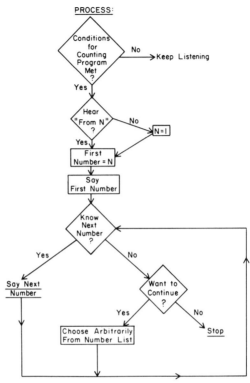

Figure 2-3. (A-C) Models of counting and counting-on. (The particular connections and list memberships included throughout Figure 2-3 are chosen purely for purposes of illustration. Also, in the process, N is defined as any integer.) (A) Model I. Parts A-C from "The Development of Numerical Understandings," in H. Reese & L. P. Lipsitt (Eds.), *Advances in Child Development and Behavior Vol. 16.* Copyright 1982 by Academic Press. Reprinted by permission.

This model resembles Greeno et al.'s in that the representation includes no particular structure beyond "next" connections. The process is also uncomplicated. First, a starting point is chosen. Then children say the next number if they can recall it, and continue for as long as they have "next" connections. When they reach a number for which they do not have a "next" connection, they either arbitrarily choose a next number or stop.

As Figure 2-3B illustrates, the representation and process used by Model II children (those who stopped between 20 and 99) are hypothesized to be considerably more complicated. Within the representation, numbers can be tagged as members of two lists: the digit repetition list and the rule applicability list. The numbers 1 through 9 are the ones that most often will be on the digit repetition list, although

(B)

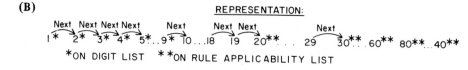

REPRESENTATION:

*ON DIGIT LIST **ON RULE APPLICABILITY LIST

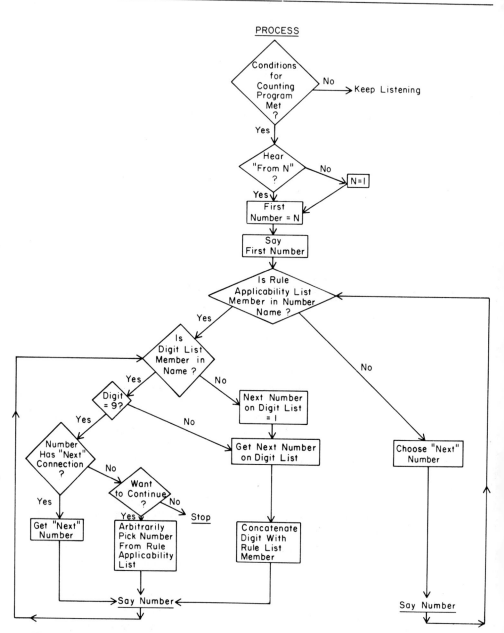

Figure 2-3. (B) Model II.

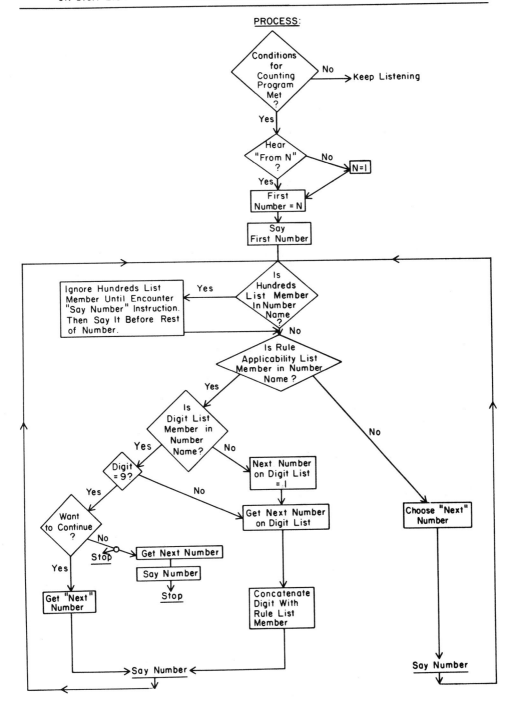

Figure 2-3. (C) Model III.

some children's lists will be slightly longer or shorter. Decade names starting with 20 can be on the rule applicability list.

The Model II process operates on this representation as follows. Suppose that a girl is asked to count. For the first 19 numbers she follows a process identical to that of Model I, since none of the numbers contains a rule applicability list member. However, 20 is on her rule applicability list, so the program branches to the reader's left.

The first question in this part of the program is whether there is a digit list member in the number name. The name 20 does not contain any digit list member, so the next number on the digit list is set equal to 1. One is retrieved as the next number on the digit list and is concatenated with 20 to produce 21. The girl says "21" and again considers whether there is a digit list member in the name. Now there is a digit list member, 1. Since the digit does not equal 9, she retrieves the next number on the digit list, 2, concatenates it with 20 to produce 22, and says "22." This process continues until she says "29," at which point the digit equals 9. Since the number 29 has a specific "next" connection in the Figure 2-3 representation, she says "30" and repeats the cycle.[2]

When the girl reaches 39, her representation has no "next" connection. This is an important choice point that accounts for many of the distinctive phenomena in the 20-99 group's counting. The girl must decide whether or not to continue. If she decides not to go on, she stops at the 9 number, in this case 39. Otherwise, she arbitrarily picks a number from her rule applicability list. This could result in an omission, if the number is too far advanced; in a repetition, if it is not far enough advanced; or, fortuitously, in the correct answer. After the choice of the rule applicability list member, the girl continues until she reaches a 9 number at which she decides to stop.

The Model III representation (Figure 2-3C) incorporates only two changes from that of Model II: the addition of the hundreds list, and the completion of the rule applicability list. The Model III process also resembles that of the previous model. It proceeds identically until it reaches 100. Then, the child notes that there is a hundreds list member in the number. She ignores the hundreds list member for purposes of *forming* subsequent numbers, but remembers to add it for purposes of *saying* them. Remembering to do this may be of more than trivial difficulty; young children who could count beyond 100 often momentarily forgot the hundreds term at one or more points in their counts (e.g., "125, 26, uh, I mean 126"). This is one reason why within the Model III process, the instruction to remember to say the hundreds name is separated from the point at which children actually say it.

Model III children can continue counting for a very long time. Such factors as fatigue and boredom seemed as likely as lack of knowledge to determine their stopping points. Therefore, Model III includes a slightly altered stopping rule. When

---

[2] The decision to call this list the rule applicability list rather than the decade name list may cause some immediate confusion but should lead to greater clarity in the long run. The set of numbers could not accurately be called the decade name list because 10 is a decade name yet cannot be concatenated with digits to form other numbers. What distinguishes 20, 30, and successive decade names is precisely that with them, the generative *rule* is *applicable*—hence the name *rule applicability list members*.

children's desire to continue becomes sufficiently slight, they stop at the next point at which the job would be complete—either at the next 9 or at the next 0 (e.g., at 129 or 130).

These three models account for the major features of the counting of children who stopped within the corresponding ranges. First, consider stopping points. Model I does not imply any particular distribution of stopping points, because there is no obvious way of predicting which "next" connections will be missing. Model II predicts that stops will occur at numbers ending in 9. Children stop because the number ending in 9 does not have a "next" connection. Model III suggests that stops should occur at either a 0 or a 9, points at which the job is complete.

Now, consider omissions and repetitions. The omissions and repetitions of greatest interest were those involving entire decades. Model I has no mechanism that would lead to such departures from the standard order. In Model II, they occur when children arbitrarily pick a higher or lower number from the rule applicability list after reaching a number ending in 9 that does not have a "next" connnection. Model III again predicts no such omissions and repetitions.[3]

The frequency and types of nonstandard numbers produced by the three models also differ. Children who used Model I would not be expected to generate nonstandard numbers. Model II children who had just begun to use the digit repetition list would produce such numbers if the boundaries of their digit lists were too high. For example, rather than the digit repetition list ending at 9, as in Figure 2-3B, it might end at 11, so they might say "29, 20-10, 20-11." Children who used Model III presumably would have overlearned the digit list, but might have difficulty remembering the recursive procedure for forming numbers with hundreds list members.

Finally, consider the counting-on data. Model I includes no mechanism for children to count-on if they are started beyond their counting range. Model II does include such a mechanism; children would count-on to the end of the decade from any number that they recognized to include a rule applicability list member and would continue to the following decade if the "next" connection was known. Model III generates behavior similar to Model II, except that at times the model would count-on beyond the highest decade it had reached previously. This would be attributable to Model III children's having stopped counting previously because of lack of motivation rather than lack of knowledge. With the single exception of the moderate-expertise children's difficulty in proceeding to the next decade in the counting-on situation, these predictions matched the major features of the preschoolers' counting and counting-on behavior. (For a discussion of the likely causes of the one exception, see Siegler and Robinson, 1982.)

---

[3]The decision to connect each member of the rule applicability list to the preceding 9 number rather than to the preceding rule applicability list member was not arbitrary. We tested several 5-year-olds' ability to count by 10s, a skill that they presumably would have if successive decade names were linked together. Specifically, the experimenter asked children to count by 10s, prompted them by saying "10, 20," and then asked them to continue. None of the children was able to count in this way, although all had previously counted by 1s beyond 30. Thus, it seemed likely that the children's interdecade connections were between 9 numbers and the next rule applicability list member, rather than between successive rule applicability list members.

Preschoolers' Knowledge of Numerical Magnitudes

Existing Research on Adults and Children. Another central aspect of children's knowledge of numbers is their knowledge of numerical magnitudes. Research in this area was greatly stimulated by Moyer and Landauer's (1967) finding that comparing the magnitudes of digits of discrepant sizes (e.g., 4 and 8) took less time than comparing the magnitudes of digits of similar sizes (e.g., 4 and 5). At the time, this symbolic distance effect must have appeared quite surprising, because the experiment was replicated at least five times within the next 5 years (Aiken & Williams, 1968; Fairbank, 1969; Knoll, cited by Moyer & Bayer, 1976; Parkman, 1971; Sekuler, Armstrong, & Rubin, 1971).

As Moyer and Landauer noted, however, the psychophysical literature provides a well-documented analog to the symbolic distance effect. Psychophysicists long ago discovered that the more discrepant on some dimension the magnitudes of two stimuli are, the faster they can be compared on that dimension. Another well-known psychophysical phenomenon also proved to be present in the numerical comparisons; the smaller the size of the smaller stimulus, the quicker the judgment (e.g., 2 and 4 can be compared more quickly than 4 and 6). This is usually called the min effect.

Two broad classes of models have emerged to account for adults' numerical comparisons: analog and discrete. The central assumptions underlying analog models are that representations of all types of magnitudes preserve continuous information about physical size, and that these analog values are compared directly, perhaps through some type of random-walk process (e.g., Moyer & Dumais, 1978). In contrast, the central assumption underlying discrete models is that magnitudes are grouped into categories, each of which carries a semantic code (e.g., large, small) and that it is the codes which are compared (e.g., Banks, Fujii, & Kayra-Stuart, 1976). Substantial bodies of data have been collected supporting each type of model, although it is our impression that discrete models have been most consistently in accord with data on *numerical* comparisons.

Despite the large amount of work on adult's understanding of numerical magnitudes, little is known about how such understanding develops. Both of the developmental studies that we located had serious methodological shortcomings that rendered doubtful the conclusions that the investigators drew (see Siegler & Robinson, 1982, for details). This lack of knowledge is unfortunate, not only because of the inherent place of magnitudes within children's understandings about numbers, but also because developmental research has substantial potential to illuminate general issues within the magnitude comparson literature. As Banks (1977) pointed out, almost all magnitude comparison studies have involved one of two types of stimulus materials: overlearned material, such as letters and digits; and arbitrary material, such as different-colored sticks or nonsense syllables. Neither of these types of material seems ideally suited to studying acquisition processes. In the first case, acquisition is already complete; in the second, the material being acquired is inherently unrepresentative of the semantically rich material that people learn about in the world outside the laboratory. Studying children's acquisition of knowledge of numerical magnitudes could overcome both problems. The materials are semantically rich (Lehman, 1979), yet can be studied at a point where they are not entirely mastered.

Preschoolers' Numerical Magnitude Comparisons. To obtain a more detailed picture of preschoolers' knowledge of numerical magnitudes, the same children who participated in the counting-on experiment were brought back to the experimental room. They were presented with the standard numerical comparison task for the 36 possible comparisons of the digits 1-9. The procedure was repeated on four occasions.

The period from 3 to 5 years proved to be one in which considerable development occurred in children's ability to compare digit magnitudes. Three-year-olds were correct on 56% of their comparisons, 4-year-olds on 81%, and 5-year-olds on 90%.

Both the size of the minimum number and the distance between the two numbers proved predictive of 4- and 5-year-olds' error patterns. This finding raised the issue of what representations of numerical magnitudes might underlie the children's performance. One method that can be used to address such questions is multidimensional scaling. The input to the scaling algorithm that we used (KYST) was the percentage of errors that children made on each of the 36 problems. The output was an arrangement of the nine digits in a one- or two-dimensional space.

The most striking result of the multidimensional scalings was that the numbers did not fit especially well into the compressive logarithmic function generally believed to characterize representations of numerical magnitudes in adults and older children. Rather, they seemed to fall into clusters, with quite small distances within clusters and quite large distances between them. Consider, for example, the data of the 4-year-olds shown in Figure 2-4A. There are some reasons for preferring the two-dimensional representation over the one-dimensional one—notably that the stress declines from .24 to .11—but even the one-dimensional representation does not closely resemble the hypothesized logarithmic spacing. Rather, the numbers seem to arrange themselves into four clusters: (1), (2,3), (4,5), and (6,7,8,9).

This finding motivated us to reanalyze Sekuler and Mierkiewicz's (1977) reaction time data with 6-year-olds (Figure 2-4B). Again, note that the results do not fit especially well the logarithmic function postulated previously. Rather, the numbers fall into a few clusters.

In order to test the impression of clustering in our own error data, we next performed hierarchical clustering analyses (using the diameter method; see Johnson, 1967). The results for the 4-year-olds are shown in Figure 2-4C. As can be seen in the patterns of ovals (stimuli within the smallest number of ovals are the most similar), the clusters are quite similar to those revealed impressionistically.

The emergence of two distinct dimensions in the multidimensional scaling solutions implied that the difficulty of the magnitude comparison problems was determined by the two numbers' being in the same or in different clusters, rather than by the distance between clusters. To test this hypothesis, a regression analysis was performed using between- versus within-cluster status as a predictor of the relative difficulty of the 36 comparison items. The cluster membership variable accounted for 63% of the variance in the number of errors, not that different from the 73%

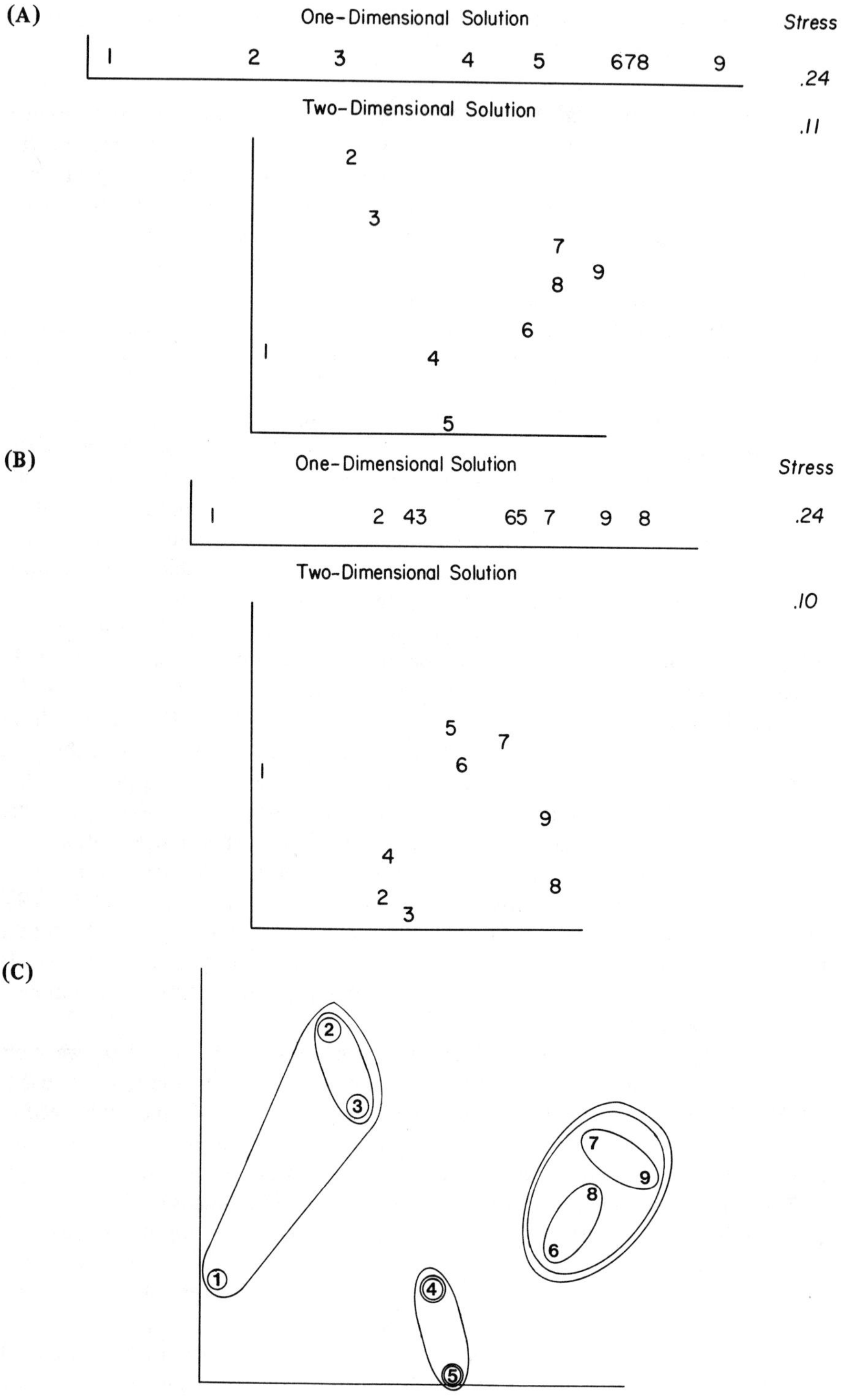
(A)
One-Dimensional Solution
Stress
1 2 3 4 5 678 9
.24
Two-Dimensional Solution
.11
2
3
7
9
8
6
1
4
5
(B)
One-Dimensional Solution
Stress
1 2 43 65 7 9 8
.24
Two-Dimensional Solution
.10
5
7
6
1
9
4
8
2
3
(C)
2
3
7
9
8
6
1
4
5

that could be accounted for by using absolute distances between each pair of digits in the scaling solution as the predictor.

Thus, several sources of evidence were consistent with the notion that young children represent digit magnitudes in terms of a few clusters. It must be noted, though, that all of these sources of evidence involved the end products of magnitude comparisons. Thus they involved a process as well as a representation. To obtain more direct evidence about children's representations of numerical magnitudes, we thought it important to determine (a) what verbal labels children attached to the digits; (b) whether the labels were related to their magnitude comparison performance; and (c) if labels and performance were related, whether teaching children a new clustering scheme would influence their pattern of errors in comparing magnitudes. The two experiments reported next addressed these questions.

Verbal Labeling of Numbers. In both Trabasso's (1977) and Banks, Fujii, and Kayra-Stuarts's (1976) discrete category models, people were said to attach a semantic code to each stimulus being compared. The only empirical support for this claim was that it was consistent with the semantic congruity effect. Siegler and Robinson (1982) examined this claim by presenting the same group of preschoolers with the following instructions:

> Today I'm going to ask you some questions about the numbers from 1 to 9. Some of these are big numbers, some are little numbers, and some are medium numbers. I'm going to say a number, and you need to tell me if the number is a big number, a little number, or a medium number.

The experimenter asked about the nine numbers in random order.

Given this procedure, even the 3-year-olds demonstrated some knowledge of numerical magnitudes. The mean value of the numbers that they termed small was 3.14; of the numbers that they labeled medium, 5.15; and of the numbers that they labeled big, 6.00. This does not imply that there was no development in skill at applying the labels. By age 5, the mean values of numbers assigned the small, medium, and large labels were 2.16, 5.12, and 7.75, respectively.

Next, Siegler and Robinson considered whether children's labeling could have been useful on the magnitude comparison task. They found that inserting children's labels into a simple comparison process (select labels for each number with probabilities indicated by the labeling experiment; if one number has a greater label, it is larger; if the labels are equal, again choose labels from the same probability distribution) yielded 58% correct answers for 3-year-olds, 75% for 4-year-olds, and 80% for 5-year-olds. Thus, the 4- and 5-year-olds' labels were potentially useful on the numerical comparison task; if the children used them, they would have performed at a level well above chance.

Figure 2-4. Multidimensional scaling solutions for magnitude comparison data.
(A) Scalings of 4-year-olds' errors (our data).
(B) Scalings of 6-year-olds' solution times (data from Sekuler & Mierkiewicz, 1977).
(C) Hierarchical clustering of 4-year-olds' errors (our data).
From "The Development of Numerical Understandings," in H. Reese & L. P. Lipsitt (Eds.), *Advances in Child Development and Behavior Vol. 16.* Copyright 1982 by Academic Press. Reprinted by permission.

The number of correct answers predicted by the foregoing measure of the quality of each child's labels also proved to be closely related to the number of correct answers the child had produced on the numerical comparison task. Across the three age groups, the correlation was $r = .80$. The correlations were also substantial within the three age groups, ranging from $r = .55$ to $r = .73$. The labels also predicted the relative difficulty of the individual problems. Illustratively, they were found to account for 66% of the variance in 4-year-olds' number of errors on the 36 problems.

Thus, the labeling experiment demonstrated that the labels children applied to numbers logically could have led to above-chance performance in the magnitude comparison context, that the labels were correlated with individual differences in the percentage of correct answers on the comparison task, and that the labels predicted the relative difficulty of the comparison problems.

A central question remained, however: Was the children's labeling part of the process by which they compared magnitudes, or did performance on the one task simply predict performance on the others? This issue was addressed in the next experiment.

Effects of Teaching a Labeling Strategy. If children's labels were functionally involved in the magnitude comparison process, then teaching them a specific set of labels for the numbers might be expected to influence their later comparisons. In particular, children who used the labeling scheme that they were taught would be expected to be more successful on between-category comparisons (defined in terms of that labeling scheme) than on within-category ones. A control group that was not taught this particular labeling scheme would be expected to show a smaller between-category versus within-category difference, because they would be less likely to use this set of labels. In addition, if children previously had selected labels independently for each number, then instructing them in the use of an entire set of labels would reduce their percentage of incorrect answers (as will be explained in detail in the models that follow). The primary purpose of the training experiment was to test these predictions.

The children who participated were 4-year-olds who attended a day-care center. Those in the labeling training group were taught that 1, 2, and 3 were little numbers, that 4, 5, and 6 were medium-size numbers, and that 7, 8, and 9 were big numbers. Those in the control group were asked the size of each number but were not taught a particular labeling scheme. The next day, children were brought back to the experimental room and presented with the 36 standard magnitude comparison problems.

The 10 children in the training group learned the labels quickly. Nine did not make an error after the third trial block. The training in labeling greatly reduced the number of errors that the children made on the subsequent magnitude comparison task. Children who were trained to apply the labels were correct on 96% of the comparisons, as opposed to 79% correct answers among children in the control group. The labeling training also changed the distribution of children's magnitude comparison errors. Children in the training group made 65% of their errors on the nine items involving within-cluster comparisons. By contrast, children in the control group made only 29% of their errors on the same nine items.

Three Models of Numerical Magnitude Comparison. Figure 2-5 depicts three models that would generate magnitude comparison performance of the types we observed. First consider Model I (Figure 2-5A). The representation is based directly on the 3-year-olds' performance in the labeling experiment. Read vertically, this matrix indicates the probability that each number was assigned each categorical label. Read horizontally, the matrix indicates the probability that each category included each member. When asked whether a number is small, medium, or large, Model I children simply retrieve labels with the probabilities indicated in the representation. When asked to compare magnitudes, however, the children do not utilize any of the knowledge from the representation; they simply guess, thus producing chance-level comparison performance.

Next consider Model II, hypothesized to underlie the moderately expert performance (60-95% correct) of the majority of 4-year-olds (Figure 2-5B). Model II incorporates one major change from Model I: Its magnitude comparison process makes use of the categorical information. As shown in Figure 2-5B, when children are presented with a magnitude comparison problem, they generate a label for each number. The choices of labels are independent for the two numbers, and occur for each number with the probabilities shown in the columns of the representation. If the labels differ, children choose as bigger the number associated with the larger label. If the labels are identical, children regenerate labels for each number until the labels differ. Note that regardless of the particular probabilities assigned to the labels, this type of model almost inevitably leads to errors. Unless the child creates at least $N - 1$ distinct categories for the N numbers in the comparison set, he or she will always have some probability of assigning the larger label to the smaller number.

Model III, intended to characterize the near-perfect performance of most of the 5-year-olds, incorporates number-label links corresponding to those that appear in Model II. However, another hierarchical level is superimposed on the links: overall categorical organizations. As shown in Figure 2-5C, the child's representation includes several divisions of the nine numbers into categories. Each time a magnitude comparison problem in presented, the child chooses one of the categorical organizations with the probability shown in the representation. Choosing an organization determines the assignment of labels to numbers. If the labels differ, the child chooses the number attached to the larger label as being bigger. If the labels are identical, the child again chooses a categorical organization. The cycle continues until a categorical organization is chosen that assigns different labels to the two numbers being compared.

Finally, Model II-III, a hybrid of Models II and III, produces the performance of the trained 4-year-olds in the training experiment (Figure 2-5D). The representation includes the Model II probabilities of each number's being assigned each label, and also the one categorical organization that the children were taught in the training procedure. The process starts with the Model III approach, in which a categorical organization is selected. Because the only categorical organization that the 4-year-

(A)

Representation

(Empirically derived probabilities of each number being assigned to each category)

Category	Number								
	1	2	3	4	5	6	7	8	9
Smallest	.6								
Small	.2	.25	.42	.08	.25	.08	.17		.08
Medium	.2	.58	.42	.92	.58	.67	.50	.67	.67
Big		.17	.17		.17	.25	.33	.33	.25

Process

For Labeling

Choose Label For Number

For Magnitude Comparison

Guess

(B)

Representation

Category	Number								
	1	2	3	4	5	6	7	8	9
Smallest	.7								
Small	.2	.72	.61	.22	.06			.06	
Medium	.1	.28	.33	.67	.72	.67	.56	.27	.44
Big			.06	.11	.22	.33	.44	.67	.56

Process

For Labeling   **For Magnitude Comparison**

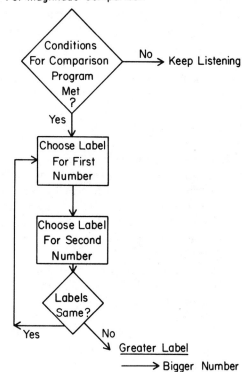

Figure 2-5. Models of magnitude comparison.

(A) Model I. (Here and in Figure 2-5B, the probabilities for the numbers 2-9 are the group-level probabilities that children in the labeling experiment (3-year-olds in Figure 2-5A, 4-year-olds in Figure 2-5B) assigned each label to each number. The Figure 2-4 scaling and clustering results suggested that the number 1 was in a separate "smallest" category not tapped by the labeling procedure; therefore, hypothetical probabilities have been assigned to the number 1.)

(B) Model II.

Parts A-D from "The Development of Numerical Understandings," in H. Reese & L. P. Lipsitt (Eds.), *Advances in Child Development and Behavior Vol. 16.* Copyright 1982 by Academic Press. Reprinted by permission.

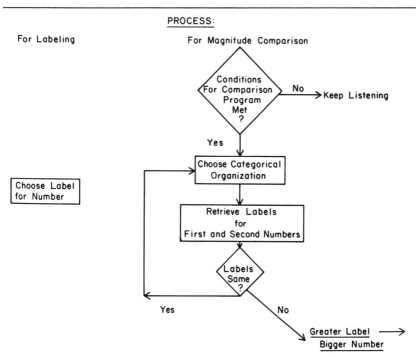

Figure 2-5. (C) Model III. The probabilities of each number being assigned to each label were chosen to correspond roughly to the labeling experiment probabilities that the 5-year-olds assigned each label to each matching number. An exact matching was impossible, because in the labeling experiment the children were asked to assign labels to numbers independently, but within this model, category boundaries are dependent on each other. [Note: Figure 2-5 (D) appears on the following page.]

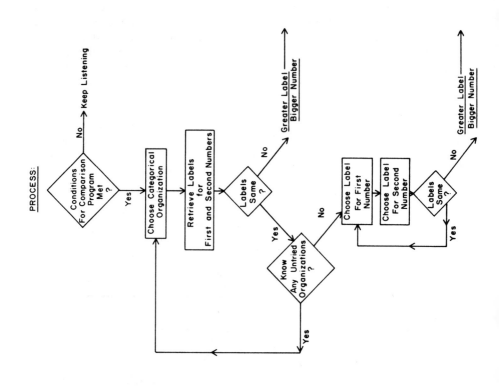

Figure 2-5. (D) Model II-III.

olds know is the one they were taught, they use it to assign labels to the numbers. If this procedure assigns different labels to the numbers, the children answer correctly. If it assigns the same labels, however, they would not know any alternative organizations, and therefore would revert to the Model II process of assigning labels to each number independently until the labels differed.

These models give rise to the types of magnitude comparison performance, labeling, and learning that were observed in the three experiments. Model I prescribes the 3-year-olds' behavior in a rather direct way. As implied by the Figure 2-5A probabilities, these children can assign labels to the numbers that have some correspondence to the numbers' magnitudes. However, they do not use this knowledge in comparing the magnitudes; instead they simply guess, producing the roughly chance predictions performance that was observed.

Model II predicts a considerably lower error rate and a distribution of errors that is linked to the characteristics of the problems. Averaged across all 36 problems, the model generates 84% correct answers, similar to the 81% that was observed. The symbolic distance effect emerges because numbers that are farther apart are less likely to be assigned incorrectly ordered labels. The min effect emerges because the distribution of labels changes more rapidly at the small end of the scale. This distribution of labels, in turn, probably arises from the children's having more knowledge about the smallest numbers and therefore classifying them in a more differentiated fashion. The labeling experiment results of accurate labeling of numbers as small, medium, and large arises from the children's choosing labels for the numbers in accord with the Figure 2-5B probabilities.

Model III predicts that no errors should occur, because within each categorical organization, the category boundaries are correctly ordered and nonoverlapping. The effects of categorization will continue to be seen in solution times, however. Between-category comparisons will on average arise earlier in the comparison process when the digits are farther apart and when the minimum number's magnitude is small. Sekuler and Mierkiewicz's data on 6-year-olds and older children are in accord with these predictions.

Finally, Model II-III, the model of the trained children's knowledge, produces performance similar to Model III on the between-category comparisons and similar to Model II on the within-category ones. The superior performance predicted by this model on, and only on, the between-category problems explains both why trained children made fewer errors overall than untrained ones, and why the bulk of the few errors they made were within-category errors.

Preschoolers' Knowledge of Addition

Existing Research. Young children's knowledge of addition has been the subject of far more research than their knowledge of counting or numerical magnitudes. Perhaps the best known model of the addition process, Groen and Parkman's (1972) min model, is based on a chronometric approach. Within this model, the adder chooses the larger of the two numbers and then increments it by one a number of times equal to the smaller number. The only factor contributing to differences among problems in solution times is the number of increments dictated by the minimum number.

The min model fit Groen and Parkman's data quite well except on ties, problems where both children's and adults' solution times were nearly constant over all of the items tested. These data led Groen and Parkman to amend their model so that ties were reproduced directly from "fast-access memory" while other problems were reconstructed by the incrementing process.

Groen and Parkman's model and alternatives to it that have been proposed (Svenson, 1975; Ashcraft & Battaglia, 1978) have been based primarily on chrono-metric data (for a review, see Ashcraft, 1982). Another source of evidence about the addition process comes from clinical descriptions. These descriptions suggest that children use a variety of strategies on addition problems. Ilg and Ames (1951), for example, observed that some children decompose the problem 3 + 14 into 14 = 10 + 4; 3 + 4 = 7; 10 + 7 = 17. In other clinical descriptions, children have been said to rely on 5s, 10s, and ties as reference points from which to calculate answers; to move their feet rhythmically to help them count; to count on from the larger num-ber; and to count on from 1 (Hebbeler, 1976; Yoshimura, 1974). Although most of these descriptions of addition strategies are anecdotal, the reports have been persis-tent enough to leave little doubt that young children employ a variety of methods in adding.

Considered as a group, these studies reveal a cleavage between the types of models that have been formulated and many of the phenomena that have been observed. The models of addition—Groen and Parkman's, Ashcraft and Battaglia's, and Svenson's—all have been designed to depict *the* strategy people use. The detailed observations of addition have revealed a large number of distinct strategies that people use on particular problems. The discrepancy suggests that the chronometric data on children's addition may reflect an averaging over different strategies rather than a consistent adherence to any one strategy. Above and beyond determining how children execute any particular addition strategy, we need to learn how they choose among alternative approaches.

Preschoolers' Addition Strategies. Considering the possibility that children use a variety of addition strategies raises many questions. Which strategies are used most frequently? What are their accuracy and temporal characteristics? Are choices of strategies systematically related to the particular numbers involved in problems? Does variable strategy usage help children add more accurately and/or more quickly than using the same strategy at all times? If so, why? To address these questions, Siegler and Robinson (1982) videotaped 3-, 4-, and 5-year-olds in the process of adding each of the 25 problems that result from combining addend (1-5) and augend (1-5). The children were the same ones who earlier counted and com-pared magnitudes.

As in the previous experiments, the period from age 3 to age 5 proved to be one of substantial development. Three-year-olds were correct on 20% of the addition problems, 4-year-olds on 66%, and 5-year-olds on 79%. Scrutiny of the videotapes revealed that children adopted at least four approaches to solving addition problems: the counting fingers strategy, the fingers strategy, the counting strategy, and (for want of a better name) the no-visible-strategy approach. The four strategies differed in their visible and audible manifestations, accuracy, temporal characteristics, and types of errors with which they were associated.

When using the counting fingers strategy, children put up the fingers on one hand, then put up the fingers on the other hand, and then counted the two sets of fingers. As shown in Table 2-3, the strategy was used moderately often, was very slow, and produced accurate performance. When errors occurred, they were most often close misses.

When using the fingers strategy, children put up their fingers but showed no evidence of counting them. The fingers and the counting fingers strategies produced similarly accurate performance, but the time needed to execute the fingers approach was shorter. Errors on the fingers trials, like those on the counting fingers trials, were usually close misses.

When using the counting strategy, children counted aloud but without any visible referent. In all cases these counts started from 1. The strategy was associated with moderately long solution times and was the least accurate and the least often used of the four strategies. Errors were often quite distant from the correct answer.

The fourth category was a catchall for those trials on which the children did not engage in any visible or audible behaviors prior to answering; these trials were grouped as "no visible strategy." This approach was the most frequently used, the second least accurate, and the most rapidly executed strategy. The accuracy data fell into a distinctly bimodal distribution. Sixteen of the 30 children performed at high accuracy rates when they used no visible strategy; they were correct on 86-100% of trials. The other 14 children were much less accurate, ranging from 13% to 67% correct. Both the high-accuracy and the low-accuracy children executed the approach rapidly, and both groups' errors often were far from the correct answer.

The most striking finding of the experiment involved the connection between strategy use and problem difficulty. As shown in Figure 2-6, on each problem the percentage of errors was closely related to the percentage of trials on which one of the three visible strategies was used ($r = .91$). The relation actually was attenuated slightly by the tendency of children more frequently to solve problems on which they used a visible strategy. If only the percentage of errors on no-visible-strategy trials is used to estimate difficulty, the correlation between frequency of visible strategy use and problem difficulty increases slightly to $r = .92$.

Using the visible strategies more often on the more difficult problems proved to be highly adaptive. Performance was more accurate on 24 of the 25 problems when visible strategies were used than when they were not. Moreover, the frequency of use of visible strategies on the 25 problems correlated $r = .73$ with the gain in accuracy on each problem from using a visible strategy.

These results answered two of our original questions. First, use of visible strategies was indeed related to the characteristics of the addition problems, with the more difficult problems eliciting a greater frequency of strategy use. Second, employing such visible strategies aided children's performance, with the greatest benefits accruing on the most difficult problems. Left unanswered, however, was the question of how children chose which, if any, strategy to use on a problem.

One possibility was that children were consciously aware of problem difficulty

Table 2-3 Characteristics of Arithmetic Strategies

Strategy	Trials On Which Strategy Was Used (%)	Mean Solution Time (sec)	Correct Answers (%)	Errors Where Answer Was Within One of Correct Sum(%)
Counting fingers	15	14.0	87	70
Fingers	13	6.6	89	80
Counting	8	9.0	54	44
No visible strategy	64	4.0	66	41

Note: From "The Development of Numerical Understandings," in H. Reese & L. P. Lipsitt (Eds.), *Advances in Child Development and Behavior Vol. 16.* Copyright 1982 by Academic Press. Reprinted by permission.

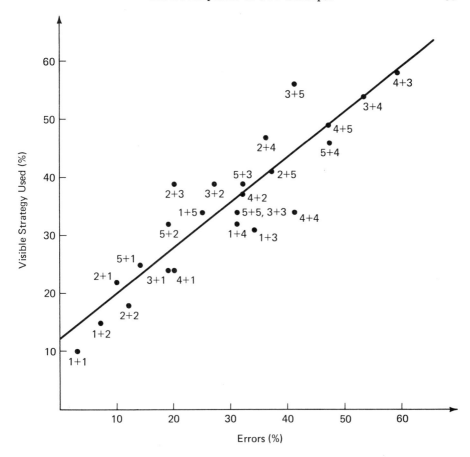

Figure 2-6. Percentage of errors on arithmetic problems as a function of addend and augend size.

and employed a visible strategy only when they judged the problem too difficult to solve without one. This might be labeled the metacognitive hypothesis. The metacognitive hypothesis is based on an implicit model of the strategy-choice process in which problem difficulty gives rise to judgments of problem difficulty, which in turn give rise to use of visible strategies when needed.

This model implies that problem difficulty and judgments of problem difficulty should be highly correlated, especially given the observed high correlation between problem difficulty and visible strategy use. To test this prediction, we asked a group ($N = 12$) of 5-year-olds, students at a nursery school very similar to the one at which the original experiment was run, to label each of the 25 problems as easy, hard, or in-between.

The difficulty ratings correlated only moderately with the actual difficulty of the problems as estimated by the errors of our sample, the errors of Knight and Behrens's (1928) sample, and the solution times of Groen and Parkman's (1972) sample (correlations ranging from $r = .31$ to $r = .50$). It might be argued that these relatively low correlations could have been due to our obtaining the performance and difficulty ratings data from different samples. However, the correlations were much higher on other intersample comparisons: between the percentages of errors on the 25 problems in our and in Knight and Behrens's samples, between the percentage of errors on these problems in our sample and the solution times in Groen and Parkman's sample, and between the percentage of errors on Knight and Behrens's sample and the solution times in Groen and Parkman's sample (correlations ranging from $r = .72$ to $r = .89$). Thus, the data lent little support to the view that children's judgments of problem difficulty were responsible for the relation between strategy use and problem difficulty.

A Model of Strategy Choice in Addition. Another possibility was that the correlation between visible strategy use and problem difficulty was a by-product of the solution process. One model that would give rise to such a correlation is displayed in Figure 2-7. The representation consists of a matrix of augends and addends together with the sums for each problem. Next to each sum is a number (in parentheses) that is not present in any child's representation, but that is important within the model. This is the joint probability that the child recalls the correct answer to the problem and is sufficiently confident of this answer to advance it without resorting to a visible strategy. This joint probability will differ for each child and for each situation that a given child finds himself in. The probabilities in Figure 2-7 were the group-level likelihoods within the present experiment that on each addition problem, 4- and 5-year-olds used no visible strategy and recalled the answer correctly.[4] This matrix is similar in principle to the tabular structures used to represent addition facts in network retrieval theories of mental arithmetic (See Figure 4-2 in this volume).

The process that is applied to this representation begins with the setting of a confidence criterion by which children decide whether they are sure enough of an answer to give it. Then they try to recall the answer to the problem. If their confidence in the recalled answer exceeds the criterion, they say it. Otherwise, they augment their representations of the augend and addend. They can do this externally, by putting up their fingers, or internally, by forming some type of imaginal representation. If their confidence in an answer at this point exceeds the criterion, they give it. Otherwise, they count their fingers or the imaged objects and state the last number of the count as their result.

This model gives rise to the four approaches that we observed. If children answer at the first "Recall" point in the process, they will not have used any visible strategy. If they put up their fingers but answer without counting them, they will have used the fingers strategy. If they image objects corresponding to augend and addend and then count aloud, they will have used the counting strategy. If they put

---

[4] "Recall" is used here in quite a loose sense. It is entirely possible that on some of the trials where children did not use a visible strategy and answered correctly, they used the min approach described by Groen and Parkman or some other strategy (see Siegler & Robinson, 1982, for an extended discussion).

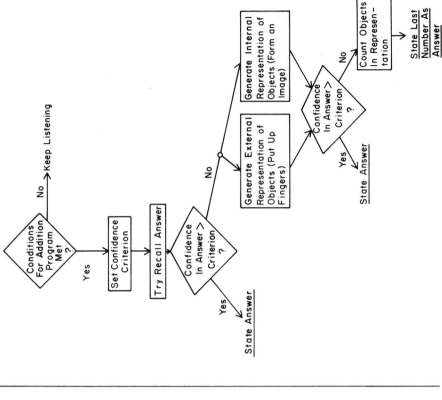

PROCESS:

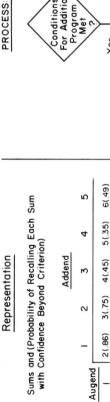

Representation

Sums and (Probability of Recalling Each Sum with Confidence Beyond Criterion)

	Addend				
Augend	1	2	3	4	5
1	2(.86)	3(.75)	4(.45)	5(.35)	6(.49)
2	3(.68)	4(.69)	5(.49)	6(.28)	7(.26)
3	4(.58)	5(.40)	6(.35)	7(.09)	8(.13)
4	5(.55)	6(.23)	7(.07)	8(.36)	9(.15)
5	6(.68)	7(.52)	8(.34)	9(.08)	10(.38)

Figure 2-7. Model of strategy choice in addition. The probabilities in parentheses represent the percentage of trials on which children used no visible strategy and answered correctly. From "The Development of Numerical Understandings," in H. Reese & L. P. Lipsitt (Eds.), *Advances in Child Development and Behavior Vol. 16.* Copyright 1982 by Academic Press. Reprinted by permission.

up their fingers, count them, and answer after counting, they will have used the counting fingers strategy.

The model also accounts for the relative solution times and accuracy rates of the four strategies. It predicts straightforwardly that the no-visible-strategy approach should be the fastest, the fingers approach the next fastest, and the counting and counting fingers approaches the slowest. All of the processing steps necessary to execute each of the faster strategies are included within the steps necessary to execute the slower ones. Predictions of relative accuracy also can be derived, albeit not quite as directly. Both the overall low accuracy and the bimodal distribution of accuracies of the no-visible-strategy approach follow from the view that some children used this approach because they set loose criteria for deciding when they knew the answer, and others used it because they did not need external aids in order to retrieve the correct answer. The high accuracy of the counting fingers strategy would have been expected, since 4- and 5-year-olds are very adept at counting the 2-10 objects required by the problems (Gelman & Gallistel, 1978). Several factors may have contributed to the high accuracy of the fingers approach: pattern recognition of the number of fingers that were put up, kinesthetic cues associated with putting up particular sets of fingers, and longer search time than that typical of the no-visible-strategy approach.[5] Finally, the relative inaccuracy of the counting approach is consistent with Kosslyn's (1978) finding that children have difficulty maintaining a clear image for as long as it took to execute this strategy, an average of 9 seconds.

Perhaps the central feature of the model is that it accounts for the correlation between problem difficulty and strategy use. Children do not need explicit knowledge about problem difficulty in order to produce the relation. Instead, at each step in the solution process, children consider whether their confidence in an answer exceeds the level demanded by their criteria. The more difficult the problem, the less likely it is that this will occur at an early point. Thus, children are led to take increasingly effortful steps to solve the more difficult problems. In a sense, they use internal strategies when they can and external ones when they must.

Conclusions: The Development of Numerical Knowledge

What knowledge of numbers might produce these numerical skills? The three models shown in Figure 2-8 correspond to the knowledge that we hypothesize is most often possessed by 3-, 4-, and 5-year-olds, respectively.[6] A cursory examina-

---

[5] To understand why kinesthetic cues associated with raising one's fingers might be helpful for recalling a sum, consider what would happen if your eyes were closed and someone lifted one or more fingers on each of your hands. With at least some combinations, the number of fingers raised might well "feel" like 2, 4, or 10, for example. Whether children are helped by such information is an open question, but the kinesthetic cues offered at least one explanation for the superior accuracy of the fingers approach.

[6] The models in Figure 2-8 are intended to provide descriptions of the modal tendencies among 3-, 4-, and 5-year-olds, but should not be taken to imply a lockstep progression among the three skills or a perfect correlation between age and skill. Empirically, each skill possessed a moderately high correlation with age and a moderately high correlation with the other two skills. Age correlated $r = .64$ with percentage of correct answers on the numerical comparison problems, $r = .68$ with percentage of correct answers on the addition problems, and $r = .49$

tion of the models reveals two features: They are quite forbidding looking, and they appear similar to each other. Because of the models' forbidding appearance, we will describe one of them, Model II, at some length. Because of the similarities across the three models, we will characterize two of them, Models I and III, by comparing them with Model II.

The Model II representation is organized as a three-level hierarchy. Numbers as a class are at the top of the hierarchy, then categories of numbers (e.g., small numbers), and finally individual numbers (e.g., 6).

Numbers as a class can be operated on by several processes: they can be counted, their magnitudes can be compared, they can be added and (presumably) subtracted. That children treat numbers as a class distinct from other classes was evident in what they did not do as much as in what they did. No child ever gave a nonnumerical answer to an addition problem or used any nonnumerical term in counting. When children used nonstandard numbers in their counting strings, they were always combinations of standard ones. Therefore, we believe that several processes that can operate on numbers are attached to numbers as a class rather than to particular groups of numbers or to individual numbers. (The details of these processes are omitted from Figure 2-8 because of considerations of space; they are shown earlier in the chapter in the figures indicated.)

At the middle level of the hierarchy are categories of numbers, ordered by magnitude. Both the number conservation data reported in Siegler (1981) and the magnitude comparison data reported in the present investigation suggest that these categories possess psychological reality for young children. Illustratively, the conservation operators that are applied to small numbers differ from those that are applied to large ones (Figure 2-1B). Each category is linked both upward to the class of numbers and downward to individual numbers. The particular probabilities linking the categories to the individual numbers are based on those that appeared in the Figure 2-5B representation—the empirically derived probabilities that 4-year-olds assigned each label to each number.

The lowest level of the hierarchy involves individual numbers. In addition to being tied to the category labels, numbers can be tied to each other by "next" connections. Some numbers also are labeled as members of the digit repetition and rule applicability lists. The smaller ones are involved in addition facts that the children are more or less confident of knowing. Although our experiments did not tap other information about individual numbers, informal discussions with preschoolers suggest that they possess additional knowledge about them. For example, a 4- year-old told us that 1 is the number that she starts counting with, that it is the

---

with how high children counted. Across the three age groups, the percentage of correct answers on the addition task correlated $r = .80$ with the percentage of correct answers on the numerical comparison task, the percentage of correct answers on the comparison task correlated $r = .60$ with the highest number counted on the counting task, and the percentage of correct answers on the addition task correlated $r = .65$ with the highest number counted on the counting task. The correlations between pairs of tasks were also fairly high within age groups, averaging $r = .54$ for the nine within-age correlations. Overall, 27 of the 39 children (70%) who performed all three tasks would have been assigned to the same aggregate model by virtue of their performance on each of the three individual tasks.

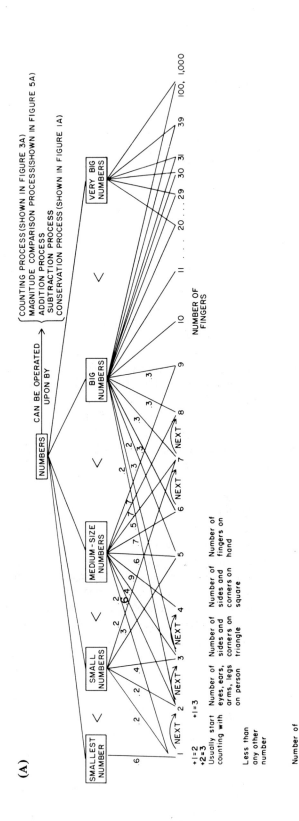

Figure 2-8. (A-C) Integrative models of preschoolers' knowledge of numbers. (A) Model I. Parts A-C from "The Development of Numerical Understandings," in H. Reese & L. P. Lipsitt (Eds.), *Advances in Child Development and Behavior Vol. 16.* Copyright 1982 by Academic Press. Reprinted by permission.

(B)

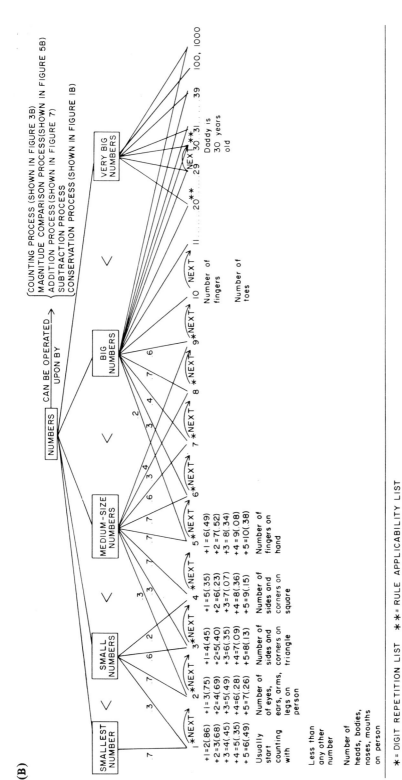

Figure 2-8. (B) Model II.

(C)

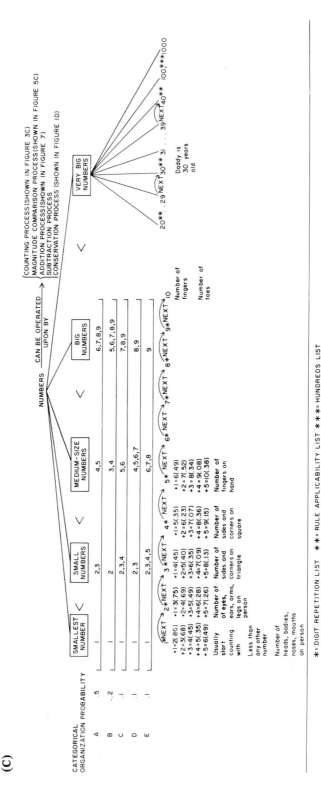

Figure 2-8. (C) Model III.

number of heads, bodies, noses, and mouths on a person, and that it is the smallest number.

The Model II depiction of moderately skilled performance provides a vantage point for considering the more and less advanced knowledge depicted in Model III and Model I. First, consider some properties that are hypothesized not to change in this age and skill range. The three-level hierarchical form of the representation is constant across models. Also relatively constant are many of the particular connections within and across levels of the hierarchy. Even in Model I, the larger numbers are more often associated with the larger categories; even in Model I, some of the "next" connections between digits are present; even in Model I, some facts linking individual numbers to other semantic properties (e.g., people have two hands) are known. Development in these (although not all) aspects of the representations appears to be a gradual, incremental process.

At the other extreme, development can be seen in sharpest relief in the processes that children apply to their representations. These processes change greatly for counting, comparing, and conserving between Models I and II, and the processes for counting and comparing undergo large changes between Models II and III as well. The pattern is reminiscent of the often-expressed speculation that development entails at least as great a growth in what children can do with information as in the amount of information they possess (Bruner, 1973; Piaget, 1972; Simon, 1972).

How can we evaluate the quality of these models? Empirically, they predict in detail preschoolers' counting, comparing, conserving, and adding. Model II can again be used to illustrate. When counting, the model stops at 9s, skips and repeats decades, forms nonstandard numbers if the boundary of its digit list is too high, and counts on at least to the next 9 from points within or beyond its spontaneous counting range. When comparing magnitudes, it errs most often on problems with large minima and small splits, assigns labels that correspond reasonably well to the relative magnitudes of numbers, and learns from instruction that imposes an overall categorical organization on the numbers. When performing number conservation problems, it answers small-number problems correctly but judges large-number ones by the relative lengths of the rows. When adding, it usually recalls the answers to the easiest problems without using visible strategies, and uses visible strategies on more difficult problems. Thus, the model mimics a considerable range of preschoolers' behaviors in manipulating numbers.

A second virtue of the models is the quality that Klahr and Wallace (1976) termed *developmental tractability*. For most of the changes between models, we can easily imagine how the more advanced form could grow out of the less advanced one. In counting, children first learn the "next" connections that are the only relations that bind the small integers they encounter; then they add information about the cyclical patterns inherent in the next higher numbers; and eventually they extend the list membership notion to include the much larger numbers. In learning about numerical magnitudes, children first obtain a rough sense of magnitudes that allows them to assign numbers to categories having some correspondence to the numbers' sizes; then they learn how to use the categorical information to compare magnitudes; and finally they impose overall categorical organizations that subsume the connections between individual numbers and categories. In learning about number conservation, children first quantify only in limited situations, then quantify in all situations, and finally obtain knowledge about transformations that eliminates the need to quantify. In adding, children first memorize solutions to specific problems, and then learn supplementary reconstructive strategies to use on problems where they cannot retrieve the answer. Thus, children build on what they already know to construct increasingly successful approaches.

The models' separation between representations and processes proved useful for specifying the source of this developmental tractability. Modeling approaches that focus solely on processes, such as the rule assessment approach, might have revealed as much about developmental changes in the preschool period, but probably would not have revealed the developmental constancies that also were present. The representation-process distinction also suggested a basis for intertask linkages, such as the use of categories in both conservation and comparison (see Siegler and Robinson, 1982, for discussion of these linkages). In sum, the format's flexibility seems well adapted to characterizing the multiple facets of conceptual understanding.

Characterizing both representations and processes also can help to resolve conflicting claims about children's conceptual understanding that have arisen in the literature. The format's flexibility allows rival views to be placed in a common framework, thus enabling direct comparisons to be made. Recent studies of children's concepts of life (Richards, 1981; Richards & Siegler, Note 1) illustrate this function.

Children's Concepts of Life

The research in this section alternates its focus among existing verbally stated theories of children's life concepts, more formal models based on these theories, and experiments designed to test the predictions of the theories. The research is organized into four parts. In the first part we describe several existing theories of children's understanding of life. These theories differ in many ways, and establishing similarities and differences among them proves difficult. Therefore, in the second section we characterize each of the theories more formally in the language of representations and processes. These characterizations help us derive specific empirical predictions from the theories. The predictions are tested in the third section, a series of five experiments on children's life concepts. The first three experiments concern what objects children believe are alive. In these experiments we examine children's rules for labeling objects alive, their prototypic living things, and the influence of situational factors on their rules for inferring life. The last two experiments examine the attributes that children ascribe to living things. Here we focus on the attributes that children associate most closely with life and how children use information about attributes to infer whether objects are alive. In the fourth section we examine the implications of the five experiments for the competing theories of the development of the life concept, and formulate new models that incorporate the experimental results within the framework of one of the existing theories.

Existing Research on Life Concepts

The earliest extensive account of children's knowledge of life was reported by Piaget (1929). He postulated a four-stage progression leading to conceptual mastery. Children in Stage I (up to 6 years of age) judge as alive things that are active or that perform a function. This includes people, animals, bicycles, and ovens. Stage II children (roughly ages 6 to 8 years) attribute life only to things that move. Stage III children (roughly ages 8 to 12 years) attribute life only to things that move autonomously: people, other animals, and celestial objects such as the sun and moon. Stage IV children attribute life either to animals alone or to both plants and animals.

Many investigators have attempted to replicate and extend Piaget's experiments. The result has been a fairly large literature (for a recent review, see Brainerd, 1978), but one from which few conclusions can be drawn. Perhaps the only point of general agreement is that children at times attribute life to inanimate objects. Russell (1940a, 1940b), Huang (1943), Huang and Lee (1945), Klingensmith (1953), Klingberg (1957), and Laurendeau and Pinard (1962) have all replicated Piaget's findings on this point. Beyond this finding there is little consensus. Huang and Lee (1945) and Laurendeau and Pinard (1962) questioned Piaget's emphasis on the role of motion in children's attributions of life. Russell (1940a, 1940b) and Laurendeau and Pinard (1962) questioned the age norms that Piaget assigned to the four stages. Huang and Lee found that children attribute life to nonliving objects more often than they attribute the correlates of life to the same objects (Piaget reported the opposite). Klingensmith (1953) suggested that children's misattributions were due to their confusing *alive* with *lively*. Huang and Lee (1945) and Laurendeau and Pinard (1962) suggested that children basically understand the life concept, but that in some circumstances they base judgments on other cues.

These disagreements may have arisen because investigators have asked children different questions and asked the questions about different objects. Many of the variations were triggered by uncertainties about Piaget's orginal procedures and his stage classification criteria. Within Stage IV, Piaget included children who thought that both plants and animals were alive and children who thought that only animals were. Piaget did not indicate whether Stage II and III children attribute life to things that *can move* or to things that *are moving*; some of his examples are consistent with each interpretation. The only distinction between Stages III and IV is in children's understanding of celestial bodies; it is unclear whether Stage III children reason less maturely or simply have less information about a narrow class of phenomena. Thus, it is not surprising that some investigators have included celestial bodies and plants in their stimulus sets and that others have not. Nor is it surprising that investigators have emphasized different features of objects in asking their questions. The variability in questions and stimuli would not have been harmful—in fact would have been valuable—if the goal had been to reveal multiple aspects of children's understandings of life. Because the goal has been to determine whether children did or did not understand *the* life concept, however, the work has not led to any clear conclusion. Instead, each investigator has developed a distinct theory about children's concept of life. Even comparing the theories is difficult.

To penetrate beneath these surface differences, and to identify points of agreement as well as disagreement, it may be helpful to characterize Piaget's and other
investigators' theories within a common framework. The framework that we will
use depicts both children's representation of the life concept and the processes that
operate on those representations. The representational language is based on Anderson's (1976) ACT System.

Representation. In the present model, as in ACT, information in memory is
represented in terms of nodes and links that are connected to form propositions.
Nodes are entities; links are relations among entities. For example, in the proposition "Bill has a ball," Bill and ball would be represented by nodes and the possessive
"has a" by a link connecting the two nodes. Links between nodes are strengthened
by association. Each link has a resting strength, which corresponds to the ease with
which it can be accessed. These resting strengths are determined by the number of
encounters the child has had with that proposition.

Figure 2-9 illustrates the modeling language. Each proposition is represented by
an oval and is defined by the nodes to which it connects and by the types of connecting links. Subject and predicate relations are designated by the labels "S" and
"P." Unqualified links connecting two nodes indicate "All S are P." If two nodes
are connected by subject-predicate links extending in both directions, then all of
the instances of each and only those instances are the other. Thus, the Figure 2-9
model of Piaget's Stage I indicates that all animals are active things, that all ovens
are active things, and that all active things and only those things are alive.

Another type of proposition is illustrated in the Figure 2-9 model of Piaget's
Stage IV(b). The proposition "Some active things are alive" is designated by the use
of a subset node (X). This construction signifies that there exist some entities that
are both self-moving and alive. Figure 2-9B also illustrates the union relation (U). In
the latter, the union of plants and animals constitutes a separate node, plants
and animals.

Activation plays a key role in the functioning of the semantic network. Processes
operate only on currently active propositions. Attending to a proposition activates
its components. For example, asking a child "Are dogs alive?" would activate the
nodes "dog" and "alive." Once a given node or link is activated, it may activate
related material. Activation of a link always activates the node connected to it.
Activation of a node may activate any link connected to it; links become active
if they are strong relative to other links connected to the node. One danger within
such a system is that activation might spread until the entire system was active;
therefore, a damping mechanism is postulated that deactivates nodes and links that
have not been activated sufficiently recently.

Processes. A child faced with a categorization task of the nature "Is S P?" is
hypothesized to follow the general question-answering process shown in Figure
2-9B. The child first activates the nodes corresponding to S and P in his propositional network. Then he searches through the activated links connected to these
nodes for specific relations. When one of these relations is found, the child answers.

(A)

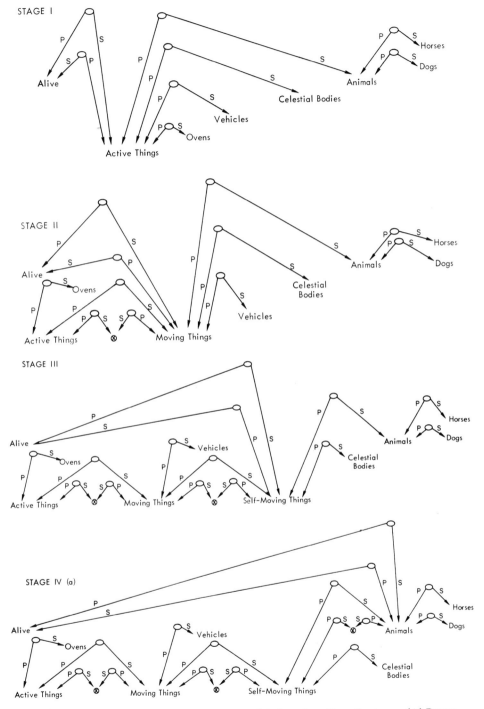

Figure 2-9. **(A-B)** Propositional network models based on Piaget's stages. (A) Representation: Stage I, Stage II, Stage III, Stage IV.

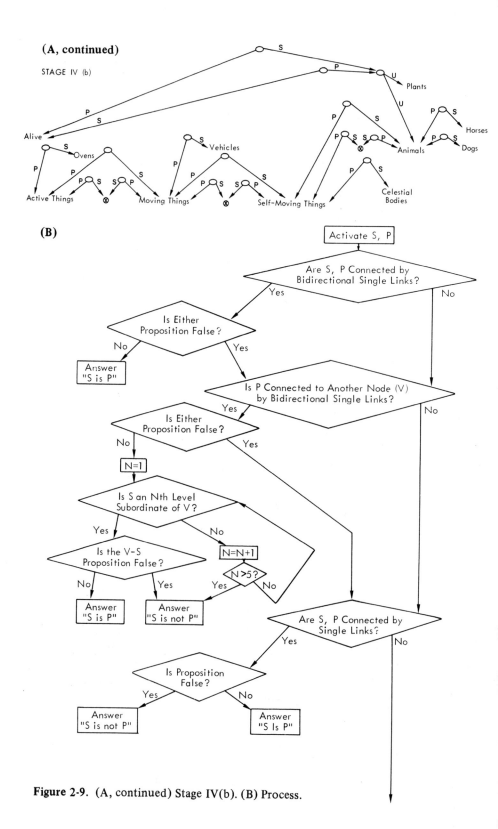

Figure 2-9. (A, continued) Stage IV(b). (B) Process.

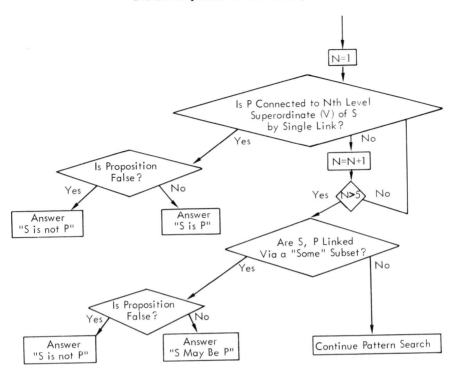

Figure 2-9. (B, continued)

The child first checks to see if S is connected to P via unqualified single-link connections extending in both directions. If so, and if neither proposition is marked false, the child answers, "S is P."

If this relation is not present, the child checks whether P is connected to another node (V) by links extending in both directions. The presence of both the proposition "P is V" and the proposition "V is P" indicates that only V is P. When these two propositions are present, and neither is marked false, the child searches to see if S is a first-level subordinate of V, that is, if it is connected to V by the link "All S is V." If so, he answers, "S is P." Illustratively, if a child were asked "Are flies alive?" and his representation included the relations "Flies are animals," "Animals are alive," and "Alive things are animals," he would answer that flies are alive. If "P is V" and "V is P" relations are present and S is not a first-level subordinate of V, the child searches through successive levels of subordinates of V. For example, flies might be subordinate to insects and insects to animals. If the child fails to find a match, he concludes that S and V are unrelated, and answers, "S is not P." In Figure 2-9B, the search termination point has been designated arbitrarily as anything beyond a fifth-level subordinate of V. In practice, the cutoff level for a given search may vary greatly from individual to individual and from situation to situation.

If P is not connected to any node by single links extending in both directions, the child next checks whether an unqualified "S is P" relation is present linking the subject and predicate he was asked about (e.g., *dogs* and *alive*). If it is, the child checks to see if the relation is marked false. He answers "S is P" unless it is marked false, in which case he answers "S is not P."

The child next tests if an *N*th-level superordinate of S is linked to P via a single link (e.g., "Dogs are animals; animals are alive"). Again, this "V is P" relation results in the answer "S is P" if the relation is not marked false, "S is not P" if it is.

In the final test illustrated in Figure 2-9B, the child checks whether S and P are connected via a "some" link, and whether the proposition is marked false (e.g., "There are plastic things; there are alive things; no things are plastic and alive"). If so, the child asnwers, "S is not P." If the "some" relation exists and is not marked false, the child answers, "S may be P."

A number of more obscure patterns might provide partial information concerning whether S is P. They are not illustrated here for reasons of brevity, and because the frequency of their use is hypothesized to be very low even among adults.

Characterizing Children's Knowledge of Life in Terms of Representations and Processes

Depicting children's knowledge as models that include representations and processes provides a basis for comparing alternative theories of conceptual development. Therefore, we have translated four prominent theories of children's understanding of *alive* into such a form. The four models are presented in the first section below. After this, we describe a series of five experiments intended to distinguish among the models. Following the descriptions of these experiments, we propose an inclusive model that incorporates the results of the new experiments as well as previous findings.

A Model Based on Piaget's Theory. Figure 2-9 is our translation of Piaget's theory. Figure 2-9A illustrates the representations of alive associated with each of his four stages, and Figure 2-9B illustrates the question-answering process common to all of the stages. In the Stage I representation (Figure 2-9A), the "alive" node is connected to the "active things" node by unqualified links extending in both directions. Thus, all active things, and only those things, are considered to be alive. Rounding out the representation are propositions relating objects to action, such as "Animals are active things" and "Ovens are active things." Note that plants are omitted from Figure 2-9A. Piaget belived that although Stage I children connect plants and the attributes of plants (has roots, etc.), they do not connect plants and life.

The process (Figure 2-9B) indicates how children of all ages answer questions of the form "Is S P?" We will illustrate its workings in the context of a Stage I child answering the question "Are dogs alive?" After activating the "dogs" and "alive" nodes in the representation, the child discovers that "dogs" and " alive" are not connected by single links extending in both directions, that "alive" is connected to another node ("active things") by links extending in both directions, that "dogs" is not a first-level subordinate of "active things," but that it is a second-order subordinate of them. Since none of the propositions is labeled false, the child concludes, "Dogs are alive." Note that if Stage I children are asked if an oven is alive, they reach an affirmative conclusion via the same process.

The Stage II and III models are quite similar to that for Stage I. The only differences are in the representation. The change from Stage I to Stage II is limited to the addition of an unqualified bidirectional link between "moving things" and "alive" and a qualification of the link between "active things" and "alive" to "Some active things are moving things." (Our initial assumption is that the motion node here and in the models of the other three theories corresponds to being capable of motion.) Between Stages II and III, an unqualified bidirectional link between "self-moving things" and "alive" is added and the relation between "moving things" and "alive" is qualified from "all" to "some." Thus, in determining which things are alive, the Stage II child should answer affirmatively to things that are subordinate to the "moving things" node, and the Stage III child should answer affirmatively to things that are subordinate to the "self-moving things" node.

In Stage IV, the repeated association between life and animals and the lack of association between life and other moving things has its effect: The child constructs two new propositions, signifying that all animals, and only animals, are alive. The link between self-moving things and life is qualified to a "some" relation so that it is consistent with the new propositions. This level of understanding is illustrated in Figure 2-9A as Stage IV(a). Piaget also suggested an alternative to this rule, represented as stage IV(b). The Stage IV(b) child has developed propositions linking a set including all animals and plants with life. When asked which things are alive, the Stage IV(a) child should pick animals, whereas the Stage IV(b) child should pick animals and plants. Thus, in this model, changes from each stage to the next stem from changes in the attribute tied to the "alive" node by an all-and-only link.

A Model Based on Huang and Lee's Theory. We can contrast these models, derived from Piaget's theory, with a model based on Huang and Lee's theory (Figure 2-10A). Whereas Piaget's views of Stages I to IV(a) suggests an appropriate process operating on fundamentally flawed representations, our model of Huang and Lee's theory suggests small flaws in both representation and process interacting to produce errors in a few situations. Their description implies a process (Figure 2-10A) much like the appropriate one shown in Figure 2-9B but with the potential to conduct too narrow a search if a strong emphasis has been placed on some attribute that is unconditionally linked to the subject. Consider the process attempting to answer the question "Are cars alive?" If the attribute "movement" was primed, and movement was connected to cars by the unqualified link "All cars move," the process first would try to answer the "Are cars alive?" question by finding an unqualified link between movement and alive. If such a link existed, the process would produce the answer "Cars are alive" before it ever conducted the usual search process. To characterize the shortcoming anthropomorphically, the Figure 2-10A process is overly sensitive to context and a little too impulsive.

This impulsivity in the question-answering process is not inevitably fatal in answering "Is S P?" questions, and would not cause difficulty in the present case if not for a related flaw in the representation of "alive." In the Figure 2-10A representation, certain links that should be "some" connections are unqualified. In particular, the link connecting "moving things" and "alive" indicates that all moving things are alive. This flaw, like that in the process, is quite small, and neither would

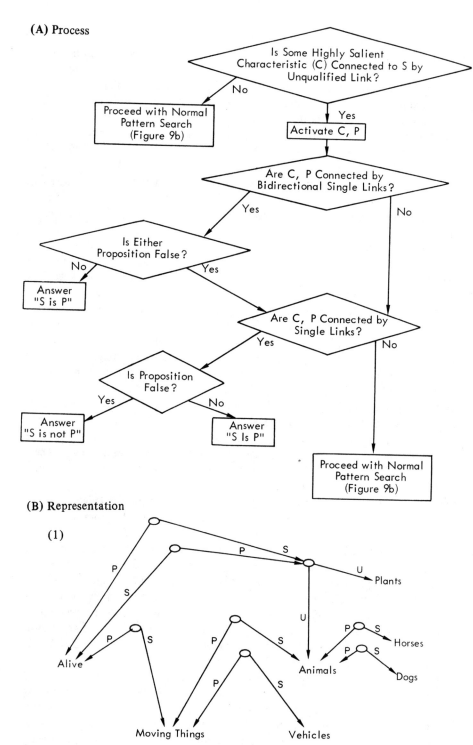

Figure 2-10. Propositional network models
(A) Question-answering process suggested by Huang and Lee.
(B) Life concept representations suggested by (1) Huang and Lee, (2) Klingensmith,
(3) Laurendeau and Pinard.

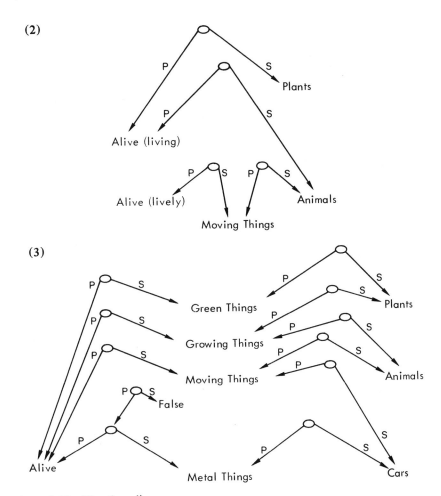

(2)

Plants

Alive (living)

Alive (lively)   Animals

Moving Things

(3)

Green Things   Plants

Growing Things

Moving Things   Animals

False

Alive   Cars

Metal Things

Figure 2-10. (Continued)

produce any behavioral effect without the other. If only the flaw in the representation existed, the process always would ask first about a bidirectional single-link
relation, and when it found such a link between "alive" and the "plants/animals"
node, would use it to produce the correct answer. It would never get to the "all"
link between "moves" and "alive." Similarly, if only the difficulty in the process
were present, priming the attribute of movement would not lead to an incorrect
answer, since the relation between life and its imperfectly qualified properties (e.g.,
movement) would be qualified by a "some" relation. On not finding an unqualified
connection between the primed attribute (movement) and life, the process would
proceed through the correct Figure 2-9B process. Again, no error would result. Only
the interaction of the flaws in the representation and process leads the system astray.
Developmental improvements would be due to children changing the "Moving
things are alive" link to a "Some moving things are alive" link, to their more consistently following the appropriate question-answering process even when contextual
cues highlighted a property associated with the subject, or to both changes.

A Model Based on Klingensmith's Theory. Klingensmith's theory can be depicted more simply. He suggested that the concept of life consisted of two subconcepts, corresponding to "living" and "lively" (Figure 2-10B). As in the Piagetian model, the correct Figure 2-9B process operates on a flawed representation. In Klingensmith's model, children associate alive (living) things with animals and plants and they associate alive (lively) things with motion. When faced with the task of determining what things are alive, children could activate either of the nodes labeled "alive." Errors would be due to their activating the wrong sense of *alive* at the beginning of the Figure 2-9B process. Developmental change would arise from the child's realizing that the term *alive* corresponded to "living" rather than "lively" in ordinary, nonmetaphoric uses.

A Model Based on Laurendeau and Pinard's Theory. Figure 2-10C is the representation implied by Laurendeau and Pinard's theory of the life concept. Whereas Piaget suggested that young children identify life with motion, Laurendeau and Pinard suggested that they identify life with a large number of attributes. The attributes of animals and plants, rather than animals and plants themselves, are linked to alive. In our representation of their theory, the concept of life consists of a number of unqualified single-link propositions connecting life with attributes associated with life (e.g., green, moving) that in turn are linked to animals and plants. Although this model uses the same process suggested for the Piagetian model, the resulting behavior differs. For example, if children are asked "Is a car alive?" they first activate the nodes corresponding to "car" and "alive." Because cars are linked to life by several first-level superordinates, children choose which-

Table 2-4 Predicted Answers for Each Problem Type for Children Using Each Rule on the Concept of Life

Problem Types		Rules			
Object	Motion State	I	II	III	IV
Person	Was still	No	Yes	Yes	Yes
Person	Was moved	Yes	Yes	Yes	Yes
Person	Moved self	Yes	Yes	Yes	Yes
Animal	Was still	No	Yes	Yes	Yes
Animal	Was moved	Yes	Yes	Yes	Yes
Animal	Moved self	Yes	Yes	Yes	Yes
Tree	Was still	No	No	No	Yes
Tree	Was moved	Yes	No	No	Yes
Plant	Was still	No	No	No	Yes
Plant	Was moved	Yes	No	No	Yes
Vehicle	Was still	No	Yes	No	No
Vehicle	Was moved	Yes	Yes	No	No
Vehicle	Moved self	Yes	Yes	No	No
Object	Was still	No	No	No	No
Object	Was moved	Yes	No	No	No

ever superordinate relation they activated first. The particular choice depends both on the resting strengths of the attribute-life links and on momentary attentional factors. Thus, a child might conclude either that cars are alive because they are moving things or that cars are not alive because they are metal things. Developmental improvement would result from qualifications being placed on relations between life and its attributes. For example, the relation between motion and life might be altered to a "some" relation.

Describing these theories in a common representational language clarifies their similarities and differences. Every model predicts that even young children will classify animals as alive. All also postulate that young children will connect motion with life. The models differ, however, in their particular connections between motion and life, in when that connection should influence performance, and in one case, in the question-answering process that would operate on the representation of alive. The specific differences in predicted performance will be discussed in the context of five experiments that we conducted on children's concepts of life.

Five Experiments on Children's Concept of Life

Which Objects are Alive?

Experiment 1: Judgments of Life Status. Ability to classify objects as living or not living is one important aspect of the life concept. To determine how children perform such classifications, we employed the rule assessment methodology (Siegler, 1976; 1981). Children were shown pictures of objects and asked if each was alive. Based on the centrality of motion status and of the type of object in previous theories, we hypothesized four rules that children might use on this task. In Rule I, children judge to be alive objects that are moving. In Rule II, they judge to be alive objects capable of motion. In Rule III, they believe that animals are alive but that plants are not. In Rule IV they believe that both animals and plants are alive.

The next step was to design a problem set in which different beliefs about the role of motion and the type of object would produce distinct patterns of responses. Children were asked about the life status of exemplars of the following classes: people, other animals, trees, other plants, vehicles, and other objects. Exemplars of these six categories were described verbally either as being stationary, as being moved by an external agent, or (where physically possible) as moving autonomously. The physically possible combinations of type of object and motion state resulted in the 15 types of problems listed in Table 2-4. As can be seen, these types of problems yielded distinct answer patterns for each of the rules described earlier, as well as for a number of other rules. For example, a child who thought that things that *are* moving are alive would answer correctly about animals, people, plants, and trees that were moving autonomously or being moved and also would answer correctly about objects and vehicles that were stationary, but would answer incorrectly about animals, people, plants, and trees that were stationary, objects that were being moved, and vehicles that were moving autonomously or being moved.

Four instances of each of the 15 problem types were presented, each consisting of a picture and a one-sentence story. For example, on one item children were shown a picture of a dog and told, "The dog sat waiting for its master. Was the dog alive?" These questions were presented to 4- and 5-year-olds and to 6- and 7-year-olds. To be classified as using a rule, a child needed to answer at least 50 of the 60 problems as predicted by that rule.

The four models predict different behaviors on this task. The model based on Piaget's theory predicts that the younger children should use motion-based rules, and that older children should report that animals or animals and plants are alive. The model based on Huang and Lee's theory predicts that children of all ages should consider animals or animals and plants alive, since the context does not especially emphasize any attribute of the objects. The model based on Laurendeau and Pinard's theory is consistent with a wide range of findings, from constant usage of a motion rule (if the resting strength of the link between motion and life is stronger than that of any other link) to exclusive reliance on the type of object (if the resting strength of the link tying animals or aminals and plants to life is strongest). The model based on Klingensmith's theory also would be consistent with a wide range of findings, depending on the relative strengths of the links to "living" and "lively."

As shown in Table 2-5A, all 32 children met the rule usage criteria. Only one child used a rule based on the motion state of the objects—the other 31 children were found to be using our Rule III or IV. That is, almost two-thirds of the children believed only people and animals were alive; the others (with one exception) believed that plants as well as people and other animals were alive. These results were consistent with the models based on Huang and Lee's theory, not at odds

Table 2-5 Number of Children Using Each Rule in Each Age Group

Age Group	Rule Used			
	Motion	People and Animals	People, Animals, Plants, and Trees	No Rule
A. Recognition of Life States Experiment				
4- and 5-year-olds	1	12	3	0
6- and 7-year-olds	0	8	8	0
B. Motion Emphasis Experiment				
4- and 5-year-olds	10	3	1	2
6- and 7-year-olds	0	9	7	0
8- and 9-year-olds	0	0	16	0

with the models based on Laurendeau and Pinard's and Klingensmith's theories, and directly at odds with Piaget's hypothesis that young children would equate alive with active, moving, or capable of motion.

Experiment 2: Prototypic Instances of Life. Another aspect of conceptual understanding is the concept's extension: the objects that are included within it. Piaget's model (Figure 2-9A: Models I, II, and III) predicts that depending on the child's age, the life concept's extension should be anything that is active, that moves, or that moves autonomously. Huang and Lee's model (Figure 2-10A) predicts that the extension should be animals and plants (assuming that no attribute has been strongly primed). Klingensmith's model (Figure 2-10B) predicts that for young children, the extension should be living or lively things. Laurendeau and Pinard's theory (Figure 2-10C) predicts that for young children, any object having attributes associated with life should be a possible extension.

To test these predictions, we asked children to name things that are alive. We assumed that children would answer such questions through a process akin to that depicted in Figure 2-9B. That is, they would base answers on the quality of the link between the predicate (alive) and either the objects themselves or superordinates of the objects (e.g., animals). For example, if there was an unqualified bidirectional link between alive and animals, the children would name only animals as exemplars of alive things. Within a superordinate category, strength of association between instances and the superordinate was assumed to guide the choice of instances; in the foregoing example, items most closely associated with animals would be chosen. Subjects of a wide age range participated in this study: 4- and 5-year-olds, 6- and 7-year-olds, 8- and 9-year-olds, 10- and 11-year-olds, and adults.

Two major results emerged. First, more than 99% of answers fell into one of five categories: people, other animals, trees, other plants, and parts of living things. The prototypic living things were known quite early: Cats, dogs, fish, and birds

Table 2-6 Number of Individuals in Each Age Group Mentioning at Least One Member of Each Category

	Category				
Age Group	People	Animals	Plants	Parts of Living Things	Wrong Answers
4- and 5-year-olds	12	16	2	0	2
6- and 7-year-olds	12	16	5	0	1
8- and 9-year olds	14	16	15	3	1
10- and 11-year-olds	15	16	15	5	2
Adults	16	16	13	5	3

were among the five most frequently mentioned living things from age 6 to 7 years onward. Table 2-6 lists the number of subjects in each age group who mentioned at least one member of each of the six categories of objects studied in Experiment 1 plus parts of living things. As can be seen in the table, participants almost never mentioned inanimate objects, moving or nonmoving, as living things.

Second, the items that children listed changed both quantitatively and qualitatively with age. As Table 2-6 shows, the number of children mentioning plants and trees increased with age, as did the number mentioning parts of living things. Older children and adults also named significantly more animals and significantly more plants and trees than the younger children, with the bulk of the increase coming between the ages of 7 and 9.

These results are in close accord with those of the first experiment. Initially children believe that people and other animals are alive. Following this, they add plants to the list of living things. Finally, they add parts of living things to their lists.[7] Objects that move but that are not plants or animals do not seem to be considered alive.

Experiment 3: Effects of Emphasizing Motion. In the first experiment, only 1 of the 32 children relied on objects' motion states in judging whether they were alive. No one judged on the basis of whether the object was capable of motion. In the second experiment, children almost never cited objects capable of motion but nonliving as alive. One reason for the disparity between the results of Piaget's studies and the results of these two experiments may be the type of data on which the investigator relied. The conclusions of our experiments were based on judgments and citations of exemplars. Piaget's conclusions were based largely on children's justifications of their answers.

Judgments and citations of examples on the one hand and explanations on the other might diverge for two reasons: (a) The children might not be aware of the method they used to judge and choose examples; or (b) they might be aware of the method they used, but not believe that it constituted a suitable justification. Within the second class of accounts, it seemed possible that the method of asking questions may have influenced children's justifications. Consider a child's position in the experimental situation. She is asked whether dogs are alive and answers yes. Then the experimenter asks her, "How do you know that dogs are alive?" Perhaps she would answer that dogs are animals and that animals are alive. Alternatively, she might not advance this explanation because she interprets the question as "What property of dogs makes you think they are alive?" Within such an uncertain situation, the child might hazard several tentative answers; even subtle signs of approval by the experimenter for a motion justification might have a large effect. Several of Piaget's (1929) protocols illustrate that children indeed were not overly confident of their judgments and that they tentatively advanced a number of explanations of them.

---

[7]It can be argued that since parts of living things are not viable in isolation, the performance of 8- to 9-year-olds was superior to that of older children and adults. On the other hand, it is perfectly logical to say that the heart, brain, and so on of a living creature also are alive as long as it is understood that they remain part of that living creature.

To test the interpretation that under such conditions the phrasing of questions could exert a large influence, we manipulated the degree to which our questions emphasized objects' motion states. Children were presented with the same objects as before but heard appended to the questions a tag phrase emphasizing motion. For example, after being presented with the picture of the dog, children were asked, "The dog sat waiting for its master. Was the dog alive *while it was sitting still?*" The tag phrase called attention to and summarized the motion state of the object. We presented the same 60 pictures as in Experiment 1, varying only the tag phrase in the question. The participants were 4- and 5-year-olds, 6- and 7-year-olds, and 8- and 9-year-olds.

The model based on Huang and Lee's theory suggested that such priming of motion would have a large effect, since the priming would lead young children to search for connections between motion and life and to respond that moving things were alive if they found such connections. The models based on Laurendeau and Pinard's and Klingensmith's theories also suggested that priming the connection between motion and life might increase the likelihood that the motion-alive link or the lively interpretations would be used, depending on the resting strengths and the degree of priming. The model based on Piaget's theory did not predict any obvious role of context.

The number of children who used each rule under these motion-emphasis conditions is presented in Table 2-5B. All of the 8- and 9-year-olds reported that people, animals, plants, and trees were alive and that other objects were not. Slightly less than half of the 6- and 7-year-olds used this rule; the other 6- and 7-year-olds judged only people and animals to be alive. Thus, motion emphasis had no effect on the answers of these two age groups. In contrast, motion emphasis clearly affected the 4- and 5-year-olds' answers. The majority of them used a rule in which objects were alive when they were moving and not alive when they were stationary. This result is consistent with the argument that a motion emphasis in Piaget's procedures may have led to his detection of motion-based rules among the youngest children tested.

The results of these three experiments allow us to evaluate the models of young children's life concepts shown in Figures 2-9 and 2-10. The Figure 2-9A models were clearly inconsistent with the data. Even 4- and 5-year-olds did not base judgments of life on whether things were active, on whether they could move, or, in ordinary circumstances, on whether they were moving. This age group's prototypic living things were all animals, again contrary to the model. Thus, the Figure 2-9 models could be rejected. The experimental results did not contradict the Figure 2-10B and 2-10C models, but gave no support to large parts of them. The Figure 2-10B model indicated that children could interpret "alive" as either living or lively, but there was no evidence that children ever used the latter interpretation. Not one child cited brooks, musical pieces, or dances as living things. Similarly, of all of the links between life and its attributes in Figure 2-10C, young children used only the links between animals and life and, when motion was emphasized, the link between motion and life. Although young children may well connect numerous attributes with life, the data demand that the links between life and animals be distinguished from others.

The model that fit most consistently and parsimoniously with the data is the one depicted in Figure 2-10A, the model based on Huang and Lee's theory. This model predicts all of the major findings obtained with the 4- and 5-year-olds. It indicates that such young children ordinarily will judge only animals as alive, but that they will classify on the basis of motion if the context emphasizes this attribute. The general thrust of the model, that the young children's knowledge of alive was basically accurate but had a few specific flaws, also seemed in accord with the data. Therefore, this model was chosen as the foundation on which we would build in the next experiments.

Children's Inferences of Life from Its Attributes

Experiments 1-3 focused on prototypic living things and on links between familiar objects and life. Experiments 4 and 5 focus on another aspect of the life concept: connections between it and other attributes. The result of Experiment 3 demonstrated that connections between one such attribute, motion, and life could mediate classifications of familiar objects as alive. In Experiment 4 we examine which attributes children associate most closely with life. In Experiment 5 we examine how children use knowledge of attributes to classify novel objects as alive or not alive.

Experiment 4: Attributes Characteristic of Living Things. We performed Experiment 4 to investigate children's associations between life and various attributes. We asked children of ages 4 and 5, 6 and 7, 8 and 9, and 10 and 11 and adults to name attributes that made things that are alive different from things that are not. Subjects were asked to stop after 5 minutes or after they listed eight answers.

The total number of attributes reported increased with age, as did the overlap in the particular attributes reported. On average, the 8- and 9-year-olds listed more than twice as many attributes as did children in the two younger groups. The 10- and 11-year-olds reported about the same number of attributes as the 8- and 9-year-olds but the answers of individual children overlapped to a greater degree.

The five attributes of life most often mentioned by children of each age are listed in Table 2-7. Only one of the five attributes most often mentioned by the 4- and 5-year-olds and by the 6- and 7-year-olds was true of plants: in the former case, that living things die, and in the latter case, that living things eat. By contrast, three of the attributes mentioned by 8- and 9- and 10- and 11-year-olds and four of the attributes mentioned by adults were true of both plants and animals.

Thus, the experiment revealed two trends in children's knowledge of life's attributes. First, at the age at which most children begin to report that plants as well as animals are alive, they also begin to report many more attributes of life than previously. Following this, the children's answers become less idiosyncratic and begin to apply to both animals and plants.

Experiment 5: Inferring Life from Its Attributes. The previous experiment demonstrated that children have considerable knowledge of attributes that are associated with life. Our final experiment was designed to determine whether chil-

Table 2-7 The Five Most-Mentioned Attributes of Life for Each Age Group

4- and 5-Year-Olds	6- and 7-Year-Olds	8- and 9-Year-Olds	10- and 11-Year-Olds	Adults
1. Moves	1. Moves	1. Moves	1, 2. Moves, Eats	1. Eats
2. Someone told me	2. Talks	2. Eats	3. Breathes	2. Reproduces
3, 4, 5. Talks	3, 4. Eats	3. Talks	4. Grows	3. Dies
I just know	Makes Noise	4, 5. Breathes	5. Has feelings	4. Grows
Dies	5. Walks	Are different colors		5. Moves
Walks	Dead things lie down			
	Dead things are extinct			

dren can use knowledge of these attributes to infer life status, and whether they view as differentially predictive attributes that are necessary and sufficient indicators of life, attributes that are sufficient indicators of life, and attributes that are only correlated with life.

On our task, the experimenter described attributes of an unknown object and children needed to decide if the object was alive. Six attributes that varied in their relations to life were sampled: growth, reproduction, vision, rootedness, movement, and capacity to make noise. The first and second attributes are necessary and sufficient attributes of life. The third and fourth are sufficient but not necessary indicators. The fifth and sixth are merely attributes of some living things.

Participants in this experiment were instructed to imagine that they were the commander of a spaceship searching a distant planet for life. They would receive radio descriptions of objects that were found by explorers on the planet's surface, and their task was to decide if each object was alive. The 60 possible pairs of attributes (each of the six attributes could be described as present or not present; the same attribute was never said to be both present and not present on a given trial) were given to the participants. For example, they might be told, "We've found something that moves and that doesn't make noise: do you think it is alive?" Participants were 4- and 5-year-olds, 6- and 7-year-olds, 8- and 9-year-olds, and adults.

To compare the strengths of associations between life and the six attributes, we computed a life attribution score for each attribute. This score was the percentage of yes answers when the attribute was described to the child as being present minus the percentage of yes answers when the attribute was described as being absent. The more strongly an attribute is associated with life, the greater its life attribution score should be.[8]

The life attribution scores for each age group are listed in Table 2-8. The 4- and 5-year-olds attributed life to entities said to have any of the five other attributes more often than to things said to have roots. Between the ages of 4 and 5 and 6 and 7, the importance attached to growth and having roots increased substantially. The 6- and 7-year-olds attributed life to growing things more often than to things having the other five attributes. The 8- and 9-year-olds attributed life to growing things more often than to anything else, and to things that reproduce more often than to things having the remaining attributes. Adults attributed life more often to objects that grow or reproduce than to objects that had other attributes.

The results of this experiment suggested that children as young as 8 and 9 years of age have stronger associations between life and its necessary and sufficient attributes than between life and attributes that are only sufficient for or correlated with it. The importance of one necessary and sufficient attribute, growth, was grasped even by 6- and 7-year-olds. No evidence was found that children or adults

---

[8]This quantitative index did not allow us to determine whether children or adults viewed any one type of attribute as qualitatively distinct from the others. One indirect indication that they did not view the three types of attributes as qualitatively distinct was that few children invariably concluded that the object was alive when a necessary and sufficient attribute was present; however, this may have been due to the children's not being sure whether earthly relations necessarily applied in outer space.

differentiate between attributes correlated with life and attributes that are sufficient indicators of life.

Conclusions: The Development of Life Concepts

From the results of these five experiments, and from our analyses of previous theories of children's life concepts, we constructed the overall depiction of development shown in Figure 2-11. These models are elaborations of the Figure 2-10A model, our translation of Huang and Lee's theory, which fit more naturally with the results of Experiments 1-3 than did the other models. The depiction includes four parts, representing the understandings of typical 4-, 6-, and 8-year-olds and of adults.

The proposed model of a typical 4-year-old's life concept is presented in Figure 2-11A. The core of this model is identical to that shown in Figure 2-10A. The major change from that model is the addition of varying link strengths for the associations between life and life's attributes. For purposes of simplicity, these connections are depicted as four levels of link strength. The strengths are based on the results of Experiment 5. Life attribution scores below .10 are translated as implying no links, scores between .10 and .49 are considered indicative of weak links, scores between .50 and .59 are considered indicative of medium-strength links, and scores of .60 or more are considered indicative of strong links. Since only the rank orders of the absolute link strengths are important for the models, the arbitrariness of the cutoff points did not seem to pose serious problems. Note that whereas several propositions link the attributes of animals to life, no propositions link plants or the attributes of plants to life. In none of the experiments did most 4- and 5-year-olds demonstrate knowledge that plants are alive.

The 4-year-olds' process for answering "Is S alive?" questions is the one suggested by our translation of Huang and Lee's model (the process portion of Figure 2-10A).

Table 2-8 Life Attribution Scores for Each Attribute by Individuals from Five Different Age Groups

Age Group	Attribute (%)					
	Moves	Has Eyes	Has Babies	Makes Noise	Has Roots	Grows
4- and 5-year-olds	42	31	45	27	10	36
6- and 7-year-olds	49	44	40	33	36	61
8- and 9-year-olds	45	38	50	32	33	68
10- and 11-year-olds	56	33	60	33	31	65
Adults	41	40	71	33	37	64

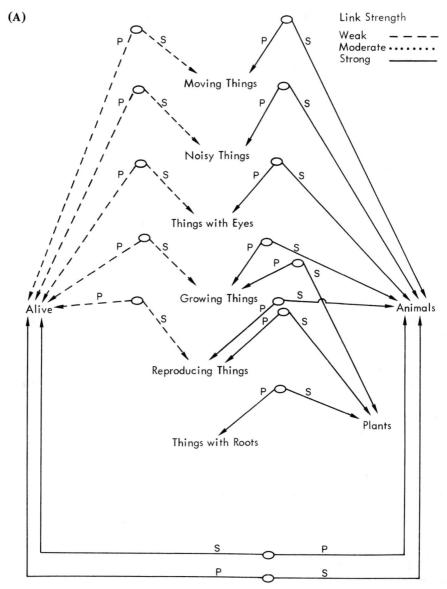

Figure 2-11. (A-D) (A) Propositional network memory model for the 4-year-old's concept of life.

In most circumstances, 4-year-olds search for a proposition that connects life to the subject of the question. They discover that life is connected to animals via unqualified links extending in both directions. If the subject of the question is an animal, the children respond that it is alive; otherwise, they respond that it is not alive. However, in one circumstance 4-year-olds follow a different procedure. If their attention is strongly drawn to an attribute that is connected by an unqualified link

(B)

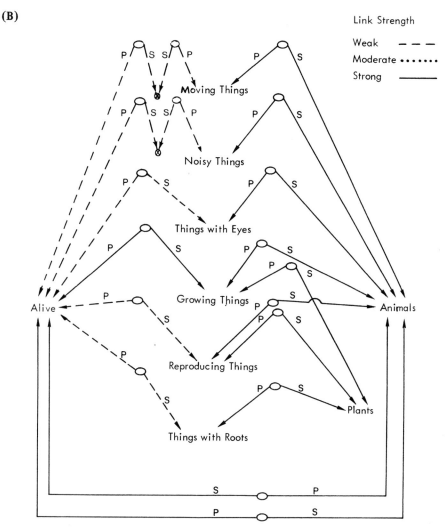

Figure 2-11. (B) Propositional network memory model for the 6-year-old's concept of life.

to the subject of the question, they abandon the normal search process. Instead, they determine whether the emphasized attribute is connected to life by an unqualified link. If they find such a connection, as they would in the case of motion in Figure 2-10A, they answer immediately. Otherwise, they fall back on the more typical question-answering process and answer according to whether the object is an animal.

Contrast this model to the Figure 2-11B model of a typical 6-year-old's concept of life. The relation between life and growth has become stronger than the relations between life and other attributes. A weak relation between the attribute of having roots and life has been established (both of these changes are based on the life

(C)

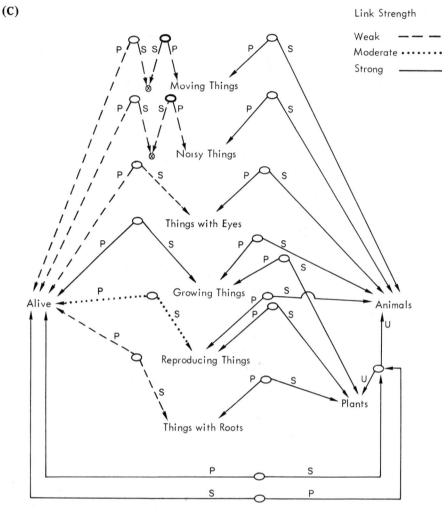

Figure 2-11. (C) Propositional network memory model for the 8-year-old's concept of life.

attribution scores in Experiment 5). Children no longer deviate from the standard question-answering process and have modified the link between motion and alive to a "Some moving things are alive" relation. The Figure 2-11B model implies that both greater consistency in the question-answering process and qualification of the motion-alive link are responsible for the dramatic decrease in the effects of motion emphasis between ages 4 and 6 (Experiment 3). Either change alone, however, would produce the same behavioral effect. At present we have no empirical basis for choosing among the three possibilities.

The structure of memory for a typical 8-year-old is characterized in Figure 2-11C. This model includes several changes. The propositions "Animals are alive" and "Living things are animals" have been altered to read "Animals and plants are alive"

(D)

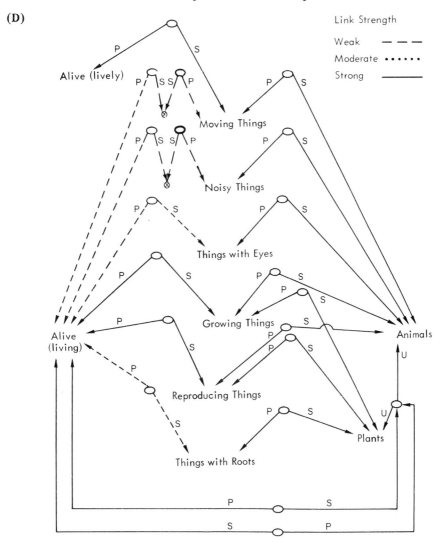

Figure 2-11. (D) Propositional network memory model for the adult's concept of life.

and "Living things are animals and plants." This change is based on the increased likelihood of 8-year-olds' classifying plants as alive and of their citing at least one plant as a living thing (Experiments 2 and 3). In addition, the link between life and reproduction has increased in strength, although it still is not as strong as that between life and growth (Experiment 5). The effects of these changes on the children's behavior are marked. Eight-year-olds not only report that plants as well as animals are alive, but also list as prototypic qualities of living things attributes that apply to plants as well as animals (Experiment 4).

Finally, consider the adult model (Figure 2-11D). One addition to this model is the metaphorical sense of alive, suggested by Klingensmith. Although we do not know the age at which people know metaphorical as well as literal meanings, it is clear that at least some adults know and make use of both. Second, the link between reproduction and life has continued to increase in strength, so that now it is as strong as that between growth and life (Experiment 5).

The four models in Figure 2-11 present a preliminary characterization of how changes in the representation of "alive" might combine with an increasingly consistent execution of the standard question-answering process to account for the behavior of children of different ages. The models account for developmental changes in children's rules for classifying objects as alive, in their choices of prototypic living things, in the effects of emphasizing motion on their rules for attributing life, in knowledge of life's attributes, and in inferences about life status from information about attributes. Only through the use of multiple tasks tapping the life concept was the construction of such detailed and extensive models possible.

General Conclusions

In this section we focus on two themes that have recurred frequently in the chapter: the value of depicting knowledge in terms of representations and processes, and the multifaceted nature of conceptual understanding.

The Representation-Process Distinction

Characterizing children's knowledge as a combination of representations and processes offers a number of advantages. It allows us to describe aspects of knowledge that are constant over development as well as aspects that change. It encourages us to model quite complicated ideas that would be difficult to express as either representations or processes alone. It has heuristic value. Below we discuss these qualities.

Depicting both representations and processes often reveals developmental constancies as well as changes. One simple explanation for this quality would be to equate the constancies with one side of the model, probably the representation, and the changes with the other side, probably the process. Any such equation is almost certain to be wrong, however. As Newell (1972) noted, in any representation-process pair, the representation is the more slowly changing part *at the time the process is active.* However, this does not imply that information in the representation changes more slowly developmentally. In many domains of development, children rapidly increase the information that is most naturally depicted as part of their representation while continuing to employ the same process. For example, children learning the capitals of the 50 states would rapidly expand their links between state names and capitals but probably would maintain the same question-answering process. In addition, as Newell (1972) also noted, information that serves as the process in one context often is the representation in another. Illustratively, the descriptions of processes in this article will enter the knowledge bases of readers and readers will be able to perform a variety of processes on them.

Thus, there is no one-to-one correspondence between the part of the model and the rate of development. Such an equation cannot account for the utility of models that include representations and processes in revealing both developmental constancies and changes. Instead, it seems likely that breadth and specificity are the qualities that result in such models' revealing constancies as well as changes. Theoretical formulations that are explicit about both representations and processes tend to be sufficiently broad and sufficiently specific that they reveal many aspects of children's knowledge relevant to performance. Almost always, some of these aspects change with development and others do not. At times, as in most of the current work on numbers, the most dramatic changes are in the processes; at other times, as in the work on attributes of life, the changes are most dramatic in the representation; at yet other times, as in the models of counting, large changes occur in both representations and processes.

The goal of formulating complete models may be the key to revealing both similarities and differences across age groups. Developmentalists inherently are interested in changes, and thus often may be tempted to slight those understandings that do not change with age. Building models that incorporate as many features involved in task performance as possible (e.g., models depicting both representations and processes) forces us to be more evenhanded in our treatment of constancies and changes.

Another advantage of portraying knowledge as representations and processes is that such portrayals allow us to discover and model new phenomena. This characteristic can be illustrated with reference to the research on the life concept. Proceeding at a purely verbal level, we might have summarized the first three experiments as indicating that 4- and 5-year-olds ordinarily judge only animals to be alive, but that contextual emphasis can lead them to judge on the basis of motion status. However, the numerous connections in the network representations between animals and their attributes caused us to question which attributes in addition to movement children might rely on to judge life. Examination of the representation suggested a hypothesis: Children would judge on the basis of attributes connected to animals by unqualified links, but not on the basis of attributes connected to animals by "some" links. This hypothesis may be incorrect, but it seems more likely to us than either of the two alternatives that we generated: (a) Movement is the only quality on which preschoolers will judge life; and (b) preschoolers will judge life on the basis of any quality emphasized by contextual cues. Although we could have generated the present hypothesis without the depiction of representations and processes, historically we did not do so, and the "all" and "some" links within the representation directly stimulated our formulation of the idea. (We were looking at the models when we thought of it.) In general, modeling representations and processes may aid analysis of complex phenomena because such models summarize our current conclusions in an easily accessible visual form and thus facilitate comparing and combining different parts of our thinking.

The models of how children attribute the presence of life to objects also were broadened by our attempts to describe both representations and processes. Initially we did not try to model how children answered questions, since it seemed only tangentially relevant to their concepts of life. Once we tried to model the question-answering process, however, we realized that small deficiencies in that process could be as critical in producing flawed judgments as deficiencies in the representation of the life concept. The models of the question-answering process suggested that preschoolers might encounter difficulty with many other concepts when the context spotlighted some attribute connected to the subject of the question by an unqualified link. Again, we would have been unlikely to generate the hypothesis without modeling both representations and processes.

The Multifaceted Nature of Conceptual Understanding

The present investigations of the development of knowledge about numbers and life reinforced our belief that researchers must focus on many aspects of concepts in order to understand conceptual development. Some of the tasks that we presented to children were closely comparable to tasks that often have been considered *the* measure of understanding of that concept. Others of the tasks have received little or no prior attention. In retrospect as in prospect, trying to formulate a principled argument for why the first group of tasks is superior to the second strikes us as futile.

Not only is the relative utility of the tasks difficult to evaluate, the tasks also cannot be viewed as yielding equivalent information. The overall representations included some information useful across more than one task (e.g., the division of numbers into categories) but also many task-specific components. Different levels of understanding of individual tasks (e.g., initial, intermediate, and advanced understanding of numerical magnitude comparison) were clearly related; relations spanning different tasks (e.g., magnitude comparison and addition) were less evident. From the vantage point of the present studies of numbers and life, it still seems that there is no single age at which children master a concept and no single order in which they master any but the most widely separated concepts.

This perspective has led to our present research strategy: to sample diverse areas included in a concept, to build models of the development of understanding of each of those areas, and to integrate the individual models into a comprehensive depiction of what children know about the concept. Our strategic bet is that building extensive models of children's understanding, and progressively integrating new experimental results into the models, will help research on conceptual development to cumulate. This strategy is expensive; all of the experiments reported in this chapter focus on only two concepts. Given the multifaceted nature of conceptual development, however, such an expensive strategy may be necessary.

Reference Notes

1. Greeno, J. G., Riley, M. S., & Gelman, R. *Young children's counting and understanding of principles.* Unpublished manuscript.
2. Richards, D. D., & Siegler, R. S. The development of the concept of life. In preparation, 1982.

References

Aiken, L. R., & Williams E. N. Three variables related to reaction time to compare digits. *Perceptual and Motor Skills, 1968, 27,* 199-206.

Anderson, J. R. *Language, memory, and thought.* Hillsdale, N.J.: Erlbaum, 1976.

Anderson, J. R. Arguments concerning representations for mental imagery. *Psychological Review*, 1978, *85*, 249-277.

Ashcraft, M. H. The development of mental arithmetic: A chronometric approach. *Developmental Review*, 1982, *2*, 213-236.

Ashcraft, M. H., & Battaglia, J. Cognitive arithmetic: Evidence for retrieval and decision processes in mental addition. *Journal of Experimental Psychology: Human Learning and Memory*, 1978, *4*, 527-538.

Banks, W. P. Encoding and processing of symbolic information in comparative judgments. *The Psychology of Learning and Motivation*, 1977, *11*, 101-159.

Banks, W. P., Fujii, M., & Kayra-Stuart, F. Semantic congruity effects in comparative judgments of magnitude of digits. *Journal of Experimental Psychology: Human Perception and Performance*, 1976, *2*, 435-447.

Beilin, H. Cognitive capacities of young children: A replication. *Science*, 1968, *162*, 920-921.

Bever, T. G., Mehler, J., & Epstein, J. What children do in spite of what they know. *Science*, 1968, *162*, 921-924.

Braine, M. D. S. The ontogeny of certain logical operations: Piaget's formulation examined by nonverbal methods. *Psychological Monographs*, 1959, *73*, no. 5 (Whole No. 475).

Brainerd, C. J. *Piaget's theory of intelligence.* Englewood Cliffs, N.J.: Prentice-Hall, 1978.

Brainerd, C. J. *The origins of the number concept.* New York: Praeger, 1979.

Brown, A. L. The construction of temporal succession by pre-operational children. In A. D. Pick (Ed.), *Minnesota Symposium on Child Psychology* (Vol. 10). Minneapolis: University of Minnesota, 1976.

Bruner, J. S. *Beyond the information given: Studies in the psychology of knowing.* New York: Norton, 1973.

Bryant, P. E. *Perception and understanding in young children.* New York: Basic Books, 1974.

Fairbank, B. A. *Experiments on the temporal aspects of number perception.* Unpublished doctoral dissertation, University of Arizona, 1969.

Flavell, J. H. Stage-related properties of cognitive development. *Cognitive Psychology*, 1971, *2*, 421-453.

Fuson, K. C., Richards, J., & Briars, D. J. The acquisition and elaboration of the number word sequence. In C. Brainerd (Ed.), *Progress in cognitive development* (Vol 1). New York: Springer-Verlag, 1982.

Gelman, R. The nature and development of early number concepts. *Advances in Child Development and Behavior*, 1972, *7*, 115-167.

Gelman, R., & Gallistel, C. F. *The child's understanding of number*. Cambridge, Mass: Harvard University Press, 1978.

Ginsburg, H. *Children's arithmetic: The learning process*. New York: Van Nostrand, 1977.

Groen, G. J., & Parkman, J. M. A chronometric analysis of simple addition. *Psychological Review*, 1972, *79*, 329-343.

Hebbeler, K. *The development of children's problem-solving skills in addition*. Unpublished doctoral dissertation, Cornell University, 1976.

Huang, I. Children's conception of physical causality: A critical summary. *Journal of Genetic Psychology*, 1943, *63*, 71-121.

Huang, I., & Lee, H. W. Experimental analysis of child animism. *Journal of Genetic Psychology*, 1945, *66*, 69-74.

Ilg, F., & Ames, L. B., Developmental trends in arithmetic. *Journal of Genetic Psychology*, 1951, *79*, 3-28.

Johnson, S. C. Hierarchical clustering schemes. *Psychometrika*, 1967, *32*, 241-254.

Klahr, D., & Wallace, J. G. *Cognitive development: An information-processing view*. Hillsdale, N.J.: Erlbaum, 1976.

Klingberg, G. The distinction between living and not living among 7-10-year-old children, with some remarks concerning the so-called animism controversy. *Journal of Genetic Psychology*, 1957, *90*, 227-238.

Klingensmith, S. W. Child animism: What the child means by "alive." *Child Development*, 1953, *24*, 51-61.

Knight, F. B., & Behrens, M. S. *The learning of the 100 addition combinations and the 100 subtraction combinations*. New York: Longmans, Green, 1928.

Kosslyn, S. M. Imagery and cognitive development: A teleological approach. In R. S. Siegler (Ed.), *Children's thinking: What develops?* Hillsdale, N.J.: Erlbaum, 1978.

Laurendeau, M., & Pinard, A. *Causal thinking in the child*. New York: International Universities Press, 1962.

Lehman, H. *Introduction to the philosophy of mathematics*. Totowa, N.J.: Rowman & Littlefield, 1979.

Miller, S. A. Nonverbal assessment of conservation of number. *Child Development*, 1976, *47*, 722-728.

Moyer, R. S., & Bayer, R. H. Mental comparison and the symbolic distance effect. *Cognitive Psychology*, 1976, *8*, 228-246.

Moyer, R. S., & Dumais, S. T. Mental comparison. *The Psychology of Learning and Motivation*, 1978, *12*, 117-155.

Moyer, R. S., & Landauer, T. K. The time required for judgments of numerical inequality. *Nature (London)*, 1967, *215*, 1519-1520.

Newell, A. A note on process-structure distinctions in developmental psychology. In S. Farnham-Diggory (Ed.), *Information processing in children*. New York: Academic Press, 1972.

Parkman, J. M. Temporal aspects of digit and letter inequality judgments. *Journal of Experimental Psychology*, 1971, *91*, 191-205.

Piaget, J. *The child's concept of number*. New York: Norton, 1952.

Piaget, J. Intellectual evolution from adolescence to adulthood. *Human Development*, 1972, *15*, 1-12.

Piaget, J. *The child's conception of the world*. St. Albans, Great Britain: Paladin, 1973. (Originally published in 1929.)

Pollio, H. R., & Whitacre, J. Some observations on the use of natural numbers by preschool children. *Perceptual and Motor Skills*, 1970, *30*, 167-174.

Richards, D. D. *Children's concept learning: The child's concept of life*. Unpublished doctoral dissertation, Carnegie-Mellon University, 1981.

Rothenberg, B. B., & Courtney, R. G. Conservation of number in very young children. *Development Psychology*, 1969, *1*, 493-502.

Russell, R. W. Studies in animism, II: The development of animism. *Journal of Genetic Psychology*, 1940, *56*, 353-366. (a)

Russell, R. W. Studies in animism, IV: An investigation of the concepts allied to animism. *Journal of Genetic Psychology*, 1940, *57*, 83-91. (b)

Sekuler, R., Armstrong, R., & Rubin, E. Processing numerical information: A choice time analysis. *Journal of Experimental Psychology*, 1971, *90*, 75-80.

Sekuler, R., & Mierkiewicz, D. Children's judgments of numerical inequality. *Child Development*, 1977, *48*, 630-633.

Siegler, R. S. Three aspects of cognitive development. *Cognitive Psychology*, 1976, *8*, 481-520.

Siegler, R. S. The origins of scientific reasoning. In R. S. Siegler (Ed.), *Children's thinking: What develops*? Hillsdale, N.J.: Erlbaum, 1978.

Siegler, R. S. Developmental sequences within and between concepts. *Monographs of the Society for Research in Child Development*, 1981, *46*, no. 2 (Whole No. 189).

Siegler, R. S., & Robinson, M. The development of numerical understandings. In H. Reese & L. P. Lipsitt (Eds.), *Advances in child development and behavior*. New York: Academic Press, 1982.

Simon, H. A. On the development of the processor. In S. Farnham-Diggory (Ed.), *Information processing in children*. New York: Academic Press, 1972.

Svenson, O. Analysis of time required by children for simple additions. *Acta Psychologica*, 1975, *39*, 289-302.

Trabasso, T. The role of memory as a system in making transitive inferences. In R. V. Kail, Jr., & J. W. Hagen (Eds.), *Perspectives on the development of memory and cognition*. Hillsdale, N.J.: Erlbaum, 1977.

Yoshimura, T. *Strategies for addition among young children*. Paper presented at the 16th annual convention of the Japanese Association of Educational Psychology, 1974.

3. Gene-Culture Linkages and the Developing Mind

Charles J. Lumsden

What is the nature of the mechanism that has created human mental development in its particular form, rather than in any other? Investigations conducted during the past several years (Lumsden & Wilson, 1980a, 1980b, 1981) indicate that a study of the answers to this question is the key to a characterization of human nature that is more complete and appropriate than has hitherto been possible. Each of the disciplines of the social sciences is ultimately shaped by its perception of the core properties of human behavior. If these properties could somehow be specified in a manner that generates laws of mind and cultural organization, even in crude form, the contents of the constituent disciplines might be reformulated to some degree and explained by a common theory. If, in addition, the biology and evolutionary origins of the core properties can be sufficiently well understood, a network of causal explanation could be devised that bridges the social sciences and human sociobiology—the discipline that deals with the biological foundations of social behavior in *Homo sapiens*.

Such theory construction has been hampered by a reluctance on the part of social scientists to incorporate the relevant findings of modern biology, especially from population genetics, the neurosciences, and sociobiology. Biologists for their part have contributed relatively little to the social and cognitive sciences because of inattention to the properties of mind and cultural diversity. In analyzing the great circuit that runs from the genetic blueprint through all the steps of ontogeny to culture and back again, the central piece—the development of the individual mind—has been largely ignored.

Sociobiology has hitherto attempted to link human genes and behavior in a direct manner. Using the basic principles of population genetics and ecology, researchers have sought to explain and predict the environmental conditions under which dominance systems, altruism, pair bonding, parental care, homosexuality, play, and other forms of social behavior are most likely to arise during the course of genetic evolution (for recent overviews see Markl, 1980, and Wilson, 1975). The method has been notably successful in the study of animals, which display more invariant, "instinctive" behavior. It has been successful to only a limited degree in the analysis of human behavior. New insights have been provided concerning very general human activities, such as incest avoidance, polygamy, family organization, and territorial defense (Alexander, 1979; Barlow & Silverberg, 1980; Chagnon & Irons, 1979; Markl, 1980; Symons, 1979; van den Berghe, 1979; Wilson, 1975). Thus sociobiology has gained some recognition in the social sciences during the past decade because of an increasing awareness of (1) the evidence for a genetic basis of the cognitive and emotional properties underlying complex human behavior (see, e.g., Lumsden & Wilson, 1981, chaps. 1 and 6), and (2) its effectiveness in explaining the origin and biologically adaptive significance of some pancultural forms of behavior.

However, conventional sociobiology (Wilson, 1975) has not yet accounted for the properties of the human mind, including especially the activities of cognition and their ontogenetic development. Nor has it begun to provide a more fundamental understanding of culture. These failures have led many social scientists and philosophers to doubt whether human thought and social behavior possess a biological foundation beyond the most general capacity to learn and create culture (Bock, 1980; Harris, 1979; Montagu, 1980; Sahlins, 1976). They question whether students of human biology will ever be able to bridge the natural, behavioral, and social sciences in any but a trivial fashion. As a result they consider the existing gaps between these disciplines to be permanent discontinuities, grounded in epistemology and reinforced by the unique status of the human mind. We suggest that the gaps are instead transient epiphenomena to be filled by understanding a largely unknown evolutionary process in which mental development and cultural history are shaped by biological imperatives while biological traits are simultaneously altered by genetic evolution in response to cultural events. Elsewhere, we have referred to this interaction as *gene-culture coevolution* (Lumsden & Wilson, 1981).

An explicit analysis of gene-culture coevolution seems especially worth attempting in cognitive-developmental theory for the following reason. Most features of human nature are difficult to generalize by direct perception or by analysis of their behavioral manifestations, because of their variable, often evanescent, expression. There are, however, suggestive precedents; for example, it is also difficult to formulate the laws of heredity by direct perception of variability within populations, or the laws of demography by the repeated censusing of many populations. A different, complementary approach therefore seems to be indicated. Human nature and its development, like human heredity or demography, might be better understood by analyzing the mechanism that generates them. One can therefore ask: What is this process, how does it work, and how did it originate? We suggest that the mechanism is in fact gene-culture coevolution (Lumsden & Wilson, 1980a, 1980b, 1981). In this chapter I report what we perceive to be some of its most general and fundamental properties, emphasizing in particular its treatment of mental development.

We suspect that a successful application of gene-culture coevolutionary theory in the manner described here will replace the heredity-versus-environment controversy in developmental psychology with a program of research that makes increasingly explicit the biology of the developing mind.

Many writers have made important contributions to the problem of coevolution during the past 10 years. They have variously stressed the similarity in the outcomes of genetic and cultural evolution (Durham, 1978; Emlen, 1976), the sometimes competitive nature of the two modes of change (Richerson & Boyd, 1978), the potential of the coevolutionary process to shape learning capacity (Feldman & Cavalli-Sforza, 1976), and the diversity of animal societies that employ some form of social transmission combined with timetables of behavioral development (Bonner, 1980; Mundinger, 1980). But there has hitherto been no attempt to systematically analyze the substance of cognitive science and developmental psychology from the viewpoint of modern evolutionary biology, and in doing so to search for the organic processes that create human nature and link genes to culture. Nor has there been an effort to derive exact patterns of cultural diversity from the biological properties of mental development. In briefest terms, the essential unsolved problem is the reconstruction of the full circuit of gene-culture coevolution, step by step, in sufficient detail to incorporate structure and variation in cognition and development, among both individuals and cultures.

Cultural Inheritance

The Culturgen

For the purposes of cognitive and behavioral studies it is useful to define a *society* as a group of individuals belonging to the same species and organized in a cooperative manner; the diagnostic criterion is reciprocal communication that facilitates cooperative behavior, extending beyond mere sexual activity (see also Wilson, 1975). A key property of *culture* used in the method of gene-culture theory (Lumsden & Wilson, 1980a, 1981) is its source as the resultant of the artifacts, behaviors, institutions, and mentifacts (Huxley, 1958) transmitted through the environment among members of a society, and the holistic patterns they form. (*Mentifacts* are mental constructs having little or no direct correspondence to real objects, people, or events. Hence, for example, myth telling and totems can be interpreted as the outward manifestations of the mind's sanctifying, group-binding activities; see Lenski & Lenski, 1970; Rappaport, 1971.)

It has been conventional in anthropology and the other social sciences to use static terms, such as *culture trait*, to refer to this array of cultural entities. In order to capture the dynamic, generative role that they actually play in mental development and the sustenance of social form, we have suggested the term *culturgen,* from the Latin *cultur(a),* culture, + *gen(o),* produce; it is pronounced "kulterjen." Although the concept of a culturgen cannot yet be specified in complete detail, a minimal representation sufficient to begin the formulation of testable gene-culture theories (Lumsden & Wilson, 1982a, 1982b) envisages a culturgen as an equivalence class of feature clusters associated with one or more artifacts, behaviors, or menti-facts, such that the clusters in the class either share without exception one or more attribute states, or share a consistently recurring range of such states within a poly-thetic set. Sometimes, as in the adoption versus rejection of a particular ritual or sexual custom, the relevant culturgens are readily denumerable by an external observer and are few in number. Alternatively, the variation among possible cultur-gens can be continuous (as, e.g., in the array of all conceivable color classifications) and the culturgens are inferred only with greater difficulty.

The Three Modes of Transmission

It is possible in principle for the effects of culturgens on individuals in an evolv-ing system to belong to one or the other of three classes. The first is pure genetic transmission, in which the culturgens that will affect mental development are pre-specified by the genes (hence, an entirely genetic culture that depends on learning and even on teaching is a theoretical possibility). The second is pure cultural trans-mission, in which no innate constraints limit the choice of culturgens that in competition with others can be used by the developmental mechanism (the tabula rasa state). The third is gene-culture transmission, in which innate rules of epi-genesis, underwritten by the genes and modulated by culture, discriminate among multiple culturgens and are more likely to use some rather than others during the assembly of the mind. The three possibilities are illustrated in Figure 3-1.

Human Cognitive Development Is Innately Biased

Contrary to an impression widely held among biologists and social scientists, most and possibly all forms of human culture and psychological development are sustained by gene-culture transmission rather than by pure cultural transmission. Detailed studies have been conducted of the development of choice among very dis-tinct culturgens, and they have almost always yielded data indicative of the presence of epigenetic rules in which an innate bias favors certain stimuli and developmental branch points over others. We have found it useful for the purposes of gene-culture theory to sort these epigenetic rules into two classes. The *primary epigenetic rules* are developmental mechanisms that affect the structure and function of the more automatic processes that lead from initial sensory filtering to perception. Examples are a neonate preference for sugar combined with a significant aversion to salty and bitter flavors (Chiva, 1979; Cowart, 1981; Maller & Desor, 1974); the innate discri-mination of four basic hues (blue, green, yellow, red—Bornstein, 1981; Bornstein, Kessen, & Weiskopf, 1976) and a greater ease of learning color classifications clus-tered on these color modes (Berlin & Kay, 1969; Kay & McDaniel, 1978; Mervis & Rosch, 1981; Rosch, 1973); and infant phoneme discrimination, affecting later speech structure (Eilers, Wilson, & Moore, 1977).

The *secondary epigenetic rules* shape the mechanisms of higher cognition, such as the processes of feature extraction, valuation, and decision making. Cases include infant preference for certain kinds of visual patterns (Fantz, Fagan, & Miranda,

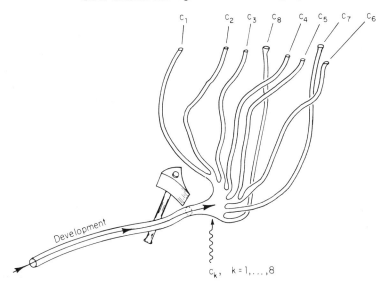

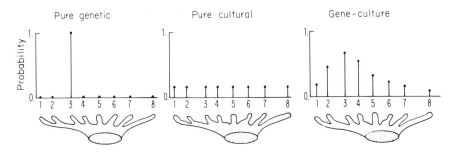

Figure 3-1. A hypothetical fragment of a pathway of cognitive development, showing the three possible modes of cultural transmission. *Top*: The effect (indicated by the wavy line) of one or more culturgens, c_k, causes the pathway to split into alternate courses, k, of development (in this hypothetical example, $k=1, \ldots, 8$). "Cutting" the branches where they stem allows the characteristics of the three transmission modes to be visualized. *Bottom*: In pure genetic transmission, innate constraints prespecify the effective culturgen (in this case c_3). In pure cultural transmission, no innate constraints bias the course of development. In gene-culture transmission, innate epigenetic rules discriminate among the culturgens and are more likely to use some rather than others to direct the course of mental development.

1975; Hershenson, Munsinger, & Kessen, 1965); neonate oculomotor orientation to normally composed facial features (Freedman, 1974; Mauer & Barrera, 1981); smiling and other specific forms of nonverbal communication (Eibl-Eibesfeldt, 1979); nonverbal signals used in mother-infant bonding, resulting in long-lasting effects on later maternal care (DeCasper & Fifer, 1980; Klaus, Jerauld, Kreger, McAlpine, Steffa, & Kennell, 1972); sexual differences in the carrying of infants and other larger objects (Lockard, Daley, & Gunderson, 1979; Salk, 1973); the fear-of-stranger response (Morgan & Ricciuti, 1973); the predisposition to acquire phobias against certain dangerous objects, such as heights, running water, and snakes, but not others, including electric sockets and guns (Marks, 1969); critical parameters of human cognition, such as short-term memory capacity and storage and retrieval times from long-term memory (Newell & Simon, 1972; Simon, 1979); the acquisition of certain linguistic knowledge structures rather than others (Chomsky, 1980; Wexler & Culicover, 1980); the development of sexual feelings toward siblings (Shepher, 1971; Wolf, 1966, 1968, 1970; Wolf & Huang, 1980); understanding about numbers (Gelman & Gallistel, 1978; Keil, 1981) and logic (Keil, 1981; Osherson, 1976); and the proliferation of ontological knowledge in long-term memory (Keil, 1979, 1981).

The distinction between primary and secondary rules is crude and somewhat arbitrary. Nevertheless, it is a natural and refinable taxonomy, and has proved an adequate means by which the basic relevant processes of cognitive development can be connected to evolutionary theory for the first time (Lumsden & Wilson, 1980a, 1980b, 1981, 1982a, 1982b).

That the epigenetic rules have a genetic basis is strongly indicated by the circumstance that so many are relatively inflexible and appear early in childhood. In addition, pedigree analysis and standard comparisons of fraternal and identical twins, in some cases strengthened by longitudinal studies of development, have yielded evidence of genetic variance in many categories of cognition and behavior investigated by these means, including some that either constitute epigenetic rules or share components with them. These categories include color vision, hearing acuity, odor and taste discrimination, number ability, word fluency, spatial ability, memory, timing of language acquisition, spelling, sentence construction, perceptual skill, psychomotor skill, extroversion and/or introversion, homosexuality, proneness to alcoholism, age of first sexual activity, timing of achievement on Piagetian developmental tests, some phobias, certain forms of neurosis and psychosis, electrophysiological activity of the brain, and others (for reviews see Loehlin & Nichols, 1976; Lumsden & Wilson, 1981; McClearn & DeFries, 1973; Vogel, 1981; R. S. Wilson, 1978). Single genes have been identified that affect certain cognitive abilities selectively (Ashton, Polovina, & Vandenberg, 1979), as well as the ability to discriminate certain odorants (Amoore, 1977). Also, it has become apparent that mutations at a single genetic locus can result in profound but highly specific changes in the architecture and operation of brain tissues such as mammalian neocortex (Caviness & Rakic, 1978; Rakic, 1979). This phenomenon is strikingly manifested in the mutant mouse strains reeler, weaver, and staggerer (Figure 3-2). In each type of animal, a single genetic change results in the reorganization of the neural circuitry in the cerebellum and a number of other brain regions. These alterations modify behavior at the level of locomotion, and in the case of reeler they have been linked to such higher level processes as choice and decision (Bliss & Errington, 1977).

Despite this combined mass of empirical data, it might be objected that on a priori grounds the case of pure cultural transmission is the more plausible because it dispenses with a clutter of innate constraints, relying instead on the information-carrying capacity of culture to equip a developmental process encumbered only by

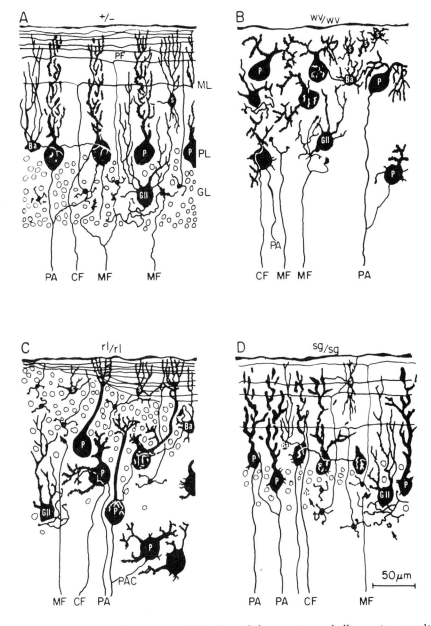

Figure 3-2. Changes in the neuronal circuitry of the mouse cerebellar cortex, result-ing from mutations at a single locus. The induced behavior patterns are diagnostic for the genetic change. *A*, normal; *B*, homozygous weaver; *C*, homozygous reeler; *D*, homozygous staggerer. (Ba = basket cell, CF = climbing fiber, G = granule cell, GII = Golgi type II cell, MF = mossy fiber, P = Purkinje cell, PA = Purkinje cell axon, PF = parallel fiber, S = stellate cell.) Modified from Caviness and Rakic 1978); reproduced from Lumsden and Wilson (1981).

the most general, domain-universal of constraints on storage and processing. Such a viewpoint would be unwarranted. Physiological equalization of preferences among culturgens and the neutralization of innate biases requires a genotype that embodies the capacity for complex fine-tuning mechanisms. Pure cultural transmission can be sustained only with precise controls that depend on an extreme, specialized set of innate epigenetic rules to lock the organism into the tabula rasa state.

The Leash Principle and Directed Cognition

The conclusions about the existence of innate biasing epigenetic rules are consistent with the recent theoretical demonstration that the tabula rasa state of pure cultural transmission is unstable in evolutionary time (Lumsden & Wilson, 1981). During the process of gene-culture coevolution a population of tabula rasa organisms, even if present initially, is very likely to evolve rapidly into a condition where the tabulae rasa have been replaced by organisms equipped for gene-culture transmission. In a cultural species the genetic fitness of an organism is affected not only by its genotype but also by its cultural heritage as expressed by the set of culturgens that affect development. The genetic fitness is influenced by the pathway of enculturation that the organism follows, and is enhanced by any tendency of mental epigenesis to use culturgens with greater relative fitness. The innate epigenetic rules of gene-culture transmission provide this capability, guiding the organism to incorporate or respond to sets of relatively advantageous culturgens more often than sets of relatively deleterious culturgens.

Consider, in contrast, a population of tabula rasa organisms, which alter the degree of influence over development exercised by specific culturgens without reference to the consequences for genetic fitness. The developmental field is unbiased by innate constraints. The population exists in an environment that will in general contain both adaptive and less advantageous culturgens, but it is unable to distinguish between them. Moreover, its members are susceptible to cultural programming that could at whim shape their preferences to favor deleterious culturens. Over a period of generations the population is unstable against invasion by genetic mutants that program innate biases toward adaptive sets of culturgens. Because of their superior enculturation, such developmentally biased organisms outcompete the tabulae rasa, leaving more offspring generation after generation, until eventually they constitute virtually the entire population. This inference can be termed the *leash principle*: Genetic evolution operates in such a way as to keep both culture and individual cognitive development on a leash.

Some culturgens undeniably provide superior genetic fitness over others, but how is this possible? Survival and reproduction are not the products of an artifact lying in a campsite or a mentifact circulating in the recesses of long-term memory. They are fixed by explicit behavior, by muscular contraction and motion of parts of the body. The human mind intervenes to pose new strata of process and transformation between enculturation and explicit behavior. Mental activity and outward behavior are based on the knowledge structures that make up the contents of the various cognitive domains. But if it is the case that culture and the development of the human mind are sustained by gene-culture transmission, then the knowledge structures are psychological entities built up in forms governed by the epigenetic rules. When organisms are predisposed to form certain mental structures and operations as opposed to others, the result is directed cognition, a phenomenon that includes but is not subsumed by the activity of prepared learning in the sense used to describe the results of earlier studies of overt behavior in animals (Seligman, 1972a, 1972b; Shettleworth, 1972).

In principle, the achievement of directed cognition can be the result of one or more innate constraining processes. First, the canalization results in part from sensory screening, which limits perception to narrow windows opening on the vast arrays of physical stimuli impinging on the body. Second, it could result from a tendency for certain knowledge structures to take form and link preferentially with others, including those related more directly to activities in the limbic and brain reward systems, so that they are more likely to become differentially associated with particular informational, valuational, and emotive constructs. For example, bonding results from the virtually automatic positive linking of mother and infant during their initial contacts, whereas snakes, heights, and other typical subjects of human phobias are likely to acquire negative valuation and become tagged as objects of avoidance behavior. Third, canalization could result from the existence of constraints on achievable cognitive design, biasing development toward certain parameters of information processing capacity rather than others. Thus the symbol capacity of short-term memory is on the order of three to seven elements or chunks, while the comparatively infinite store of long-term memory admits new elements much more slowly than it allows them to be retrieved (Newell & Simon, 1972; Simon, 1979). The effects of these characteristics on the selection of search and computational strategies hae been documented in many areas of human reasoning and problem solving (Larkin, McDermott, Simon, & Simon, 1980; Newell & Simon, 1972; Simon, 1979, 1981). Overall, the canalization in cognitive development leads to a substantial convergence of the forms of mental activity among the members of societies and even among peoples belonging to different cultures (for reviews see Hallpike, 1979; Lumsden & Wilson, 1981; Williams, 1972). Idiosyncrasies in concept formation and all other aspects of development obviously distinguish one human being from another. But the epigenetic rules of gene-culture transmission appear to be sufficiently tight to produce a broad overlap in mental activity and behavior of all individuals and hence a convergence powerful enough to be labeled human nature (Lumsden & Wilson, 1981).

The culturally triggered knowledge structures constitute an individual's received portion of culture. With the principles that can at present be inferred from cognitive science about their ontogeny and manipulation, we are in a position to begin with the simplest forms of knowledge structures and epigenetic rules, much as the population biologist begins with the elementary rules of single-locus inheritance and gradually expands the size and complexity of the theoretical representations. This step appears to be particularly important for achieving a useful gene-culture coevolutionary theory. For human beings at least, one needs to know the role played by cognition in mediating the fitness of culturgens. Unless some answers are possible, the reciprocal relationship between genetic inheritance and cultural inheritance in mental development cannot be reliably investigated. The transformation from cul-

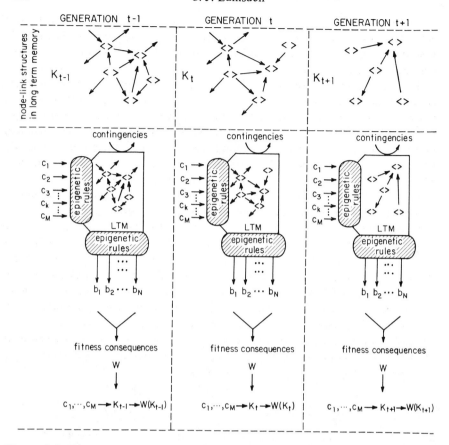

Figure 3-3. The sequence linking culture to genetic fitness through the events of cognition. Culturgens ($c_1, \ldots, c_M$) affect cognition through their formation of knowledge structures K under the influence of the epigenetic rules. The structures are represented abstractly in node-link diagram notation. The knowledge encoded in K is translated into behavioral acts ($b_1, \ldots, b_N$) by processing steps that have also been shaped by the epigenetic rules. The behavioral acts determine genetic fitness. From Lumsden and Wilson (1981).

turgens and enculturation history to genetic fitness must be characterized. Because culturgens interact with each other in their effects on development and the associated knowledge structures interact during cognition, this transformation is not trivial.

The problem can be attacked by solving it stepwise, as shown in Figure 3-3. An individual is enculturated by exposure to the culturgens of his society. This information is incorporated into the developing cognitive system under the influence of the epigenetic rules, and the resulting knowledge structures become the internalized culturgens of the individual. Other epigenetic rules influence the valuation measures and cognitive parameters. The resulting behavioral acts determine genetic fitness. It is therefore possible to speak of a fitness $W(K)$ of an individual possessing a specific cognitive design K, which consists at least of particular symbol structures encoding knowledge about the world, and information processes acting on them. Behavioral acts that result in differential survival or fecundity test not only their own evolutionary potence, but also the cognitive design, the culturgens composing it, and the epigenetic rules that guided the formation of all these elements.

In purely genetic transmission, which occurs in many lower animals, knowledge structures are inherited as hard-wired processes within the brain. In *Homo sapiens*, however, this is the case in at most a tiny fraction of behaviors, and these are primarily reflexive and autonomic in nature. Almost all of human behavior is based on knowledge that is either learned to some degree, or whose formation is otherwise triggered by the culturgens of the society. What is inherited are the epigenetic rules. These are the physiological components of mental development most directly subject to genetic evolution, and they are properly made the focus of theoretical models.

The treatment of gene-culture coevolution therefore goes far beyond conventional notions about the evolution of "a capacity for learning and culture" in its conception of the mind. The genes prescribe a rich system of epigenetic rules that, within the context of a human culture, assemble knowledge structures and ultimately an entire mind. The prescriptors of cognition and behavior comprise an intricate network of cause and effect and thus cannot be assessed as "$x\%$ genes and $y\%$ culture." The true mode of causation is fully epigenetic and not decomposable into "nature" and "nurture" in any naive additive sense. Instead, present evidence indicates that a key step required in order to understand mental development and its cultural environment is the evolutionary study of epigenetic rules.

Properties of the Epigenetic Rules

The Data

Although developmental psychology has achieved sophistication as an empirical and theoretical science, until recently epigenetic rules had not (Lumsden & Wilson, 1981) been systematically classified and described. Perhaps the principal reason for this circumstance is that in gathering data, students of cognitive development have largely neglected the possibility of innately modulated preference among multiple competing culturgens or branch points of development. They have instead more often emphasized environmental determination of preferences, using multiple stimuli selected for empirical convenience (e.g., Trabasso & Bower, 1968), or focused on a supposed universal succession of stages through which cognitive development is inferred to pass (e.g., Brainerd, 1978; Logue, 1979).

Because psychologists do not often lay out a range of options and measure the innate constraints on frequencies of choice and their effects on development, the data required to advance gene-culture theory are relatively few. However, by analyzing the published studies available to us we have concluded that the cases of primary and secondary epigenetic rules cited earlier contain sufficient evidence to be either definitive or strongly suggestive. Of these instances, six are sufficiently striking and illustrative to merit more detailed description here. (For extended discussion see the monographic treatment provided by Lumsden and Wilson, 1981.)

Taste and Smell. Food and the traditions surrounding meal preparation and consumption have been ritualized to communicate and enforce correct behavior in virtually every other facet of social life, such as greeting, courtship, hygiene, dominance, religion, conciliation, and alliance formation (Douglas, 1970; Lévi-Strauss, 1969a). There is no evidence that specific ritual forms have ever become genetically hard wired. However, the forms are clearly enmeshed in the epigenetic rules that guide chemosensory learning, and they are constrained by the rules affecting other social functions served by culinary ritualization.

Using ingestion experiments, Maller and Desor (1974) demonstrated that infants prefer a variety of sugar solutions (in the order sucrose, fructose, lactose, and glucose) over plain water through at least part of the range detectable by adults—a selectivity that continues into later life. Newborns not only prefer sweet solutions; they discriminate further among tastes that are bitter, acid, or salty, showing distinctive facial reflexes in response to each that resemble adult reactions to strong and unpleasant tastes (Chiva, 1979; Steiner, 1979). In a classic experiment that awaits definitive replication, Davis (1928) showed that three newly weaned children placed on an ad libitum cafeteria regimen quickly arrived at a nutritious and balanced diet, with the members of the experimental group converging to a remarkable degree within the array of all possible diets. Such homeostasis appears to be susceptible to genetic alterations that shift the patterns of dietary choice to new steady states. For example, the autosomal "obesity gene" *ob* in mice, when present in the homozygous state *ob/ob,* induces heavier eating, a preference for a higher proportion of fat in the diet, and less sensitivity to variations in sweetness (Mayer, Dickie, Bates, & Vitale, 1951; Ramirez & Sprott, 1979). Similarly, among human beings there exists a well-known polymorphism in the ability to taste phenylthiocarbimide (PTC), the frequency of tasters being highest in those parts of the world where natural goitrogens are endemic and apt to occur. The bitter taste of these chemicals resembles that of PTC. At least one of the anosmias, or lowered abilities of individuals to smell certain types of substances, is based on a recessive gene affecting sensitivity to pentadecalactone, which has a musklike odor (Whissell-Buechy & Amoore, 1973). Taken together, this evidence suggests that changes at specific sites in the mammalian genome can alter specific elements of the choice and preference activities involved in gustatory cognition and behavior.

Color Vision and Color Language. Many social scientists have expressed the belief that the manner in which language divides the visible light spectrum and the other perceptual fields up into meaningful categories is quite arbitrary. For example, in his text on linguistics, Gleason (1961) said, "Consider a rainbow or a spectrum from a prism. There is a continuous gradation of color from one end to the other. . . . Yet an American describing it will list the hues as *red, orange, yellow, green, blue, purple*, or something of the kind. . . . There is nothing inherent either in the spectrum or the human perception of it that would compel its division in this way." (p. 4). (See also Fishman, 1960 and Whorf, 1956.)

More recent studies have shown that these earlier expectations about the arbitrary nature of color classification are wrong. Linguistic categorizations of color are instead tied closely to the biological rules of natural color perception (Berlin & Kay,

1969; Kay & McDaniel, 1978; Ratliff, 1976; Rosch, 1973). Bornstein and his associates have provided valuable new insights into the developmental origins and primary epigenetic rules of the color classification procedure (Bornstein, 1981; Bornstein et al., 1976). In experiments involving recovery from habituation to various wavelengths of light, 4-month-old infants were found to respond to changes in the wavelength of the dishabituation stimulus as though the infant mind discriminates four categories of basic hue matching the adult categories of blue, green, yellow, and red. The infants' categorization scheme is illustrated in Figure 3-4.

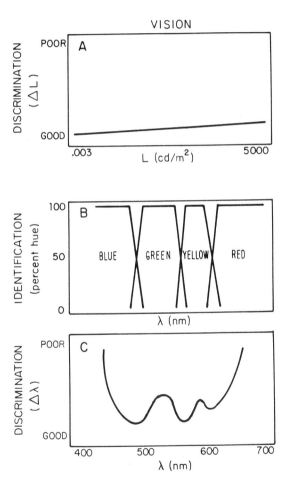

Figure 3-4. Primary epigenetic rules in color perception. (A) Luminance discrimination is a continuum and varies little as luminace changes. (B) During infancy the wavelength spectrum of visible light is perceived as though it were broken into four principal categories—blue, green, yellow, and red. (C) Wavelength discriminability varies abruptly between good and poor along the visible spectrum, with peaks roughly corresponding to the boundaries between the four hue categories. Modified from Bornstein (1979); reproduced from Lumsden and Wilson (1981).

Some progress has been made with the neurobiological mechanism of this remarkable capacity. Working with primates (the macaque monkey) whose color vision resembles that of humans, De Valois and his coworkers report the presence in the lateral geniculate nucleus of four types of color-sensitive cells: One type responds most strongly to red and is inhibited by green, another to green and is inhibited by red, another to blue and is inhibited by yellow, and another to yellow and is inhibited by blue (De Valois & De Valois, 1975; De Valois & Jacobs, 1968). The centers and boundaries of the color classes determined by the response characteristics of these cells align closely with the hue categories observed in infant and adult color classification (e.g., cf. Bornstein et al., 1976, Figure 1, with Kay & McDaniel, 1978, Figure 6).

In an earlier, classical study in comparative linguistics by Berlin and Kay (1969), native speakers of 20 languages were shown arrays of chips classified by color and brightness according to the Munsell system. The results are depicted in Figure 3-5, and demonstrate clearly that languages have evolved in a way that conforms closely to the primary epigenetic rules of color classification. The terms cluster largely into classes that correspond, on a one-to-one to one-to-three basis, to the hue categories distinguished by infants. The pattern discovered by Berlin and Kay has since been confirmed by many investigators (for reviews, see Bolton, 1978; Ratliff, 1976; and von Wattenwyl & Zollinger, 1979). Rosch (1973) found that the Dani men of New Guinea, whose color classification is rudimentary, learned a "natural" classification based on the Berlin-Kay clusters more rapidly than a scheme based on arbitrarily selected clusters. She has related this adult learning rule to the concept of prototypes, or most representative examples of a cluster, and to overlapping cluster boundaries in human semantic schemes (a recent review is provided by Mervis & Rosch, 1981). Kay and McDaniel (1978) have quantified the category overlap by using neurophysiological data and have shown that the notion of partially overlapping color clusters can be extended by means of fuzzy set theory to explain the progression during cultural evolution from simple to complex color term systems.

Kovach (1980) recently demonstrated the evolutionary potential of color cognition by means of artificial selection experiments carried out on the red-blue color preferences of chicks of the quail *Coturnix coturnix japonica*. (The color preferences of infant and adult human beings are again very similar to each other. See, e.g., Bornstein and Marks, 1982, p. 66.) Two lines diverging completely, with no overlap in color choice scores, were created in only five generations, with four to eight segregating units of inheritance estimated to underlie the lineage differences. It is apparent that in this vertebrate population epigenetic rules were altered within 10 generations by a sufficiently rigid selection protocol, and that complex aspects of development, choice, and behavior were affected by relatively small numbers of genes.

Nonverbal Communication. The motor patterns that constitute nonlinguistic communication are promising subjects for the study of epigenetic rules. Some of the signals are relatively invariant, with significant covergence in their structure and meaning occurring across cultures. Yet nearly all are also subject to modifications peculiar to the particular cultures. In his field studies of human behavior, Eibl-Eibes-

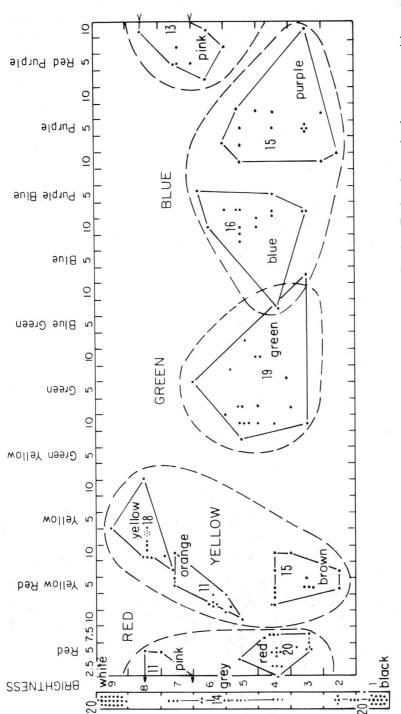

Figure 3-5. Language as constrained by the primary epigenetic rules of color classification. Each point marks the average position on a Munsell color array of a basic color term in one language, as estimated by native speakers of the language. Although 20 cultures from around the world are represented (many of which have evolved independently of one another), their color terms are clustered in a manner that corresponds to the principal colors innately distinguished by infants. Modified from Berlin and Kay (1969) by the addition of the dashed lines and the labels of the principal colors; reproduced from Lumsden and Wilson (1981).

feldt (1975, 1979) has, for example, documented varying degrees of convergence in phallic displays, eyebrow flashing, threat staring, gaze aversion, kissing, and pouting. The evidence is strong enough to leave little uncertainty that much of this behavior is human specific and distinguishes man narrowly but clearly from the other Old World primates (Lumsden & Wilson, 1981). Eibl-Eibesfeldt has also demonstrated that it is possible to trace with some rigor the development of nonlinguistic signals in children and the alterations that the signals undergo as they take on new meanings during cultural evolution.

From such studies we have concluded (Lumsden & Wilson, 1981) that a large proportion of the strategies used in nonverbal communication have been built upon the ritualizations of elementary behavior patterns, with the ritualized versions of the behavior being guided by new epigenetic rules. In some categories (such as head shaking) the elementary patterns are little more than undifferentiated motor acts serving noncommunicative acts as well. However, patterns such as smiling, other basic facial expressions, laughing, and crying appear to have been restricted to signal functions from the time of their evolutionary origin, and they were subjected to more rigid developmental constraints in the ritualization process that followed. Thus, the epigenetic rules vary among the categories of nonlinguistic communication in the pattern of their constraint, but in all cases the innate developmental biases are strong enough to limit narrowly the array of nonlinguistic signals produced during cultural evolution.

Sibling Incest Avoidance. The avoidance of incest is a pivotal subject for the social sciences. Many cultural anthropologists share the view of Lévi-Strauss (1969b) that in the practices of incest avoidance, human beings are cast free from their biological history and guided instead by idiosyncratic systems of taboos and rituals programmed by culture and functioning to maintain the network of social relations. In this instance we believe that the evidence shows the traditional conception to be incorrect.

Our line of reasoning begins with the observation that incest taboos are a cultural universal.Virtually all of the hundreds of societies studied have imposed a ban on brother-sister mating, while permitting or even encouraging it between first cousins. Only a very few, such as the Incas, Ancient Egyptians, Monomotapa of Zimbabwe, Nyanza of Zaire, and Shiluk of the Sudan, have permitted this form of pairing, and then usually only in the case of royalty or in certain noble families. Van den Berghe and Mesher (1980) point out that in all of the known incestuous arrangements, polygyny, the taking of multiple wives, is (or was) practiced by the incestuous males, resulting in a net outbreeding and an overall increase in personal evolutionary fitness. Royal women, on the other hand, were much less likely to marry downward in rank and were thus more susceptible to marriages with their siblings.

Studies by Shepher (1971) and others on the development of sexual preferences of children in Israeli kibbutzim indicate that there exists a relatively specific epigenetic rule in this cognitive domain, whereby an automatic neutralization of sexual interest emerges among people who have lived intimately together ("used the same potty") during the first 6 years of life. This epigenetic rule is not directed precisely at biological siblings. It will respond to any child with whom the young individual lives in close association, an arrangement that is likely to generate *sibling* incest avoidance when it operates within the context of the human family structure. Among the 2,769 kibbutz marriages counted by Shepher, none took place between members of the same kibbutz peer group that had lived together since birth. He did not detect a single known case of heterosexual activity, even though kibbutz adults were not opposed to peer-group sexual activity among adolescents.

Another "natural experiment" leading to similar conclusions occurred among Taiwanese families who adopted very young girls for the purposes of household work and later marriage to the hosts' sons. Such arrangements, although frequently contracted and sanctioned by the society at large, failed at a remarkable rate. In the great majority of cases the couples refused to accede to the marriage, because of probable sexual inhibition based on early domestic contact (Wolf, 1966, 1968, 1970; Wolf & Huang, 1980). When such marriages were actually undertaken they ended in separation and adultery far more often than did unions between individuals who had not been raised together. They also produced substantially fewer children than did the other marriages. The evidence suggests the existence of an innate epigenetic rule in which the resulting preference structure is strongly opposed to incestuous activity.

In American families brother-sister incest does occur, but is again relatively rare, transient, and ordinarily a source of shame and recrimination (Weinberg, 1976). The usefulness of the sociological data on industrialized societies is compromised to some extent by the differing standards that investigators (and informants) apply when judging an act to be incestuous. In taking into account the Israeli and Taiwanese data we have set a relatively robust criterion, namely, full sexual activity ending in intromission and copulation between siblings of the opposite sex.

For the epigenetic rule of sibling incest avoidance the underlying evolutionary rationale seems to be relatively clear. The well-documented result of brother-sister mating is a higher frequency of genetic deformation in the offspring (Seemonová, 1971; Stern, 1973). Thus the possession of an epigenetic rule innately biasing individual behavior away from incestuous activity is expected to confer enhanced reproductive success.

Phobias. In many animal species, individuals are innately prepared or contraprepared to learn to respond to particular conditioned stimuli in those behavioral categories most important to survival and reproduction, whereas in other behavioral categories they are typically unprepared or neutral (Seligman, 1972a, 1972b). The preparedness of human learning and the innately directed character of human cognitive development are manifested with clarity in the case of phobias, which are fears defined by a combination of a number of properties. First, they are extreme in response, often involving major reactions in the autonomic nervous system. Second, they typically emerge full blown after only one negative episode. Third, they are difficult to extinguish, persisting even when the subject is presented repeatedly with the phobic stimulus and its harmlessness is both carefully explained to and acknowledged by the subject. Finally, phobias have high specificity. The phenomena that evoke them consistently include some of the most significant dangers present in mankind's ancient environment, such as thunderstorms, snakes, closed spaces, heights, and spiders. The far more deadly artifacts of modern society, such as knives, guns, automobiles, and electric sockets are rarely effective. It appears reasonable to conclude that phobias are extreme cases of irrational fear reaction that rendered survival more likely during the genetic evolution of human epigenetic rules. As we have suggested elsewhere, "Better to crawl away from a cliff, nauseated with fear, than to casually walk its edge" (Lumsden & Wilson, 1981, p. 85).

Language. Of all the cognitive domains, that of linguistic knowledge has most often been singled out as paradigm of the manner in which the human mind differs from the minds of its primate ancestors (e.g., Hockett & Ascher, 1964). Traditional social science models have generally taken language to be the instrument through which culture imposes its idiosyncratic form on the human mind (e.g., Berger & Luckmann, 1966; Gleason, 1961; White, 1949; Whorf, 1956); but the combined evidence of psycholinguistics, neurobiology, and human genetics suggests that this extreme position should be approached with caution. Instead, it appears likely that the ontogeny of linguistic knowledge structures is the result of mental operations carried out on cultural cues under the guidance of a rich set of innate developmental constraints.

The signs of epigenetic rules operating in the domain of linguistic knowledge have been detected piecemeal by a number of investigators. Infants possess innate rules of speech perception that are adultlike and facilitate the development of language (Eimas, Siqueland, Juscqyk, & Vigorito, 1971; Liberman, Cooper, Shankweiler, & Studdert-Kennedy, 1967). Whereas variations in pitch are perceived as arrayed along a smoothly varying continuum, distinctions of voicing, like distinctions of hue, are automatically classified into categories—in this case, into phoneme clusters. For example, sounds ranging between /ba/ and /ga/ and /s/ and /v/ are clustered on the basis of perceived similarity into one or the other of these paired units. A principal component of the discrimination process is the voice onset time (VOT) for phonemes, which is the timing of the acoustical formants or energy bands relative to one another. For example, the recognition of stop and fricative consonants depends on the extent of the first formant and the direction of the second formant. The pattern of innate phoneme categorization is depicted in Figure 3-6.

The development of phoneme discrimination is channeled, moving through more than one stage during the first year of life or longer (Eilers et al., 1977). In the 11 languages surveyed by Lisker and Abramson (1964) one or more values along each VOT continuum served as reference points, dividing the continuum into two or three phonetic clusters. Ultimately a repertory of from 20 to 60 phonemes develops around these reference points, the total number varying according to culture.

Psycholinguists have pointed out the remarkable speed and precision with which linguistic knowledge develops in children of all cultures. Some have contrasted this state of affairs with the seeming absence from childhood linguistic environments of the order and completeness required for a developmentally unconstrained inductive learner to achieve competence (e.g., Wexler & Culicover, 1980, and references therein). Put briefly, there is a "paradox of the poverty of the stimulus" (Chomsky, 1980): How can linguistic knowledge develop in children when their environments apparently lack information in the requisite quantity and form?

A possible answer is that their genes provide the missing clues by way of innate

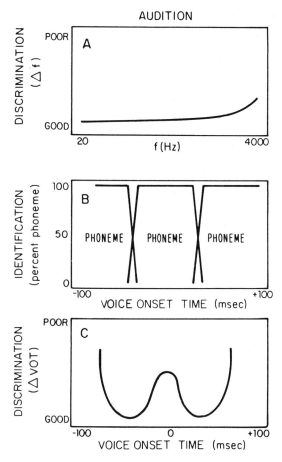

Figure 3-6. Schematic form of primary epigenetic rules in speech perception. (A) Discrimination of pitch is continuous, only slowly changing, and generally acute in the range 20 to 4,000 Hz. (B) However, phoneme classification is categorical and based on strongly varying discrimination (C) between successive energy bands, according to the time separating them (–100 to +100 msec). Modified from Bornstein (1979); reproduced from Lumsden and Wilson (1981).

developmental constraints specialized for language acquisition. These channel the assembly of linguistic knowledge to successful completion (Chomsky, 1980; Keil, 1981; Pinker, 1981), and as a corollary hold language and its cultural evolution on a leash. The most convincing demonstration of the possibility of such epigenetic rules available to us is an important recent study by Wexler and Culicover (1980), which builds on previous work in learnability theory. Their model deals with the acquisition of grammatical transformations. The child is assumed to perceive data in the relatively simple form (s, b), where s is a surface structure marker and b is a deep structure (base) marker. The markers s and b are connected in the adult language by a sequence of transformations T_k, $k = 1, 2, \ldots$, and the authors consider how an epigenetic mechanism that assembles linguistic knowledge in the child's mind can arrive at the correct set of transformations. They treat the circumstance in which the child already has a base component that can be related to a semantic representation, which in turn can be deduced from context. Hence the epigenetic mechanism has access to the surface string and its underlying deep structure, and must assemble an adequate set of transformations connecting the two.

During cognitive development the mechanism constructs, tests, and rejects transformations. The types constructed at any point in the knowledge-acquisition sequence are limited by constraints. Given an appropriate set of constraints, the child arrives at the transformations underlying the surface structure of the adult language (up to functional equivalences). Although more than 10 constraints channel development in their most realistic model, three of the more significant are the binary principle, the freezing principle, and the raising principle. The *binary principle* restricts admissible transformations to those that apply no more than one node below the level at which they cycle. Under the *freezing principle*, if a transformation maps a phrase structure node so that the structure is no longer a base structure, then that node is frozen; that is, no admissible transformation maps anything under the node. By the *raising principle*, if a transformation moves a node to a higher point in a phrase structure tree, then no admissible transformation operates on a node dominated by the raised node. Wexler and Culicover (1980) present empirical evidence of the existence and universality of these constraints in human language systems.

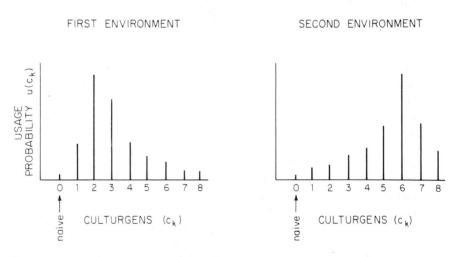

Figure 3-7. Environmental modulation of epigenetic rules. The innate design of the hypothetical epigenetic rule depicted is such that in the first environment its usage bias curve peaks on culturgen c_2 from an array of eight culturgens. In the second environment, the bias curve peaks on culturgen c_6. The pattern of response to environmental change is determined by the genetic blueprint. (The "naive" category, c_0, refers to the circumstance in which the aspect of development regulated by this epigenetic rule proceeds on a completely innate basis, independent of cultural information as embodied in the c_k.)

No data are now available that demonstrate conclusively that these or any of the postulated constraints are necessarily innate. In principle, given sufficient source data, a more generalized learner might induce the rules and proceed to acquire linguistic knowledge. However, this alternative appears to confront the same problems of stimulus impoverishment that originally led to the hypothesis of linguistic constraints. Rigorous demonstrations that learners equipped only with general, domain-universal cognitive constraints can in realistic environments achieve linguistic competence have to our knowledge not yet been forthcoming.

Linguistic theory is in a phase of rapid development, and it is possible that specific epigenetic rules will have to be rethought in the light of new developments. But already the work of Wexler, Culicover, and their associates has provided a first glimpse of the epigenetic field in one of the most complex human cognitive domains, and indicates the significant manner in which cognitive-developmental theory can lead the search for still-undiscovered epigenetic rules.

Design Principles of Epigenetic Rules

Usage Bias Curves. In our terminology, *usage* is defined broadly as one or more links in a complex chain of decisions that include the initial learning of or failure to learn certain culturgens, the frequency with which one or another culturgen triggers an associated pathway in cognitive development, the preference for one culturgen over some other upon reflection and choice by the individual, and the actual employment of particular culturgens in behavior and cognition. Thus, one can speak in workable terms of the use of culturgens by the epigenetic rules during their assembly of the mind, as well as of the use of culturgens during overt behavior. Usage bias curves give the likelihood of usage of various culturgens. Although some usage bias curves (particularly those associated with the primary epigenetic rules) are relatively rigid and do not respond to environmental context, others are flexible. An epigenetic rule can be determined by the genes in such a manner that part of its input is information about cultural and environmental context, which modulates the operation of the rule in a manner that is genetically prescribed (Figure 3-7). The ethnographic literature contains many examples of shifts in usage bias curves that are correlated with differences in habitat, nutritional and social status, and mode of production. For example, female puberty initiation rites originate most frequently in societies where a young girl continues to reside at least half the time in her mother's household, as well as in societies that depend heavily on the labor of girls and young women for the execution of sustenance activities (Williams, 1972).

The Principle of Penetrance. *Penetrance* is the propensity of an epigenetic rule to use any culturgen of a given category, irrespective of whether the choice is made among few or many. In the idealized usage bias curves depicted in Figure 3-8, high penetrance is measurable as a low frequency of individuals in the null category of no culturgen usage. A usage bias curve concentrated in the null or "naive" category reflects an epigenetic rule that functions primarily or completely on the basis of innate programming, and contributes to development in a manner that does not depend directly on the culturgens of the society.

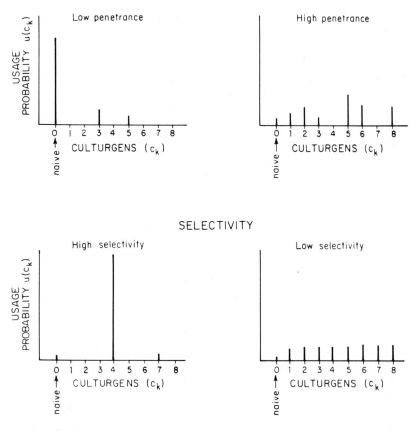

Figure 3-8. Penetrance and selectivity in usage bias curves. Penetrance is the extent to which any culturgen c_k of a given category is used by the epigenetic rule. Selectivity describes the likelihood that a given culturgen will be used by the epigenetic rule. The usage bias curves are consistently displayed by individuals of particular genotypes within specific environments. From Lumsden and Wilson (1981).

Data from developmental psychology indicate that epigenesis has least penetrance during early infancy. At later times in development, the operation of context-dependent epigenetic rules maintains high penetrance while creating a property that is conveniently termed high *selectivity*.

The Principle of Selectivity. A high degree of selectivity in the usage bias curves is revealed by a concentration of those individuals who have made a utilization choice on one or at most a few culturgens (Figure 3-8). Penetrance and selectivity are in principle evolutionarily independent; epigenetic rules and patterns of individual usage that show, respectively, one of the combinations high penetrance/high selectivity, low penetrance/high selectivity, high penetrance/low selectivity, and low penetrance/low selectivity can be readily envisaged and are theoretical possibilities that await full empirical documentation in human mental development.

The regulation of penetrance and selectivity during development can reside in the actions of three principal neural systems (Lumsden & Wilson, 1981): (1) the primary sensory receptors and coding interneurous, which determine the ease with which culturgens are initially detected; (2) the associative centers of the cerebral cortex and the attention and recall mediating centers of the hippocampus, which regulate processing capacity; and (3) the centers of the limbic system and the substantia nigra of the midbrain, which influence the processes of affect and valuation.

The Principle of Parsimony. Although the data required for rigorous testing are not yet available, it appears to us that a principle of parsimony controlled the pathway of evolution leading to the epigenetic rules in *Homo sapiens*: The evolution of innate developmental constraints terminates when cognitive development is given the least degree of selectivity that will suffice. Thus, sexual fixation is a powerful form of prepared learning that usually results in heterosexual pair bonding. However, idiosyncratic experiences during the susceptible period of development in adolescence through early maturity can redirect cognitive development in part or in whole to homosexuality or to deviant fixations such as coprolagnia, urolagnia, pedophilia, necrophilia, and fetishism. These behavior structures are difficult to alter once they are formed (Goleman & Bush, 1977; VanDeventer & Laws, 1978).

Similarly, the selectivity of sibling incest avoidance broadens to include potential mates when biologically unrelated children are raised in close contact during the first 5 to 7 years of life (Lumsden & Wilson, 1981; Shepher, 1971). In oriental populations, genes programming the early cessation of lactase production occur in high frequencies, and milk is generally avoided in oriental cuisines. But the aversion to milk appears to be based on vicarious learning via gastrointestinal distress, perhaps reinforced by cultural tradition, rather than on an innate avoidance response to milk sugar programmed to appear in childhood (Rozin, 1976).

The Principle of Transparency. When the impact of a behavior on genetic fitness depends on context, the mind is more likely to be aware of the relation and to make decisions accordingly. The more clearly the conscious mind perceives the relation, the more likely the behavior is to be highly flexible. Thus, economic behaviors affect survival and reproductive success according to the particularities of the surrounding environment and social order, relations that are intuitively understood with varying degrees of clarity and are the objects of conscious evaluation and decision making. Economic behavior is flexible, and cultures vary widely in their forms of economic organization (Boehm, 1978; Clarke, 1978; Haggett, 1972).

The contrasting mode of impact occurs when the genetic fitness varies little as context changes. Then the conscious mind is more likely to be unaware of a relation between behavior and fitness, and the tactics of cognitive development are unlikely to change across cultures. For example, the adaptive significance of sugar consumption (high caloric yield), incest avoidance (reduction of inbreeding depression), and human grammar (rapid, consistent conveyance of meaning) are understood by only the few societies that have studied them scientifically (Katz, Hediger, & Valleroy, 1974; Rozin, 1976). They are incorporated into cognitive development and into the operation of the circuit of gene-culture coevolution automatically under the guidance of strong, selective epigenetic rules.

Coevolutionary Circuits

In order to be judged of significance to cognitive-developmental theory, gene-culture studies must be capable of demonstrating the existence of the complete circuit of coevolutionary linkage in such a way that the relationships between the developing mind and genes and culture are properly described, and must establish the feasibility of elucidating the circuit's structure. An example of what can now be accomplished with this difficult problem is shown in Figure 3-9, which is drawn from one of our recent studies (Lumsden & Wilson, 1981). Alternative formulations of the circuit that are amenable to equally complete treatment have not yet been reported in the literature.

We have inferred the steps in the circuit by using information from the relevant disciplines of population genetics, neurobiology, cognitive and developmental psychology, sociobiology, and the social sciences. We envisage a sequence in which competing culturgens are introduced to a society through innovation and cross-cultural exchange, and individual members are predisposed through the epigenetic rules to use certain of the culturgens rather than others during cognitive development and subsequent behavior. The epigenetic rules affect the probabilities of culturgen usage during development and thus regulate the likelihood that a particular cognitive design will be achieved at a given time t. The behavioral effects of the design can be modeled with the usage bias curves of individual decision making, which give the transition probabilities for individual switching among alternative activities in specified environments.

In the circuit of coevolution, the genetic fitness of individuals is determined by their choice of behaviors and usage of culturgens, as well as by the concurrent choice and usage by other members of the society—in other words, by the surrounding culture. The relation between individual genetic fitness and culturgen choice is a general observation and has been explicitly documented in a wide variety of behavioral categories, including diet (Gajdusek, 1970), body marking (Blumberg & Hesser, 1975), sexual practice (Daly & Wilson, 1978), marital customs (Daly & Wilson, 1978), economic practice (Irons, 1979), and others. The fitness is the product of survivorship and age-specific fertility through the life cycle. Although the theory of gene-culture coevolution includes the study of the effects of such phenomena as genetic mutation, the introduction of new genes by population migration, and the fluctuation of gene frequencies due to small population size, we postulate that as in biological evolution in general (for review see Wilson, 1975), differential genetic fitness is a major factor in shaping the gene ensembles that prescribe epigenetic rules. When evolutionary mechanisms act through their effects on survivorship and fertility, the process is said to be *natural selection*.

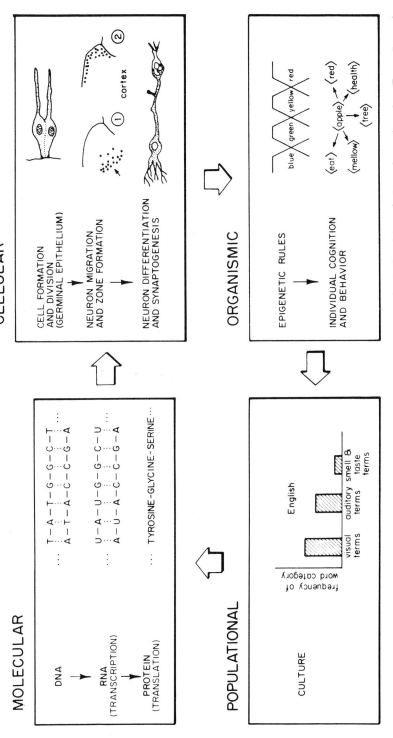

Figure 3-9. The circuit of gene-culture coevolution incorporating the essential relationships of the epigenetic rules. From Lumsden and Wilson (1981).

Thus, natural selection completes the coevolutionary circuit and places cognitive development in its correct relationship to genes and culture: The epigenetic rules (or the mind or culture, depending on the starting point chosen) create effects that reverberate around the circuit, finally to be tested by natural selection with each passage through the life cycle. The genes prescribe the epigenetic rules, which feed on culture to direct and constrain the processes of cognitive development. Individual behavior in social groups creates patterns of group action (cultural context), which are used as additional sources of information during decision making. Natural selection tests the genetic fitness of the decisions, along with the underlying genes and epigenetic rules, as well as the emitted behavior. The same process shapes all forms of epigenetic rules, regardless of whether in a given generation they mediate pure genetic transmission, pure cultural transmission, or (as we have concluded to be the case in human beings) gene-culture transmission.

From Cognitive Development to Cultural Patterns

A segment of the coevolutionary circuit that can be very usefully examined once the existence of epigenetic rules has been delineated and their role in sustaining human mental development described is the translation from cognition to cultural pattern. Success at this juncture would mean that properties of culture can be deduced from information about the core properties of human nature and its epigenesis. The theory would also then be in a position to estimate the effects that alterations in the core properties exert on culture and society. In turn, at least some epigenetic rules appear to use information about large-scale properties of culture (such as the existence of institutions of certain forms, or the net frequency of usage of a particular culturgen) in guiding mental development and individual decision making. Information about cultural patterns closes the gap in the coevolutionary circuit that is otherwise created by the input requirements of these epigenetic rules (Lumsden & Wilson, 1981).

At first sight the prospect of achieving such a step in any practical manner seems unlikely. One must account not only for the correlated activity of many developmental histories in the presence of multiple culturgens, but also for their overall cultural properties and the feedback of these patterns to cognition. In evolutionary time, multiple genotypes with different epigenetic rules and cognitive properties are involved in the culture, and to determine fitness a life-history reproduction function must be evaluated for each genotype in the interacting assembly. But by combining formal methods from social theory with techniques from population genetics, reward theory, and mathematical physics, we have been able to carry out the necessary calculations in a key case, namely, an egalitarian culture in which two culturgens feed a usage bias curve whose underlying epigenetic rule is shaped by one gene of major effect. In an egalitarian culture the network of social relationships is relatively homogeneous. Information about the activities of others modulates cognition, but each alter is evaluated in a similar manner and no single alter dominates ego's deliberations. Such egalitarianism is best approximated by human societies of hunter-gatherers, which often lack formal leaders and reach decisions via group discussion (Biesele, 1978; Lee, 1979; Lee & Devore, 1976). Most of human evolution occurred in bands resembling the hunter-gatherers in their size and, very likely, general social organization (Buys & Larson, 1979; Hage, 1976; Wobst, 1974). The cultural anthropology of the preliterate thought typical in such societies has revealed a significant tendency of the mind to chunk information into binary alternatives in the case of elementary economic decisions, myth formation, and other categories of cognition (Lumsden & Wilson, 1981, p. 53-95, 100).

The feasibility of bridging in a significant manner the gaps between individual and culture and between culture and genetic fitness in the coevolutionary circuit has therefore been established. The results indicate that the relationships among cognitive development and gene-culture linkages have some remarkable and previously unsuspected properties. The procedure we have followed is to recognize the inherently probabilistic nature of human choice and decision, together with the inevitable uncertainties about environment and social structure. These limit the precision of theoretical prediction. However, one can attempt to mathematize the theory in a manner that generates probability distributions, such as those constructed empirically by anthropologists themselves during cross-cultural surveys, and predicts the likelihood of observing given cultural patterns of behavior and organization in a specific society. (For example, in .8 of the societies .3 of the members express culturgen c_1 and .7 express c_2, where c_1 and c_2 are learnable belief systems; in .1 of the societies .5 of the members express c_1 and .5 express c_2; and so on through all possible patterns of c_1 and c_2 usage.) Thus, in deriving such frequency distributions, which we term *ethnographic curves* (Lumsden & Wilson, 1980a, 1981), we are in fact dealing with the most elementary patterns of culture, of the kind traditionally inferred by cultural anthropologists and other social scientists.

Although the full mathematical development is somewhat lengthy, the chain of reasoning can be adequately illustrated by means of a brief formal sketch. Detailed discussion can be found in Lumsden & Wilson (1981). To begin, consider a society that contains N members at time t, of whom n_1 use culturgen c_1 and n_2 use c_2 during a given interval. From the standpoint of choice, an individual life history contains a succession of decision points at which culturgen usage must be evaluated. The relevant products of the epigenetic rules for this type of activity are the culture-dependent usage bias probabilities $u_{ij}(n_1)$ that at a decision point an individual using culturgen c_i in behavior will adopt culturgen c_j given that n_1 are already using c_1. In our initial studies we have modeled the simpler domains of cognitive development, such as sibling incest avoidance, in which following a period of initial enculturation the bias curves $u_{ij}(n_1)$ do not change significantly.

Let us denote by τ_1 and τ_2 the mean lifetimes between sequential decision points for a c_1 user and a c_2 user, respectively. The quantities τ_1 and τ_2 are the means of the probability distributions for holding times in usage states c_1 and c_2. We shall model these distributions with exponential densities so that the underlying cognitive system obeys Markovian dynamics. Despite its simplicity, this approximation has proven useful in many applications to individual decision and group dynamics (e.g., Atkinson, Bower, & Crothers, 1965; Bartholomew, 1973; Coleman, 1964, 1973; Donohue, Hawes, & Mabee, 1981; Greeno, 1974; Kemeny & Snell, 1962; Lehoczky, 1980). The transition rates for culturgen switching are then $v_{ij}(n_1)$ in the individual process, where

$$v_{12}(n_1) = \tau_1^{-1} u_{12}(n_1) \qquad \text{and} \qquad v_{21}(n_1) = \tau_2^{-1} u_{21}(n_1). \qquad (3\text{-}1)$$

Culturgen usage in the society as a whole can be characterized at time t by the vector $\mathbf{n} = (n_1, n_2)$. The quantity of interest is the probability $P(\mathbf{n}, t)$, the likelihood at time t that in the society n_1 members are using culturgen c_1 and n_2 are using c_2. The set of probabilities $\{P(\mathbf{n}, t)|n_1 + n_2 = N\}$ for all possible usage patterns subject to the constraint $n_1 + n_2 = N$ is the ethnographic curve of the society.

In order to link the properties of the ethnographic curve $P(\mathbf{n}, t)$ to events at the level of the individual, we note that in any differential interval of time dt the probability of two or more simultaneous decisions is of order $(dt)^2$ and is negligible to first order. Then if the society moves from state $(n_1{}', n_2{}')$ at time t to a different state (n_1, n_2) at time $t + dt$, it can only be that

$$(n_1{}', n_2{}') = (n_1 + 1, n_2 - 1) \qquad \text{or} \qquad (n_1{}', n_2{}') = (n_1 - 1, n_2 + 1), \quad (3\text{-}2)$$

and the whole-society transition rate to or from a state $\mathbf{n} = (n_1, n_2)$ is equal to the transition rate $v_{ij}(n_1)$ for an individual, multiplied by the number of individuals in the culturgen-usage group from which the transition took place. It can then be shown (Lumsden & Wilson, 1981, pp. 118-120) that $P(\mathbf{n}, t)$ obeys the equation of motion

$$\frac{d P(n_1, n_2, t)}{dt} = (n_1 + 1)v_{12}(n_1 + 1, n_2 - 1) P(n_1 + 1, n_2 - 1, t)$$
$$+ (n_2 + 1) v_{21}(n_1 - 1, n_2 + 1) P(n_1 - 1, n_2 + 1, t)$$
$$- [n_1 v_{12}(n_1, n_2) + n_2 v_{21}(n_1, n_2)] P(n_1, n_2, t) \quad (3\text{-}3)$$

for $0 < n_1 < N$, with similar forms when $n_1 = 0$ or $n_1 = N$.

If an individual lifetime contains many points of choice and decision (as is the case in human beings), then except for a relatively brief interval of initial decay the ethnographic curve for this process is well approximated by the steady state

$$P(n_1, n_2) = P(0, N) \binom{N}{n_1} \exp \sum_{i=1}^{n_1} \ln \frac{v_{21}(i-1)}{v_{12}(i)} \qquad (3\text{-}4)$$

where

$$P(0, N) = \left[1 + \sum_{n_1=1}^{N} P(n_1, N-n_1) \right]^{-1}. \qquad (3\text{-}5)$$

When the group size N is large, these relationships can be cast into a more convenient form by using continuous variables. For two-culturgen systems a convenient measure for the cultural pattern is

$$\xi \equiv 1 - 2n_1 / N, \qquad -1 \leqslant \xi \leqslant 1, \qquad (3\text{-}6)$$

which changes by progressively smaller increments $\Delta\xi = N^{-1}$ as N increases. In the limit $\Delta\xi \to 0$ of large group size the equation of motion for the ethnographic curve is accurately modeled by the Fokker-Planck equation

$$\frac{\partial}{\partial t} P(\xi, t) = \frac{-\partial}{\partial \xi} [X(\xi)P(\xi, t)] + \frac{1}{2} \frac{\partial^2}{\partial \xi^2} [Q(\xi)P(\xi, t)], \qquad (3\text{-}7)$$

where the functions $X(\xi)$, $Q(\xi)$ are related to the individual usage bias curves by

$$X(\xi) = (1 - \xi)v_{12}(\xi) - (1 + \xi)v_{21}(\xi), \tag{3-8}$$

$$Q(\xi) = \frac{2}{N}[(1 - \xi)v_{12}(\xi) + (1 + \xi)v_{21}(\xi)]. \tag{3-9}$$

The associated steady state of the ethnographic distribution is then simply

$$P(\xi) = \frac{C}{Q(\xi)}\left[\exp\ 2\int_{-1}^{\xi}\frac{X(\xi')}{Q(\xi')}\ d\xi'\right], \tag{3-10}$$

where C is a normalization constant determined by the requirement that the total area under $P(\xi)$ be equal to unity. Generalizations of this formulation to more than two culturgens are readily achieved (Lumsden & Wilson, 1981).

It is important to note that a steady-state ethnographic curve does not mean that the society is static or unchanging in time. A society is a system in flux, in which the numbers of its members using different culturgens change. As individuals encounter choice situations and some switch culturgens, the cultural pattern moves back and forth on the usage scale $n_1 = 0, 1, 2, \ldots, N$. The ethnographic curve expresses the proportion of its history that the society spends in a particular cultural pattern. Equivalently, for this class of models it also expresses the proportion of an ensemble of very similar societies expected to be characterized at any time by a particular usage pattern.

It is possible to quantify the response of the ethnographic curves to changes in the $u_{ij}(n_1)$ and $v_{ij}(n_1)$ output by the epigenetic rules. We have shown that for a wide range of u_{ij} and v_{ij} behaviors, the ethnographic curves shift from a unimodal to a sharply multimodal form when the characteristic parameters of the usage bias curves cross a short interval (Lumsden & Wilson, 1980a, 1981). Moreover, because of the location of the quantities ln $v_{ij}(n_1)$ in the exponent of $P(n_1, n_2)$, small degrees of innate bias favoring one or the other of the culturgens can be amplified in the dependent ethnographic curve. Study of the exact models suggests that in realizable circumstances small changes in the epigenetic rules induce striking effects in the overall ethnographic pattern observable by the cultural anthropologist.

It is possible to formulate concise measures of the achievable amplification. For example, with reference to the two ethnographic curves depicted in Figure 3-10, a natural amplification factor can be defined as the relative measure

$$A \equiv \frac{P^{(1)}(n_{1,1}, n_{2,1})/P^{(1)}(n_{1,2}, n_{2,2})}{P^{(0)}(n_{1,1}, n_{2,1})/P^{(0)}(n_{1,2}, n_{2,2})}, \tag{3-11}$$

where $P^{(0)}$ is the reference curve of a group in which there is no innate bias. Let the differences $n_{1,1} - n_{1,2}$ indicated in Figure 3-11 be denoted by Δ. Then the following *amplification law* holds (Lumsden & Wilson, 1981):

$$A \equiv (v_{21}^0 / v_{12}^0)^{\Delta}, \tag{3-12}$$

where the cultural group characterized by the ethnographic curve $P^{(1)}$ has innate biases v_{ij}^0. An impression of the degree of relative amplification away from the tabu-

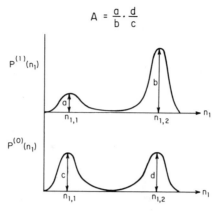

Figure 3-10. Definition of the amplification factor A for innate epigenetic biases. The values of the culturgen c_1 usage $n_{1,1}$ and $n_{1,2}$ are variable and have been placed under the modes of the ethographic curves solely for the purposes of clarity. The definition of A can be applied to ethnographic curves of arbitrary shape. From Lumsden and Wilson (1981).

la rasa state can be obtained by studying Figure 3-11, which depicts isoclines of the amplification factor A for a culture group of 25 persons. We have chosen this group size to approximate that of hunger-gatherer bands, most of which have, as far back as Pleistocene times, consisted of from 15 to 75 individuals (Buys & Larson, 1979; Wobst, 1974).

Are the epigenetic rules of human cognitive development in fact strong enough to create this type of effect? Whenever quantitative estimates can be made from data concerning the development of culturgen choice, this ratio has deviated substantially from unity—in other words, from the unbiased state. For example, in early sugar preference (Maller & Desor, 1974) the ratio is between .4/.6 and .25/.75, a bias that extends at least into childhood and affects the behavioral practices surrounding adult cuisine. In the case of greater attention to the schematic design of the human face (Freedman, 1974), the ratio has been between $\geqslant .51/.49$ and $\geqslant .6/.4$, depending on the competing designs employed. The bias leads to long-term focusing on the face, especially the eyes; the facilitation of parent-offspring bonding; and possibly the facilitation of later forms of interpersonal bonding. The distinctive position of infant holding by women, up against their left side, is preferred by a ratio of between .6/.4 and .7/.3, depending on the age of the infant (Lockard et al., 1979). (In men, infant holding appears to be unbiased with reference to the side of the body.) The proximity of the infant to the mother's heartbeat when held on the left soothes the infant and possibly contributes to mother-infant bonding. During the first 5-7 years of life, children raised in close domestic proximity avoid full sexual relationships with a bias approaching 100%. In the adult years this aversion shapes marriage patterns and cultural taboos against sibling incest. Other epigenetic rules show comparable deviations from the tabula rasa state. These conclusions, based on the data of developmental psychology, support recent and independent results from social theory that micromotives can and do have a surprisingly large impact on macrobehavior (Schelling, 1978).

Feedback to the Genes

Under the influence of the biologically grounded epigenetic rules, the members of a society create a substantial portion of their own environment in the form of culture, within which each mind develops. But the society is also a biological population in which the form of the epigenetic rules varies genetically. The relative survival and reproductive success of different genotypes depends on both the culturgens its members employ in cognitive development and in behavior, and on the surrounding culture. Thus, genetic and cultural evolution are tightly coupled, in a manner that constitutes a single coevolutionary system.

We have found that it is possible to formulate the structure of this coevolutionary system in mathematical terms, thereby allowing more incisive scrutiny of its properties. In the mathematical theory of population genetics, evolution is defined as a change with time in the relative abundance of different genes (the gene frequencies). Similarly, a coevolutionary formulation of relevance to cognitive-developmental theory must track changes with time in both the gene frequencies and the relative abundances of culturgens. The culturgens are the raw material of culture used by the epigenetic rules in assembling the mind. Thus, in place of the more familiar population-genetic equations of the form

$$p_k(t) = \begin{array}{l}\text{function of other gene frequencies} \\ \text{and environmental parameters}\end{array} \qquad (3\text{-}13)$$

for the change in time of frequency p_k of a gene G_k, we seek from the coevolutionary circuit systems of equations that reveal explicitly the coupling of genetic change to alterations in cultural form:

$$p_k(t) = \begin{array}{l}\text{function of gene frequencies,} \\ \text{culturgen frequencies, and} \\ \text{environmental properties;}\end{array} \qquad (3\text{-}14)$$

$$c_j(t) = \begin{array}{l}\text{function of gene frequencies,} \\ \text{culturgen frequencies, and} \\ \text{environmental properties;}\end{array} \qquad (3\text{-}15)$$

for genes G_k and culturgens c_j. (For convenience I have used the same symbol, c_j, to refer both to the culturgen itself and to its relative abundance in the class of culturgens of similar type. In general, the intended meaning will be clear from the context.)

The deduction of systems with the form of Equations 3-14 and 3-15 is rendered challenging not only by the complexity of the dependent phenomena, but also by the hierarchical structure of the coevolutionary circuit (recall Figure 3-9). The epigenetic rules, their operation during mental development, and the vagaries of individual decision and behavior all intervene as a network of causal linkage that couples phenomena on the level of the genes to events on the level of culture. But to formulate this linkage in a manner that takes account of its effects while placing genes and culturgens in direct juxtaposition, as in Equation 3-14, has until recently not been possible. The problem can be most clearly described by means of a commutative diagram. Let G represent the level of genetic organization, M the level of cognitive and behavioral organization, and C the level of cultural organization. We have seen that a description of the operation of the epigenetic rules provides a means of transition between G and M. Let us denote this map between the two levels as Ep, so that $Ep:G \to M$. The formalism of translation between individual decisions as

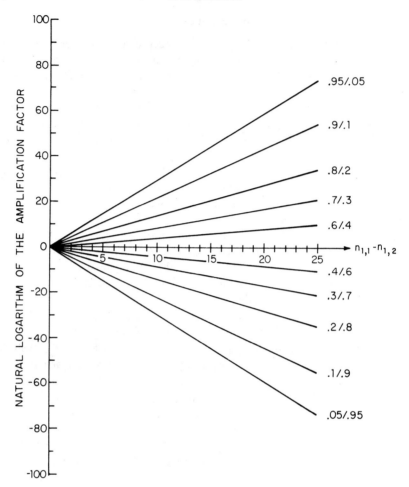

Figure 3-11. The amplification factor for the translation from individual cognitive development to cultural pattern. The isoclines of A are calculated for a society with 25 members. From Lumsden and Wilson (1981).

represented by the usage bias curves and cultural pattern as represented by the ethnographic curve $P(\mathbf{n}, t)$ provides a mapping, B, between mind M and culture C; $B: M \rightarrow C$. Thus under the combined action of Ep and B the levels $G, M,$ and C are linked:

$$G \xrightarrow{\quad Ep \quad} M \atop \Big\downarrow B \atop C$$

(3-16)

Coevolutionary systems with the form of Equations 3-14 and 3-15 will follow if it is possible to find the mapping, T, of gene-culture translation between G and C such that T is equivalent in its action to the combined operations $B \circ Ep$:

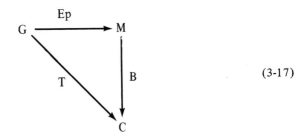

$$(3\text{-}17)$$

Recently, Lumsden and Wilson (1981) have reported methods whereby the relation between the levels G and C can be expressed in this direct manner. In order to summarize our approach, we consider again the simplest relevant case, that of a single epigenetic rule feeding on two culturgens, c_1 and c_2, and under control of a single genetic locus on a chromosome, at which the gene can take two forms A and a. Earlier in this chapter I reviewed evidence that changes in single genes can have selective and major effects on brain organization and development, on mental epigenesis, and on higher psychological functions such as choice and decision. Thus relative to the genetic locus of interest, the society is a biological population containing the three genotypes AA, Aa, and aa. Correspondingly, there are three classes of usage bias curves, represented by the transition probabilities

$$u_{ij}^{AA}(n_1), \qquad u_{ij}^{Aa}(n_1), \qquad u_{ij}^{aa}(n_1) \qquad (3\text{-}18)$$

and the transition rates

$$v_{ij}^{AA}(n_1), \qquad v_{ij}^{Aa}(n_1), \qquad v_{ij}^{aa}(n_1). \qquad (3\text{-}19)$$

All of these quantities are modulated by the pattern n_1 of overall culturgen usage. The ethnographic curve for the genotypic classes also has a more complex form than previously:

$$g(n_1^{AA}, n_1^{Aa}, n_1^{aa}, t) \; = \; \begin{array}{l} \text{the probability that, at time} \\ t, n_1^{AA} \text{ of the genotypes } AA \\ \text{are using culturgen } c_1, \text{ and so on;} \end{array} \qquad (3\text{-}20)$$

and obeys a complicated equation of motion that involves the epigenetic rules and usage patterns of all the genotypes (Lumsden & Wilson, 1981, p. 275).

It can be shown that the distribution $g(t)$ approaches a steady state, and if the social group is not too small ($\gtrsim 50$ individuals) and is not close to transition thresholds that shift the ethnographic curve from unimodality to multimodality, then $g(t)$ will in general be unimodal and sharply peaked. As a result, the pattern n_1 of overall culturgen usage will tend to lie close to its modal value, as will the distribution mean. The steady-state ethnographic curve again models $g(t)$ accurately if an individual life cycle is long enough to contain many decision points for each member, which is the general case in human societies; then $g(t)$ is for most of each generation in a form close to the steady-state solution. In turn, an analytical expression that approximates the exact steady-state curve follows from the observation that the usage pattern n_1 can with some loss in accuracy be replaced by its mean value $\bar{n}_1$. The society is thereby treated as a group of individuals rearranged from interacting with one another to interacting with a mean field of culturgen usage. After working out the probable patterns of individual usage in the presence of such a field, we find an equation relating the expected frequency of culturgen usage, $\bar{v} = \bar{n}_1/N$, directly to the frequencies p of gene A and q of gene a, where $p = 1-q$:

$$\bar{v} = \frac{p^2 v_{21}^{AA}(\bar{v})}{v_{12}^{AA}(\bar{v}) + v_{21}^{AA}(\bar{v})} + \frac{2pqv_{21}^{Aa}(\bar{v})}{v_{12}^{Aa}(\bar{v}) + v_{21}^{Aa}(\bar{v})} + \frac{q^2 v_{21}^{aa}(\bar{v})}{v_{12}^{aa}(\bar{v}) + v_{21}^{aa}(\bar{v})} . \quad (3\text{-}21)$$

The epigenetic rules appear via the usage biases in Equation 3-21, but in a manner that transforms them into a map between the frequencies of the genes and the frequencies of the culturgens. Equations directly relating the frequency of the genes to the culturgen frequencies by way of the usage bias curves, the patterns of individual decision making, and the specifics of the maturational timetables follow similarly (Lumsden & Wilson, 1981, chap. 6).

Our analysis of these pilot models involving the entire coevolutionary circuit has brought to light several noteworthy consequences of the coupling (Lumsden & Wilson, 1981). First, the tabula rasa state of pure cultural transmission is unstable. Under all plausible model conditions that we have investigated in which differential fitness benefits accrue from competing culturgens, genotypes prescribing a perfect lack of bias toward the culturgens are replaced by genotypes prescribing epigenetic rules that assemble a usage bias curve favoring the superior culturgen. This result is consistent with the general if not universal occurrence of biasing in the epigenetic rules of human behavior, as documented earlier in this chapter.

When individuals become sensitive to the usage pattern of other members of the society, the evolutionary replacement of inferior epigenetic rules closer to the tabula rasa state can be accelerated. This catalytic relationship can also be reciprocal. If sensitivity to cultural patterns is itself under genetic control, it can be enhanced by natural selection through its consistent association with the more successful culturgens.

Although biased epigenetic rules and sensitivity to usage can increase the overall rate of gene-culture coevolution, cultural transmission itself tends to slow genetic evolution *within* the coevolutionary process. The reason is that any capacity to acquire the less favorable culturgen—a property implicit in both pure cultural and gene-culture transmission—will reduce the effectiveness of natural selection below that made possible by pure genetic transmission.

Nevertheless, genetic evolution can proceed much more quickly than has been admitted in most earlier, intuitive treatments of human history. Even when the innate bias is weak in comparison with that generally observed in human developmental studies, the rate of change of gene frequency can be high enough even under mild natural selection to achieve the near replacement of one gene variant by another within as few as 50 generations, or about 1,000 years. Thus in some cultures genetic evolution might have taken place during periods of time in which relatively little culturgen innovation and social change occurred. Opportunities must have existed through both prehistoric and historical times for the genes underlying the epigenetic rules to track at least some major forms of culture and to push human mental development toward new forms of epigenetic rules favoring the more successful forms of cognition and behavior.

Finally, because of the phenomenon of usage sensitivity of the epigenetic rules and bias curves, natural selection of the genotypes is gene-frequency dependent. Its direction and intensity are determined by the number of individuals using alternative culturgens and consequently also by the frequencies of the competing gene variants that underlie the epigenetic rules. Under appropriate conditions the frequency dependence can lead to increased genetic diversity. For example, if the fitness generated by a particular culturgen begins to decline beyond a certain threshold of material benefits gained through culturgen usage, the genes favoring the usage of the culturgen may not proceed to fixation. When the postthreshold suppression is moderate, the alleles will stabilize at an intermediate frequency. When it is sufficiently strong the gene frequencies enter a chaotic regime in which they fluctuate widely. The two possibilities are illustrated in Figure 3-12.

Fitness suppression of an apparently appropriate nature is a common phenomenon in human societies. Among the !Kung San hunter-gatherers of the Kalahari desert, excessive attempts to accumulate goods and enhance personal status are met with ridicule merging in the more extreme cases into hostility. The result is the maintenance of nearly, but still less than perfectly, egalitarian societies (Lee, 1969). In economically more complex societies, role specialization and division of labor introduce another kind of suppression effect. Rising production of goods and services leads to intensifying competition, unstable markets, and ultimately a reduction in absolute benefits to the specialized producers. Higher costs in transport, storage, and processing can also play an inhibitory role. The feedback has produced a spreading out of economic and social roles, as conceived by traditional economic theory. But it might also have created a diversification of the genotypes underwriting role epigenesis and an enhanced degree of human genetic individuality.

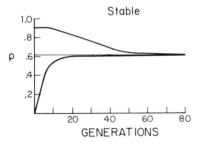 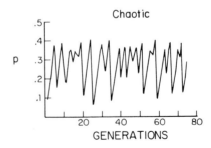

Figure 3-12. Changes in gene frequency in the suppression model of gene-culture coevolution. The symbol p denotes the frequency of gene variant A. *Left*: At lower levels of damping the trajectories of gene frequency approach a steady-state polymorphism in which both gene variants A and a are maintained in the population. *Right*: At higher levels of suppression the stable steady state breaks down and the frequencies of the gene variants A and a fluctuate chaotically in time. Similar behavior obtains for the culturgen frequencies. Modified from Lumsden and Wilson (1981).

Testing the Coevolutionary Circuit

Analysis of the gene-culture translation process demonstrates that substantial cultural diversity can be generated even by wholly inflexible rules of psychobiological development. It is therefore not the mere fact of cultural diversity per se that is of interest in the relation of cognitive-developmental theories to biological and anthropological explanations, but rather the *pattern* of the diversity, described in the theory of gene-culture coevolution by the ethnographic curves. Explicit predictions about ethnographic curves can be made from a knowledge of individual epigenetic rules and their interactions with one another. Conversely, certain conclusions about bias and likely pathways in mental development can be inferred from ordered patterns of ethnographic diversity. The empirical relation between the two levels of phenomena will constitute a stringent test of the validity of the theory of gene-culture coevolution, including its hypotheses about the nature of mental development.

The simplest and most direct conceivable test case would occur with a cognitive domain assembled by epigenetic rules that are highly biased, completely inflexible, independent of cultural context, and focused on two easily defined culturgens. The evidence available to us indicates that the phenomenon of sibling incest avoidance closely approximates this ideal set of conditions. We have recently given it particular attention (Lumsden & Wilson, 1980b, 1981).

A first approximation to the case of brother-sister incest has produced the approximate correspondence expected on the basis of gene-culture theory, although the data from both developmental studies and ethnography are not yet complete enough for us to attempt a detailed comparison of the predicted and empirical ethnographic curves. We have estimated the innate bias away from sibling incest to outbreeding to be close to absolute (the transition probability u_{21} approaches unity, where culturgen c_1 = incest avoidance and c_2 = incest behavior), and bias toward the practice of incest by an outbreeder to be close to zero (u_{12} approaches zero). Furthermore, the biases appear to be relatively insensitive to the usage pattern of other members of the society, and even to extreme degrees of social pressure in general. Thus, the $u_{ij}(n_1)$ can to a first approximation be treated as constants. Our basis for these inferences is the virtually total avoidance of full heterosexual activity in Israeli kibbutzim among unrelated young adults raised in close domestic proximity up to the age of 6 (Shepher, 1971). Their aversion to later sexual union persisted even though such behavior was approved and even encouraged by older kibbutz members. An equally impressive instance is the spectacular failure rate of the Taiwanese minor marriages, as described earlier, in which unions were contracted between sons of families and young females adopted into the families during childhood and raised with the sons in siblinglike fashion (Wolf, 1966, 1968, 1970; Wolf & Huang, 1980).

In Figure 3-13 I have depicted a set of ethnographic curves for the incest case based on different values of the u_{ij}, which are treated as constants. The actual data on brother-sister incest are too scarce and anecdotal to permit the drawing of the actual empirical curve as yet, but the scattered ethnographic accounts of a wide range of human societies (Berelson & Steiner, 1964; Murdock, 1949; van den Berghe & Mesher, 1980) suggest to us that the true curve falls closer to those generated by values of u_{21} in the range from .9 to .99 than to the other ethnographic curves displayed. A qualitative result near .99 would make pancultural avoidance of sibling incest a likely ethnographic state in societies numbering up to approximately 100 members. Moreover, the nature of the test data required from developmental and ethnographic studies has been exactly specified. Elsewhere we have conducted similar analyses of the fissioning of Amerindian villages and cyclical historical changes in women's fashions in Europe and the United States (Lumsden & Wilson, 1981).

The Significance of Gene-Culture Theory

Traditional sociobiology has made substantial progress toward explaining the forms of aggression, family structure, mate selection, and other categories of social behavior peculiar to human beings. It is methodologically sound and has stimulated new research. Yet it characterizes only the final behavioral product, which is related in some unspecified manner to the underlying genes and psychobiology. It has been able to deal with neither the mechanics of the mind nor the upward translation of human mental activity into the present diversity of cultural forms.

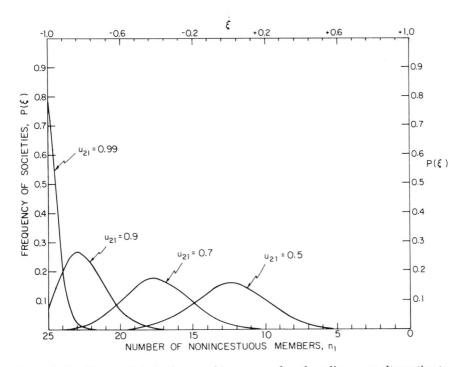

Figure 3-13. The predicted ethnographic curves of outbreeding as an alternative to brother-sister incest, within a social group of typical hunter-gatherer size (25 members). The usage bias is treated as a constant that is independent of usage patterns or other forms of social pressure; in human populations it appears to be closest to the range 0.9 to 0.99 among the values shown here. From Lumsden and Wilson (1980b).

In order that human sociobiology be carried to this next stage of explanatory capacity, it must be unified with cognitive science and the principles of cognitive-developmental theory. In short, we must insert the intervening epigenetic rules, most of which are distinctively human. The goal is an evolutionary theory of mind and culture that begins with the genes and the mechanisms that the genes create. In human beings genes do not dictate behavior; rather, they generate the organic processes of mental development, which we have termed epigenetic rules, that feed on culture to assemble the mind and channel its operation. Behavior is only one product of the mind as it deals with the events of daily life. Thus, whereas traditional sociobiology has attempted to treat the transition from genes to culture as a black box, there are in fact three major steps: from genes to the regularities of mental development, from mental development to decision and individual behavior, and from individual behavior to culture. The structures of mind are most effectively understood in terms of developmental processes, which are underwritten by genes whose frequencies are the result of the protracted interaction of behavior and selection forces working within the coevolutionary circuit. Thus to understand mind and its development fully is not just to perceive the rich detail of which it is composed, but to codify and follow it through each step in the coevolutionary circuit: from physiological time and historical change to evolutionary time and genetic change and back again.

The success of coevolutionary theory will depend ultimately on its capacity to perform three functions. First, it must derive or predict true propositions about human nature and its development that are unexplained axioms in other theories in the social sciences. Second, it should achieve a level of predictiveness and testability greater than that provided by competing modes of explanation, or at least contact the exact phenomenological models of disciplines such as economics and anthropology so as to make their underlying assumptions identical. Finally, it must suggest new questions and problems, as well as identify previously unknown phenomena of the coevolutionary process.

The particular formulation of gene-culture coevolution we have worked with must be adequately tested with reference to both its generality and its capacity to serve the human sciences by the criteria just stated. However, despite the incomplete nature of its data base and the crudity of its initial formal models, I believe that it has the advantage of incorporating a great deal of what is known about cognition and development in a manner that for the first time aligns this information with basic evolutionary biology. The formulation also establishes and analyzes for the first time the basic mechanism of the complete coevolutionary circuit. I suggest that a bridge can be constructed between the biological and social sciences by means of such methods, in a fashion that will place cognitive-developmental theories in their correct pivotal role, but without deemphasizing the uniqueness of the human species or the complexity and intrinsic interest of human thought and cultural diversity.

References

Alexander, R. D. *Darwinism and human affairs*. Seattle: University of Washington Press, 1979.

Amoore, J. E. Specific anosmia and the concept of primary odors. *Chemical Senses and Flavor*, 1977, *2*, 267-281.

Ashton, G. C., Polovina, J. J., & Vandenberg, S. G. Segregation analysis of family data for 15 tests of cognitive ability. *Behavior Genetics*, 1979, *9*, 329-347.

Atkinson, R. C., Bower, G. H., & Crothers, E. J. *An introduction to mathematical learning theory*. New York: Wiley, 1965.

Barlow, G. W., & Silverberg, J. (Eds.) *Sociobiology: Beyond nature/nurture? Reports, definitions and debate*. Boulder, Col.: Westview Press, 1980.

Bartholomew, D. J. *Stochastic models for social processes* (2nd ed.). New York: Wiley, 1973.

Berelson, B., & Steiner, G. A. *Human behavior: An inventory of scientific findings*. New York: Harcourt, Brace, & World, 1964.

Berger, P. L., & Luckmann, T. *The social construction of reality: A treatise in the sociology of knowledge*. Garden City, N. Y.: Doubleday, 1966.

Berlin, B., & Kay, P. *Basic color terms: Their universality and evolution*. Berkeley: University of California Press, 1969.

Biesele, M. Sapience and scarce resources: Communication systems of the !Kung and other foragers. *Social Science Information*, 1978, *17*, 921-947.

Bliss, T. V. P., & Errington, M. L. "Reeler" mutant mice fail to show spontaneous alternation. *Brain Research*, 1977, *124*, 168-170.

Blumberg, B. S., & Hesser, J. E. Anthropology and infectious disease. In A. Damon (Ed.), *Physiological anthropology*. New York: Oxford University Press, 1975.

Bock, K. *Human nature and history: A response to sociobiology*. New York: Columbia University Press, 1980.

Boehm, C. Rational preselection from hamadryas to *Homo sapiens*: The place of decisions in adaptive process. *American Anthropologist*, 1978, *80*, 265-296.

Bolton, R. Black, white, and red all over: The riddle of color term salience. *Ethnology*, 1978, *17*, 287-311.

Bonner, J. T. *The evolution of culture in animals*. Princeton, N.J.: Princeton University Press, 1980.

Bornstein, M. H. "Human infant color vision and color perception" reviewed and reassessed: A critique of Werner and Wooten (1979a). *Infant Behavior and Development*, 1981, *4*, 119-150.

Bornstein, M. H., & Marks, L. E. Color revisionism. *Psychology Today*, 1982, *16*, 64-66, 68-70, 73.

Bornstein, M. H., Kessen, W., & Weiskopf, S. The categories of hue in infancy. *Science*, 1976, *191*, 201-202.

Brainerd, C. J. The stage question in cognitive-developmental theory. *The Behavioral and Brain Sciences*, 1978, *1*, 173-213.

Buys, C. J., & Larson, K. L. Human sympathy groups. *Psychological Reports*, 1979, *45*, 547-553.

Caviness, V. S., Jr., & Rakic, P. Mechanisms of cortical development: A view from mutations in mice. *Annual Review of Neuroscience*, 1978, *1*, 297-326.

Chagnon, N. A., & Irons, W. (Eds.) *Evolutionary biology and human social behavior: An anthropological perspective*. North Scituate, Mass.: Duxbury Press, 1979.

Chiva, M. Comment la personne se construit en mangeant. *Communications* (Écoles des Hautes Études en Sciences Sociales–Centre d'Études Transdisciplinaires, Paris), 1979, *31*, 107-118.

Chomsky, N. *Rules and representations*. New York: Columbia University Press, 1980.

Clarke, D. L. *Analytical archaeology* (2nd ed., rev. by B. Chapman). New York: Columbia University Press, 1978.

Coleman, J. S. *Introduction to mathematical sociology*. New York: Free Press, 1964.

Coleman, J. S. *The mathematics of collective action*. Chicago: Aldine, 1973.

Cowart, B. J. Development of taste perception in humans: Sensitivity and preference throughout the life span. *Psychological Bulletin*, 1981, *90*, 43-73.

Daly, M., & Wilson, M. *Sex, evolution and behavior*. North Scituate, Mass.: Duxbury Press, 1978.

Davis, C. M. Self selection of diet by newly weaned infants. *American Journal of Diseases of Children*, 1928, *36*, 651-679.

DeCasper, A. J., & Fifer, W. P. Of human bonding: Newborns prefer their mothers' voices. *Science*, 1980, *208*, 1174-1176.

De Valois, R. L., & De Valois, K. K. Neural coding of color. In E. C. Carterette & M. P. Friedman (Eds.), *Handbook of perception* (Vol. 5). New York: Academic Press, 1975.

De Valois, R. L., & Jacobs, G. H. Primate color vision. *Science*, 1968, *162*, 533-540.

Donohue, W. A., Hawes, L. D., & Mabee, T. Testing a structural-functional model of group decision making using Markov analysis. *Human Communication Research*, 1981, *7*, 133-146.

Douglas, M. Accounting for taste. *Psychology Today*, 1979, *13*, 44-51.

Durham, W. H. The coevolution of human biology and culture. In N. Blurton Jones & V. Reynolds (Eds.), *Human adaptation and behavior*. New York: Halsted Press, 1978.

Eibl-Eibesfeldt, I. *Ethology: The biology of behavior* (2nd ed.). New York: Holt, Rinehart & Winston, 1975.

Eibl-Eibesfeldt, I. Human ethology: Concepts and implications for the sciences of man. *The Behavioral and Brain Sciences*, 1979, *2*, 1-57.

Eilers, R. E., Wilson, W. R., & Moore, J. M. Developmental changes in speech discrimination in infants. *Journal of Speech and Hearing Research*, 1977, *20*, 766-780.

Eimas, P. D., Siqueland, E. R., Jusczyk, P., & Vigorito, J. Speech perception in infants. *Science*, 1971, *171*, 303-306.

Emlen, S. T. An alternative case for sociobiology. *Science*, 1976, *192*, 736-738.

Fantz, R. L., Fagan, J. F., & Miranda, S. B. Early visual selectivity: As a function of pattern variables, previous exposure, age from birth and conception, and expected cognitive deficit. In L. B. Cohen & P. Salapatek (Eds.), *Infant perception: From sensation to cognition* (Vol. 1). New York: Academic Press, 1975.

Feldman, M. W., & Cavalli-Sforza, L. L. Cultural and biological evolutionary processes, selection for a trait under complex transmission. *Theoretical Population Biology*, 1976, *9*, 238-259.

Fishman, J. A. A systemization of the Whorfian hypothesis. *Behavioral Science*, 1960, *5*, 323-339.

Freedman, D. G. *Human infancy: An evolutionary perspective*. Hillsdale, N.J.: Erlbaum, 1974.

Gajdusek, D. C. Physiological and psychological characteristics of stone age man. *Science and Technology*, 1970, *33*, 26-33, 56-62.

Gelman, R., & Gallistel, C. R. *The child's understanding of number*. Cambridge, Mass.: Harvard University Press, 1978.

Gleason, H. A. *An introduction to descriptive linguistics.* New York: Holt, Rinehart, & Winston, 1961.

Goleman, G., & Bush, S. The liberation of sexual fantasy. *Psychology Today,* 1977, *11*, 48-53, 104-107.

Greeno, J. G. Representation of learning as discrete transition in finite state space. In D. H. Krantz, R. C. Atkinson, R. D. Luce, & P. Suppes (Eds.), *Contemporary developments in mathematical psychology* (Vol. 1). San Francisco: W. H. Freeman, 1974.

Hage, P. Structural balance and clustering in bushman kinship relations. *Behavioral Science,* 1976, *21*, 36-47.

Haggett, P. *Geography: A modern synthesis.* New York: Harper & Row, 1972.

Hallpike, C. R. *The foundations of primitive thought.* New York: Oxford University (Clarendon) Press, 1979.

Harris, M. *Cultural materialism: The struggle for a science of culture.* New York: Random House, 1979.

Hershenson, M., Munsinger, H., & Kessen, W. Preference for shapes of intermediate variability in the newborn infant. *Science,* 1965, *147*, 630-631.

Hockett, C. F., & Ascher, R. The human revolution. *Current Anthropology,* 1964, *5*, 135-147, 166-168.

Huxley, J. S. Cultural process and evolution. In A. Roe & G. G. Simpson (Eds.), *Behavior and evolution.* New Haven, Conn.: Yale University Press, 1958.

Irons, W. Cultural and biological success. In N. A. Chagnon & W. Irons (Eds.), *Evolutionary biology and human social behavior: An anthropological perspective.* North Scituate, Mass.: Duxbury Press, 1979.

Katz, S. H., Hediger, M. L., & Valleroy, L. A. Traditional maize processing techniques in the New World. *Science,* 1974, *184*, 765-773.

Kay, P., & McDaniel, C. K. The linguistic significance of the meanings of basic color terms. *Language,* 1978, *54*, 610-646.

Keil, F. C. *Semantic and cognitive development: An ontological perspective.* Cambridge, Mass.: Harvard University Press, 1979.

Keil, F. C. Constraints on knowledge and cognitive development. *Psychological Review,* 1981, *88*, 197-227.

Kemeny, J. G., & Snell, J. L. *Mathematical models in the social sciences.* Waltham, Mass.: Blaisdell, 1962.

Klaus, M. H., Jerauld, R., Kreger, N. C., McAlpine, W., Steffa, M., & Kennell, J. H. Maternal attachment: Importance of the first post-partum days. *New England Journal of Medicine,* 1972, *286*, 460-463.

Kovach, J. K. Mendelian units of inheritance control color preferences in quail chicks (*Coturnix coturnix japonica*). *Science,* 1980, *207*, 549-551.

Larkin, J., McDermott, J., Simon, D. P., & Simon, H. A. Expert and novice performance in solving physics problems. *Science,* 1980, *208*, 1335-1342.

Lee, R. B. Eating Christmas in the Kalahari. *Natural History,* 1969, *78*, 14, 16, 18, 21, 22, 60-63.

Lee, R. B. *The !Kung San: Men, women, and work in a foraging society.* New York: Cambridge University Press, 1979.

Lee, R. B., & DeVore, I. *Kalahari hunter-gatherers: Studies of the !Kung and their neighbours.* Cambridge, Mass.: Harvard University Press, 1976.

Lehoczky, J. P. Approximations for interactive Markov chains in discrete and continuous time. *Journal of Mathematical Sociology,* 1980, *7*, 139-157.

Lenski, G., & Lenski, J. *Human societies: A macrolevel introduction to sociology.* New York: McGraw-Hill, 1970.

Lévi-Strauss, C. *The raw and the cooked: Introduction to a science of mythology* (Vol. 1). New York: Harper & Row, 1969. (a)

Lévi-Strauss, C. *The elementary structures of kinship* (rev. ed.; J. H. Bell, trans.; J. R. von Sturmer & R. Needham, Eds.). Boston: Beacon Press, 1969. (b)

Liberman, A. M., Cooper, F. S., Shankweiler, D. P., & Studdert-Kennedy, M. Perception of speech code. *Psychological Review*, 1967, *74*, 431-461.

Lisker, L., & Abramson, A. S. A cross-language study of voicing in initial stops: Acoustical measurements. *Word*, 1964, *20*, 384-422.

Lockard, J. S., Daley, P. C., & Gunderson, V. M. Maternal and paternal differences in infant carry: U.S. and African data. *American Naturalist*, 1979, *113*, 235-246.

Loehlin, J. C., & Nichols, R. C. *Heredity, environment, and personality*. Austin: University of Texas Press, 1976.

Logue, A. W. Taste aversion and the generality of the laws of learning. *Psychological Bulletin*, 1979, *86*, 276-296.

Lumsden, C. J., & Wilson, E. O. Translation of epigenetic rules of individual behavior into ethnographic patterns. *Proceedings of the National Academy of Sciences of the United States of America*, 1980, *77*, 4382-4386. (a)

Lumsden, C. J., & Wilson, E. O. Gene-culture translation in the avoidance of sibling incest. *Proceedings of the National Academy of Sciences of the United States of America*, 1980, *77*, 6248-6250. (b)

Lumsden, C. J., & Wilson, E. O. *Genes, mind, and culture: The coevolutionary process*. Cambridge, Mass.: Harvard University Press, 1981.

Lumsden, C. J., & Wilson, E. O. Mind and the linkage between genes and culture: Précis of *Genes, mind, and culture*. *The Behavioral and Brain Sciences*, 1982, *5*, 1-7. (a)

Lumsden, C. J., & Wilson, E. O. Genes and culture, protest and communication. *The Behavioral and Brain Sciences*, 1982, *5*, 31-37. (b)

Maller, O., & Desor, J. A. Effect of taste on ingestion by human newborns. In J. Bosma (Ed.), *Fourth symposium on oral sensation and perception: Development in the fetus and infant*. Washington, D.C.: Government Printing Office, 1974.

Markl, H. (Ed.). *Evolution of social behavior, hypotheses and empirical tests: Report of the Dahlem Workshop on Evolution of Social Behavior, Hypotheses and Empirical Tests, Berlin, 1980*. Deerfield Beach, Fla.: Verlag Chemie, 1980.

Marks, I. M. *Fears and phobias*. New York: Academic Press, 1969.

Mauer, D., & Barrera, M. Infants: perception of natural and distorted arrangements of a schematic face. *Child Development*, 1981, *52*, 196-202.

Mayer, J., Dickie, M. M., Bates, M. W., & Vitale, J. J. Free selection of nutrients by hereditarily obese mice. *Science*, 1951, *113*, 745-746.

McClearn, G. E., & DeFries, J. C. *Introduction to behavioral genetics*. San Francisco: W. H. Freeman, 1973.

Mervis, C. B., & Rosch, E. Categorization of natural objects. *Annual Reviews of Psychology*, 1981, *32*, 89-115.

Montagu, A. (Ed.). *Sociobiology examined*. New York: Oxford University Press, 1980.

Morgan, G. A., & Ricciuti, H. N. Infants' response to strangers during the first year. In L. J. Stone, H. T. Smith, & L. B. Murphy (Eds.), *The competent infant: Research and commentary*. New York: Basic Books, 1973.

Mundinger, P. C. Animal cultures and a general theory of cultural evolution. *Ethology and Sociobiology*, 1980, *1*, 183-223.

Murdock, G. P. *Social structure*. New York: Macmillan, 1949.

Newell, A., & Simon, H. A. *Human problem solving*. Englewood Cliffs, N.J.: Prentice-Hall, 1972.

Osherson, D. N. *Logical abilities in children*. New York: Wiley, 1976.

Pinker, S. What is language, that a child may learn it, and a child, that he may learn language? *Journal of Mathematical Psychology*, 1981, *23*, 90-97.

Rakic, P. Genetic and epigenetic determinants of local neuronal circuits in the mammalian central nervous system. In F. O. Schmitt & F. G. Worden (Eds.), *The neurosciences: Fourth study program*. Cambridge, Mass.: M.I.T. Press, 1979.

Ramirez, I., & Sprott, R. L. Diet/taste and feeding behavior of genetically obese mice (C57BL/6J-*ob*/*ob*). *Behavioral and Neural Biology*, 1979, *25*, 449-472.

Rappaport, R. A. The sacred in human evolution. *Annual Review of Ecology and Systematics*, 1971, *2*, 23-44.

Ratliff, F. On the psychophysiological basis of universal color terms. *Proceedings of the American Philosophical Society*, 1976, *120*, 311-330.

Richerson, P. J., & Boyd, R. A dual inheritance model of the human evolutionary process; I: Basic postulates and a simple model. *Journal of Social and Biological Structures*, 1978, *1*, 127-154.

Rosch, E. Natural categories. *Cognitive Psychology*, 1973, *4*, 328-350.

Rozin, P. The selection of foods by rats, humans, and other animals. *Advances in the Study of Behavior*, 1976, *6*, 21-76.

Sahlins, M. *The use and abuse of biology: An anthropological critique of sociobiology*. Ann Arbor: University of Michigan Press, 1976.

Salk, L. The role of the heartbeat in relations between mother and infant. *Scientific American*, 1973, *228*, 24-29.

Schelling, T. C. *Micromotives and macrobehavior*. New York: Norton, 1978.

Seemonová, E. A study of children of incestuous matings. *Human Heredity*, 1971, *21*, 108-128.

Seligman, M. E. P. Introduction. In M. E. P. Seligman & J. L. Hager (Eds.), *Biological boundaries of learning*. New York: Appleton-Century-Crofts, 1972. (a)

Seligman, M. E. P. Phobias and preparedness. In M. E. P. Seligman & J. L. Hager (Eds.), *Biological boundaries of learning*. New York: Appleton-Century-Crofts, 1972. (b)

Shepher, J. Mate selection among second-generation kibbutz adolescents and adults: Incest avoidance and negative imprinting. *Archives of Sexual Behavior*, 1971, *1*, 293-307.

Shettleworth, S. J. Constraints on learning. *Advances in the Study of Behavior*, 1972, *4*, 1-58.

Simon, H. A. *Models of thought*. New Haven, Conn.: Yale University Press, 1979.

Simon, H. A. *The sciences of the artificial* (2nd ed.). Cambridge, Mass.: M.I.T. Press, 1981.

Steiner, J. E. Oral and facial innate motor responses to gustatory and to some olfactory stimuli. In J. H. A. Kroeze (Ed.), *Preference behaviour and chemoreception*. London: Information Retrieval, 1979.

Stern, C. *Principles of human genetics* (3d ed.). San Francisco: W. H. Freeman, 1973.

Symons, D. *The evolution of human sexuality*. New York: Oxford University Press, 1979.

Trabasso, T., & Bower, G. H. *Attention in learning*. New York: Wiley, 1968.

van den Berghe, P. L. *Human family systems: An evolutionary view*. New York: Elsevier, 1979.

van den Berghe, P. L., & Mesher, G. M. Royal incest and inclusive fitness. *American Ethnologist*, 1980, *7*, 300-317.

VanDeventer, A. D., & Laws, D. R. Orgasmic reconditioning to redirect sexual arousal in pedophiles. *Behavior Therapy*, 1978, *9*, 748-765.

Vogel, F. Neurobiological approaches in human behavior genetics. *Behavior Genetics*, 1981, *11*, 87-102.

von Wattenwyl, A., & Zollinger, H. Color-term salience and neurophysiology of color vision. *American Anthropologist*, 1979, *81*, 279-288.

Weinberg, S. K. *Incest behavior* (rev. ed.). New York: Citadel Press, 1976.

Wexler, K., & Culicover, P. W. *Formal principles of language acquisition.* Cambridge, Mass.: M.I.T. Press, 1980.

Whissell-Buechy, D., & Amoore, J. E. Odour-blindness to musk: Simple recessive inheritance. *Nature*, 1973, *242*, 271-273.

White, L. A. Ethnological theory. In R. W. Sellars, V. J. McGill, & M. Farber (Eds.), *Philosophy for the future.* New York: Macmillan, 1949.

Whorf, B. L. *Language, thought, and reality.* Cambridge, Mass.: M.I.T. Press, 1956.

Williams, T. R. *Introduction to socialization: Human culture transmitted.* St. Louis, Mo.: C. V. Mosby, 1972.

Wilson, E. O. *Sociobiology: The new synthesis.* Cambridge, Mass.: Belknap Press of the Harvard University Press, 1975.

Wilson, R. S. Synchronies in mental development: An epigenetic perspective. *Science*, 1978, *202*, 939-948.

Wobst, H. M. Boundary conditions for paleolithic social systems: A simulation approach. *American Antiquity*, 1974, *39*, 147-178.

Wolf, A. P. Childhood association, sexual attraction, and the incest taboo: A Chinese case. *American Anthropologist*, 1966, *68*, 883-898.

Wolf, A. P. Adopt a daughter-in-law, marry a sister: A Chinese solution to the problem of the incest taboo. *American Anthropologist*, 1968, *70*, 864-874.

Wolf, A. P. Childhood association and sexual attraction: a further test of the Westermarck hypothesis. *American Anthropologist*, 1970, *72*, 503-515.

Wolf, A. P., & Huang, C. S. *Marriage and adoption in China, 1845-1945.* Stanford, Calif.: Stanford University Press, 1980.

4. Working-Memory Systems and Cognitive Development

Charles J. Brainerd

It often happens that a field of inquiry comes to be so dominated by a theoretical tradition that new developments are inclined to be smothered. By the end of the Renaissance, for example, the authority of Aristotle had become so pervasive that, as Bertrand Russell remarked in his history of philosophy, "Ever since the beginning of the seventeenth century, almost every serious intellectual advance has had to begin with an attack on some Aristotlian doctrine." Much the same could be said of the effect of Newtonian mechanics on physics by the end of the 19th century, or the effect of psychoanalysis on abnormal psychology by the 1940s, or closer to home, the effect of Piagetian theory on the contemporary science of cognitive development. The enormous influence that Piaget's ideas achieved during the preceding two decades, together with the theory's almost universal scope, mean that, for the near term at least, any significant reorientation of our assumptions about cognitive development is destined to conflict with some Piagetian tenet or another.

The approach to cognitive development that I shall outline in this chapter is at variance with two such tenets, one of them general and the other specific. The general point of disagreement is an assumption that lies at the core of Piagetian theory —explicitly, the idea that cognitive development cannot be "reduced" to the development of "simpler" psychological processes such as perception, learning, and language. Over the years, this claim has been repeated in numerous articles and monographs emanating from Geneva. Perhaps the best known illustration is Piaget's first major book, *The Language and Thought of the Child*, wherein it was suggested that cognition is not synonymous with language because language development is subject to the cognitive-developmental principle of egocentrism. Research designed to show that development in other psychological domains is controlled by the stages and structures of the theory has appeared on perception (e.g., Piaget, 1967), mental imagery (e.g., Piaget & Inhelder, 1971), learning (e.g., Inhelder, Sinclair, & Bovet, 1974), and other topics.

The specific point of disagreement between the theory and this chapter is whether or not cognitive development can be reduced to memory development. The case for the negative view can be found in a series of papers (e.g., Inhelder, 1969) and two books (Piaget, 1968; Piaget & Inhelder, 1973) that were published during the late 1960s and early 1970s. The empirical centerpiece of these works is a single datum: There sometimes are long-term improvements in children's ability to remember stimuli that are related to the concrete-operational stage (seriated arrays, horizontal water levels, etc.). Although this finding is replicable (cf. Liben, 1977), hardly anyone outside Geneva regards it as presumptive evidence that stages and structures must be invoked to explain memory development. There are three principal reasons. First, the phenomenon itself, which is usually called hypermnesia in the memory literature, is well established for stimuli (e.g., pictures of household objects) that have no known connection to Piagetian stages (e.g., Erdelyi, Finkelstein, Herrell, Miller, & Thomas, 1976; Erdelyi & Kleinbard, 1978). Second, hypermnesia has been found in subject populations (university undergraduates) that are not undergoing development, at least not in the Genevan sense. Third, the existence of this phenomenon does not appear to be utterly inexplicable in terms of modern information processing concepts of memory.

The underlying thesis of this chapter is that cognitive development can, in fact, be reduced to memory development. This statement does not mean that there is a "thing" called memory development, that there is another "thing" called cognitive development, and that the latter is built up from the former as a wall is constructed from individual bits of brick and mortar. Instead, it means that memory development and cognitive development differ as do child and adult: The development of memory is the childhood of cognition; the development of cognition is the adulthood of memory. More particularly, there are three basic claims: (a) There is a target developmental data base that we seek to explain. These data, which for reasons of our own we have decided to call cognitive development, are concerned with age-related changes in performance on a certain family of complex tasks such as reading, conservation, mental calculation, perspective taking, and moral reasoning. This family of tasks is ill defined, though its members are widely believed to tap such processes as thinking, reasoning, and problem solving. (b) There is a theoretical language consisting of concepts such as "short-term storage," "encoding," and "retrieval from long-term memory" that has evolved from the laboratory study of memory. In comparison to the vague machinery of Piagetian theory, these concepts are operationally well defined. (c) The semantics of this language is sufficiently rich to be capable of explaining the facts of cognitive development as we understand them. The aim of what follows is to show that this third statement is perhaps not entirely without foundation.

The chapter proceeds in four stages. In the first section, background matters are considered. Specifically, some highly suggestive facts about the influence of memory variables on cognitive task performance are reviewed. In the second section, the history of working-memory analysis is summarized, and detailed examples are given of how working-memory models can be built and elaborated for given tasks. In the third section, research strategies for tying working-memory structures to specific aspects of children's performance are examined and the results of relevant experiments are reported. The qualitative sieve is the featured research strategy. The last section is entirely concerned with metatheoretical issues. The general question posed in that section is, Does working-memory analysis allow one to gain leverage on some of the conceptual issues that have been traditional points of reference in cognitive-developmental theory?

Effects of Memory Variables on Cognitive Development

Genevan antipathy to memory-based explanations notwithstanding, a common finding in the literature is that memory variables exert a powerful influence on a child's performance on cognitive tasks. A compelling illustration is provided by one of the simplest and most "noncognitive" of such variables, short-term memory span (the number of items that can be retrieved on an immediate recall test after one study trial).

The relationship between span length and various cognitive tasks has been studied since Ebbinhaus's time. Early work established that span length is strongly correlated with children's grades in school (Jacobs, 1887) and that mentally retarded individuals have very short spans (Galton, 1887). Also, the measurement of short-term memory span was a regular feature of early tests of intelligence (Binet & Henri, 1895). More recently, high correlations have been observed between span length and performance on modern intelligence tests (e.g., Jensen, 1964). In older children and adolescents, span length accounts for as much as 50-70% of the variance on school achievement tests such as the verbal subscale of the Scholastic Aptitude Test (SAT), the mathematical subscale of the same test, and the College Entrance Examination Board English test (see Dempster, 1981). Span length is also known to be correlated with reading disability in children (Koppitz, 1977), as are various other memory factors (Morrison & Manis, 1982; Vellutino & Scanlon, 1982), and with their levels of language development (Brown & Fraser, 1963). In adults, span length is related to several measures of text difficulty in reading (Rothkopf, 1980) and to reading comprehension (Daneman & Carpenter, 1980).

As regards the familiar thinking and reasoning paradigms associated with Piaget's concrete- and formal-operational stages, it has long been known that span length correlates with performance on such tasks. The first systematic evidence appears to have been reported by McLaughlin (1963). However, the most comprehensive findings come from a recent series of longitudinal studies by Hooper and his associates (Hooper, Swinton, & Sipple, 1976, 1979a). Hooper et al. examined the relationship between word span, digit span, and the following Piagetian measures: identity conservation, equivalence conservation, class inclusion, combinatorial reasoning, transitive inference, cardinal number, ordinal number, and eight tasks designed to measure the *groupement* structures (Piaget, 1942). The subjects were from kindergarten through Grade 9. Significant correlations, some accounting for as much as 40% of the variance, were observed between individual measures of span length (word or digit) and individual Piagetian tasks. Since the reliability of individual span-length tests is modest (see Dempster, 1981), it is likely that these correlations would have been even larger if some measure of combined word and digit span had been used.

In addition to results on span length, other findings suggest that short-term memory failures often are responsible for the errors that are observed on Piagetian measures, and therefore that the development of short-term memory accounts for large slices of the age variation in performance on these tasks. The empirical case for such a conclusion is particularly well documented for infant object permanence and children's transitive inferences.

With regard to object permanence, in the usual task (Piaget, 1954) an object to which an infant is attending is successively hidden at one or more positions. The infant is allowed to search for the object after a few seconds' delay. The Piagetian interpretation of infants' search errors is that they fail to understand that objects continue to exist when perceptual contact is not being made with them; out of sight is out of mind. But if previously encoded information (in this case, the loci of hidden objects) tends to fall out of short-term memory rapidly, the delay interval between hiding and search will cause search failures regardless of whether or not infants have the object concept. Consistent with this argument, both Bower (e.g., 1967) and Gratch (e.g., Gratch, Appel, Evans, Le Compte, & Wright, 1974) have shown that search failures decrease when the hide-search interval is shortened. Some of Bower's data suggest that infants younger than 12 months cannot usually hold information in short-term memory for intervals exceeding 5 seconds. In addition to rapid short-term memory decay, infants may be especially susceptible to proactive interference. If previously encoded information (the early hidings in a sequence) tends to interfere with the encoding of subsequent information (the last hiding), search failures will occur even though out of sight is not out of mind. Harris (1975) has reviewed evidence that proactive interference manipulations do, in fact, increase search errors on object permanence tasks. Finally, short-term memory factors other than decay rate and proactive interference have been implicated in performance on object permanence tasks (e.g., Cornell, 1981).

As for transitive inference, the basic transitivity paradigm makes use of three objects (A, B, and C) that differ by small amounts on some physical dimension (e.g., length or weight). The subjects are informed of the A-B and B-C relationships, either verbally by the experimenter or by carrying out measurements, and are required to deduce the A-C relationship. It is also common to introduce a visual illusion of some sort that runs counter to the true A-C relationship (e.g., the Müller-Lyer illusion for length or the size-weight illusion for weight). Since the A-C relationship must be deduced from the A-B and B-C relationships, it is obvious that the problem cannot be solved unless the latter relationships are encoded in the first place and are held in storage as the task proceeds. Roodin and Gruen (1970) were the first to connect short-term memory failures directly to the transitivity errors that are commonly observed during the first half of elementary school. They conducted an uncomplicated study in which kindergarten, first-grade, and second-grade children were administered two types of transitivity problems: (a) standard items of the type just described and (b) identical items with a memory hint added. The memory hint consisted of merely reminding the children of the A-B and B-C relationships just before they were asked to make a transitive inference. The results were dramatic. In Condition (a) the usual high incidence of errors was obtained. The percentages of correct inferences were 12.5%, 50.0%, and 58.3%, respectively, for kindergarteners, first graders, and second graders. Thus, normal improvement with age was observed, and at the second-grade level, the nominal lower age bound for concrete operations, only about half the inferences were correct. But in Condition (b) the percentages of correct inferences were 81.3%, 85.4%, and 89.6%, respectively, for kindergarteners, first graders, and second graders. Although one is tempted to focus on the memory hint's large effect at all age levels, note that the change was most pronounced in the youngest subjects, and more particularly, that the age trend in Condition (a) vanished when the hint was available. Within this age range at any rate, such results suggest that there are no developmental trends in the accuracy of transitive inference per se if one controls for age differences in short-term memory capacity.

The most detailed evidence about the effects of short-term memory on transitivity, or on any other Piagetian concept for that matter, come from a series of experiments by Trabasso and his associates (Bryant & Trabasso, 1971; Lutkus & Trabasso, 1974; Riley & Trabasso, 1974; Trabasso, 1975, 1977; Trabasso & Riley, 1975; Trabasso, Riley, & Wilson, 1975). One aim of this research was to evaluate process models of how serial order information is stored in memory at the time of encoding and is retrieved at the time of test to produce a transitive inference. On the whole, the data favored a model in which such information (a) is stored in a linear structure of some sort (e.g., as points on a straight line with interpoint distances being determined by the physical distance between simuli on the relevant dimension), and (b) is retrieved by scanning the linear structure from one end to the other. It is significant that this model fit the data of three age levels: children in the preoperational age range, children in the concrete-operational age range, and college students.

For present purposes, however, the most interesting datum is that, in agreement with Roodin and Gruen's (1970) findings, appropriate controls for short-term memory failure markedly improved the performance of young children and virtually erased age differences in the accuracy of transitive inference. The relevant data appear in a paper by Bryant and Trabasso (1971). Whereas Roodin and Gruen simply reintroduced the crucial information just before inference, Bryant and Trabasso used a more elegant procedure whose effect was to circumvent short-term memory deficits altogether. If, as seems unarguable from extant data, there are massive age differences in short-term memory capacity during early childhood, an obvious method of controlling for the effects of such differences on transitivity is to transfer all the critical information to a memory system that has much greater capacity, long-term memory. Bryant and Trabasso's method of achieving this result was to administer five-term problems (e.g., $A > B > C > D > E$) in which magnitude differences were perfectly correlated with the color of the objects (A = red, B = yellow, etc.). Prior to making transitive inferences, children in the 4- to 7-year-old range were given extensive pretraining on the adjacent pairs in the series—that is, they were trained until they knew the direction of the relevant *magnitude* difference between each pair of adjacent colors. When these discriminations had been learned, the experimenter requested judgments about the nonadjacent pairs (e.g., A-C, B-D, C-E). The rates of correct inferences were very high at all age levels, ranging from about three-quarters correct in the youngest subjects to essentially perfect in the oldest subjects. Similar rates of accuracy were found in a later study of retarded subjects in which the same paradigm was used (Lutkus & Trabasso, 1974). In a previous study, McManis (1969) had reported no evidence of transitivity in retarded samples until the subjects had attained a mental age of 10 or 11. However, Lutkus and Trabasso found correct response rates in the three-quarters to perfect range for retarded samples with mental ages (MAs) of 5 and 6, respectively.

Unlike Roodin and Gruen's (1970) study, there was a residual age trend, although a small one, in transitivity in the Bryant and Trabasso (1971) experiments. But the trend is not difficult to explain in memory language. Although the pretraining regimen may ensure that all subjects, regardless of age, have the relevant magnitude information in storage, it does not necessarily control for developmental differences in children's ability to retrieve information from long-term memory. Such an explanation is consistent with recent evidence from studies of young children's cued recall (e.g., Brainerd & Howe, 1982; Brainerd, Howe, & Desrochers, 1982) and free recall (e.g., Emmerich & Ackerman, 1978; Heisel, 1981) in which age differences in retrieval have been reported that are independent of age differences in storage.

A final illustration of the pervasive effects of memory variables on Piagetian logical-reasoning tasks is provided by a series of experiments on children's probability judgments that will be considered in some detail later in this chapter. In Genevan theory, probabilistic judgment and reasoning do not emerge until the formal-operational stage (see Piaget & Inhelder, 1951). The usual task that is used to measure age differences in probability judgment is a random-draws problem. At the outset, elements of two or more distinctive classes (e.g., red poker chips and blue poker chips) are placed in a container, and the container is shaken to randomize the contents. The child is then asked to predict the results of a series of random draws from the container by the experimenter. Assuming that sampling from the container is always with replacement, the correct response on each trial is to predict that an element from the most numerous set will be drawn. When such problems are administered to preschoolers and elementary schoolers, this is not the pattern of predictions that materializes. On the first trial in a sequence, children in the 4- to 8-year-old range typically predict the correct set more often than would be anticipated by chance, though by only a slight margin. (For example, if there are only two sets in the container, the correct prediction rate is about 70%.) On later trials in a sequence, these children's predictions are uncorrelated with numerousness, and instead appear to be based on complex response alternation rules. It is not until age 10 or 11 that the predictions on most trials are correct. Although this could mean that subjects are incapable of probabilistic reasoning before adolescence, it could also mean that short-term memory for the relevant numerosity information fails in young children, either in the sense of storage failure or in the sense of retrieval failure. When the procedure is modified in such a way that children are constrained both to retain numerosity information in storage and to retrieve it at the time of test, the performance of 4- to 8-year-olds becomes essentially perfect, and like

Roodin and Gruen's (1970) transitivity results, the age differences on the standard task vanish.

More generally, success on all Piaget-type paradigms requires that some specific items of background information be encoded into short-term memory, and that they be held there until the processing operations that lead to response selection can be brought to bear. On a number conservation problem, for example, a solution would not seem to be possible unless the subject encodes the fact that the two rows were equal in the first place and manages to retain this fact until the perceptual transformation has been performed and the experimenter's question has been posed. Likewise, a solution would not seem to be possible on class inclusion problems unless the cardinal numbers of the superordinate and subordinate classes have been encoded and are held in storage until after the experimenter's question has been posed.

To sum up, experience has taught us that it is not difficult to tie familiar memory variables, especially short-term memory variables, to performance on the tasks that have generated the bulk of our fact library on cognitive development. On the contrary, the strength of these memory-cognition relationships is generally much greater than relationships that have been reported for nonmemorial variables (e.g., measures of stage of cognitive development, measures of linguistic sophistication, measures of socioemotional development). Actually, as this précis of studies is intended to illustrate, it is possible in certain situations to account for all the age-related variation in cognitive performance with memory manipulations.

Results such as these are essential preliminaries to a memory-based view of cognitive development. Without them, attempts to explore the possibility that cognitive development can be reduced to memory development would be premature at best. Despite their importance, however, such results are of limited theoretical utility. They are, after all, purely descriptive. What they establish is that students of cognitive development ignore memory development at their peril. But they do not show that it is usually possible to build sensible, testable, and parsimonious models of cognitive development by relying on information processing concepts of memory. Nor do they show that it is possible to connect specific components of such models to given types of data on age-related changes. This is the business of formalized working-memory analysis.

Fundamentals of Working-Memory Analysis

History of Working-Memory Analysis, Dimly Adumbrated

The idea of analyzing performance on cognitive tasks in terms of "working-memory systems" was first given extensive consideration in the research of Baddeley and his associates (e.g., Baddeley & Hitch, 1974; Baddeley, Scott, Drynan, & Smith, 1969; Hitch, 1978a, 1978b). In these early papers, the working-memory concept was closely related to then-current models of short-term memory, more particularly to Atkinson and Shiffrin's (1968) theory of short-term storage. The general hypothesis was uncomplicated: Since the standard paradigms of the adult cognition laboratory require that certain target information be retained for brief intervals and be transformed in some manner by the subject, short-term memory factors ought to provide a productive path to understanding data from such paradigms.

At the time, however, the weight of evidence seemed to be against this hypothesis. In the medical literature, Warrington and Shallice (1969; Shallice & Warrington, 1970; Warrington, Logue, & Pratt, 1971; Warrington & Weiskrantz, 1973) had conducted some investigations of the cognitive performance of patients with severely impaired short-term memories. Impairment was defined by variables such as grossly restricted span length and poor performance on Brown-Peterson distractor tasks. Although one expects from the hypothesis that the cognitive performance of such patients should be quite defective, they performed about as well as normals. Similarly, with normal subjects, failures to implicate short-term memory in tasks such as concept identification (Coltheart, 1972) and verbal comprehension (Patterson, 1971) had been reported.

Not surprisingly, then, early research on the working-memory concept was concerned to establish a firm link between short-term memory functioning and cognitive performance. Baddeley and Hitch (1974), for example, described the aims of their experiments as follows: "First, is there any evidence that the tasks of reasoning, comprehension, and learning share a common working memory system?; and secondly, if such a system exists, how is it related to our current conception of STM?" (p. 49). The methodological focus of these early experiments was the use of concurrent processing manipulations. In the simplest instance of such a manipulation, subjects hold a near-span number of irrelevant items (e.g., nonsense syllables) in storage while they perform, say, an arithmetic test (cf. Wanner & Shiner, 1976). In a typical experiment (Baddeley & Hitch, 1974, Experiment 2), the relationship between short-term memory load and reading comprehension was studied. The reading items consisted of 32 sentences to which subjects had to respond true or false. Control subjects were shown the sentences one at a time and responded true or false to each. For experimental subjects, however, each sentence was preceded by a string of six random letters. The sentence was then presented. After the subject had responded to the sentence, he or she was given an immediate recall test for the six letters. The principal finding was that sentence response latencies were several hundred milliseconds longer in experimental subjects. Baddeley and Hitch obtained similar results for sentence response latencies when the concurrent processing manipulations involved covert rehearsal of the word *the*, covert rehearsal of the number sequence *one-two-three-four-five-six*, and covert rehearsal of a random sequence of six digits. Baddeley and Hitch also found that concurrent processing manipulations affected comprehension of prose passages.

With evidence of this sort in hand, research can proceed to the more interesting question of whether it is possible to build detailed working-memory systems to account for performance on tasks such as mental addition, sentence verification, text comprehension, probability judgment, and the like. As a rule, a preliminary working-memory system is constructed for the paradigm of interest on the basis of task considerations. Experimentation is then directed both toward identifying which components of the system, if any, are the most important ones in performance and toward articulating the conceptual structure of individual components. It is this theoretical use of working memory to devise serious explanatory models that constitutes mainstream working-memory analysis. Some practical examples of how such models are used to explain children's performance and to explain age-related changes in performance will now be considered.

Working-Memory Models of Cognitive Development

Because the objective of a working-memory model is to explain facts, not merely to offer a heuristic framework within which experimentation can proceed, it follows that the working-memory system that one constructs for a target paradigm will necessarily possess features that are unique to that paradigm. But any working-memory analysis will share some central distinctions with other such analyses. I briefly consider these shared distinctions before presenting some worked illustrations of models for specific tasks.

Conceptual Machinery. The key distinction is between storing information and processing it, with further subdivisions being possible between different forms of storage activity and different forms of processing activity. With respect to storage, although it is always possible that the information presented in a cognitive task may be transferred to long-term memory, the types of storage operations in a working-memory system are temporary. In line with existing data on temporary storage, information that is encoded into short-term memory is assumed to be consciously attended to, and therefore the subject presumably does not have to retrieve it in order to be able to use it. (Of course, the latter statement does not apply to information stored in long-term memory.) Generally speaking, cognitive tasks impose two types of storage constraints on subjects. First, there is some initial information, which includes any questions or response alternatives presented by the experimenter, that must be encoded and retained: On a transitive inference problem, the A-B and B-C relations and the experimenter's question must be stored; on a mental addition item, propositions of the form $m + n = ?$ must be stored; on conservation problems, the initial quantitative relationship between the standard and variable stimulus and the experimenter's question must be stored; on probability judgment items, the initial numerosities of the sets must be stored and then each of the experimenter's questions must be stored.

The second type of storage involves internally generated information. On certain tasks, initial stages of processing produce information that is critical to later stages of processing. Hence, this intermediate information must be held in storage until the remaining processing operations can be completed. A simple illustration of the second type of storage occurs in iterative models of mental addition and subtraction. According to such models, mental arithmetic items of the form $m + n = ?$ and $m - n = ?$ are solved by transforming the encoded representation of a problem as follows. A counter is first set to the value of the larger of two numbers in the problem (m). The counter is then either incremented (addition items) or decremented (subtraction items) exactly n times, and a solution is read out. A model of this sort is capable of finding solutions only if subjects manage to store the results of each successive iteration of the counter. Unless subjects know the total number of times that the counter has been incremented or decremented, it is obvious that they will not know when to stop and read out the solution.

On the processing side of working-memory models, a distinction is drawn between two types of processing, namely, processing that transforms stored information in some way and processing that faithfully reproduces stored information. The latter operates on the contents of long-term memory, whereas the former operates on the information that is stored in short-term memory. For simplicity, I shall refer to the second type of processing as *retrieval* and to the first type of processing as *computation*.

We have seen that cognitive tasks require that subjects transform, translate, or otherwise alter information that has been encoded into short-term memory. As a rule, the information in short-term memory consists of some crucial "background facts" (e.g., numerical equivalence of rows in number conservation, relative lengths of adjacent objects in transitivity of length, relative numerosities of sets in probability judgment) *plus the specific response alternatives that subjects must choose between*, with the latter normally being provided in questions posed by the experimenter (e.g., "Do the two rows have the same number?" in number conservation; "Which is longer, A or C?" in transitivity of length; "Am I more likely to draw an A or a B?" in probability judgment). From an abstract point of view, therefore, the subject's task is to transform the background facts in such a way that one of the available responses is delivered as a solution.

The computational operations that map background facts onto the response alternatives are not provided to the subjects; they must bring these operations with them to the experiment. Thus, a working-memory model assumes that such operations are stored in long-term memory. But having appropriate computational mechanisms in long-term memory is not all that is required in order to transform the information into solutions. It is also necessary to activate them at the proper times and in the proper sequences. This is the function of retrieval in a working-memory system. The information stored in short-term memory, including any intermediate results of initial computations, is assumed to act as a source of retrieval cues. These cues cause subjects to search their long-term knowledge banks for computational operations that are appropriate to the task at hand. Once such an operation is located, it can be retrieved to consciousness and applied to the contents of short-term memory.

The computational operations that are retrieved on cognitive tasks will obviously vary in complexity as a function of task demands. On a sentence verification task, about all that appears to be necessary is that the meanings of the individual words be properly understood. Computation is slightly more difficult in a probability judgment task, where subjects presumably must possess and be able to retrieve response rules that give the relationship between relative frequency and random sampling. Computation is still more complicated in mental arithmetic tasks involving sequences of calculations (e.g., $56 - 14 - 12 - 5 = ?$).

These examples indicate that the concept of "computational operation" is used in a very broad sense in working-memory models, ranging from knowledge of simple facts to complex calculations. The architecture of these operations in specific models depends critically on the demands of the task. It also depends critically on

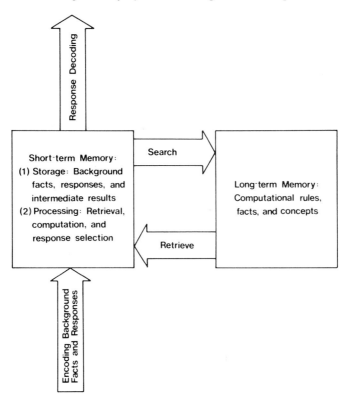

Figure 4-1. The basic diagram of how information flows through a working-memory system.

the structure of the traces that are stored in short-term memory. However, all working-memory models share the assumption that such operations are stored in long-term memory and that subjects must be able to retrieve them in order to process the contents of short-term memory.

The points considered so far can be conveniently summarized in the *basic diagram of information flow* for working-memory systems. As can be seen in Figure 4-1, the subject must first encode the background information and the response alternatives into short-term memory. A search for appropriate computational operations is then carried out in long-term memory, using the information in short-term memory as a source of retrieval cues. Computational operations are then retrieved to consciousness and applied to the contents of short-term memory to produce a response. Although these statements seem to imply that working-memory systems are intrinsically serial, it is not difficult to devise both parallel and mixed serial-parallel interpretations of structures like that in Figure 4-1 (e.g., cf. Taylor, 1976).

A last general point about working-memory systems is concerned with their capacity limitations. Short-term memory provides the "work space" where storing and processing operations are executed. Most experimental evidence points to the conclusion that short-term memory is a system with sharp capacity constraints.

Since the appearance of Miller's (1956) influential paper, it has been common to refer to the units of short-term memory capacity as chunks. It is usually assumed that a subject's short-term memory capacity is some small, discrete number of chunks, and developmental improvements in performance on short-term memory tasks (e.g., span length) are often explained on the ground that the number of available chunks increases with age.

In working-memory analysis, the units or chunks of short-term memory can be used for both storing and processing. That is, working-memory systems are believed to be flexible with respect to how many units are used for storing and processing, respectively. Such flexibility is essential because it allows subjects to fine tune working memory to accommodate the varying storing-processing requirements of different tasks. At one extreme there are tasks that place a premium on storage and require only simple processing. Sternberg-type tasks, where subjects hold several stimuli in storage simultaneously and merely scan their internal structures in order to generate responses (e.g., Murdock, 1976), are standard illustrations. At the other extreme are tasks that require complex processing of very small amounts of encoded information. Item identification problems, where subjects must identify a single stimulus (e.g., a word) in the presence of masking information (e.g., Huttenlocher & Burke, 1976; Rabbitt, 1968), are cases in point. There are still other tasks that, intuitively at least, seem to place relatively equal emphasis on storing and processing. For example, suppose that a subject is asked to calculate mentally the square root of 51 to two decimal places. Here, the initial problem must be stored, and the results of the three main steps in the calculation must be stored. But subjects must also execute three multiplication operations and two subtraction operations in proper sequence.

Despite the flexibility of working memory with respect to the allocation of work space to storing and processing, the capacity restrictions of short-term memory impose a ceiling on the number of operations that can be executed. The general rule is that the combined storing-processing load, measured in terms of the number of chunks that must be activated, cannot exceed the total number of chunks available in subjects' short-term memories. Thus, cognitive tasks become susceptible to error as their combined storing-processing loads approach the chunk ceiling. It is easy to think of examples of adult cognitive tasks in which subjects are unable to perform above chance levels, although they are quite capable of carrying out each of the storing and processing operations that are involved. If the problem "What is the product of 496 and 55,784: 27,668,864 or 27,868,864?" were posed in a mental calculation experiment, it is unlikely that most subjects, even mathematicians, would be correct more than half the time. Yet, the fact that these same subjects would probably not have any difficulty with "What is the product of 22 and 17—374 or 364?" shows that they can store numerical information and subject it to arithmetical processing. (The effect of short-term memory load on adults' mental calculation has been studied by Hitch, 1978a, 1978b.) Insofar as development is concerned, the fact that there may be age-related changes in the capacity of working-memory systems, changes that are independent of children's ability to store given types of information and to process it in given ways, will be seen to have considerable theoretical significance later on.

The discussion in this subsection can be summarized by observing that working-memory distinctions provide investigators with several conceptual degrees of freedom that can be brought to bear on the problem of explaining age change data. The principal ones are the following.

1. *Encoding failure.* On a particular task, it may be that children below a certain age do not usually possess operations for encoding the critical information into short-term memory; they cannot form the proper traces. Certainly, age-related trends in encoding are common findings in experiments on memory development, with developmental interactions in the effects of item concreteness on encodability being one well-researched illustration (for reviews, see Pressley, 1977; Reese, 1977). In the study of concept development there is ample evidence that young children do not understand the relational language used on Piagetian tasks in the same way that adults do (e.g., Palermo, 1974). Hence, Piaget's clinical method, as well as other heavily verbal paradigms, have often been criticized on the ground that children may not understand the terminology (e.g., Braine, 1959, 1962; Siegel, 1978, 1982). These familiar "linguistic confusion" criticisms are, from the standpoint of working memory, special cases of encoding failure hypotheses. An equally familiar example of an encoding failure hypothesis is the notion that children are often distracted by salient irrelevant cues on tasks such as conservation (e.g., Boersma & Wilton, 1974) and class inclusion (e.g., Wohlwill, 1968). As the linguistic and attentional examples were intended to suggest, there are two basic varieties of encoding failure, namely, the subject lacks the necessary encoding operations for the critical information (e.g., "does not understand the language") or fails to encode the critical information despite being able to do so (e.g., "is distracted by misleading cues").

2. *Storage failure.* Suppose that children possess the necessary encoding operations and execute them properly—that is, the critical background facts and the response alternatives are correctly encoded into short-term memory. This does not guarantee that the traces will remain in storage until processing has been completed. There are two obvious sources of such storage failure: (a) simple temporal decay (short-term memory is generally regarded as a very labile system) and (b) retroactive interference from subsequently encoded information. (There is a third, less obvious source, retroactive interference from processing, that is more properly considered under the heading of space constraints.) Hence, it is always possible that traces carrying information that is essential to solution may fall out of storage between the time they were originally encoded and the time of response selection. A hypothetical example comes from the aforementioned studies of transitivity. In this research, children are often screened for their understanding of relational phrases such as *longer than*, *shorter than*, or *heavier than* in order to ensure that they understand the terminology. Moreover, the information about the A-B and B-C relationships is presented in such a way that it is highly salient. If the same subjects then have difficulty making transitive inferences because the A-B and B-C relationships are unavailable, it seems more likely that this is due to storage failure than to encoding failure.

3. *Computational (software) failure.* Even if children encode the critical information properly and hold it in temporary storage, their long-term memories may simply not contain the software that is necessary to convert the information into correct responses. In this connection, we may speak of two categories of computational failure. On the one hand, children may not possess procedures that are capable of operating on information of the sort that is stored in short-term memory. A possible illustration occurs with preschool children who are quite capable of encoding and retaining numerical relationships (cf. Brainerd, 1981a, 1981b), but who may not yet possess the iterative software that will convert such information into solutions to mental arithmetic problems. When this first type of computational failure occurs, subjects must either guess or select responses by processing irrelevant information. The other category of computational failure refers to situations in which children possess software that operates on the target information in short-term memory, but the software generates the wrong response selections. Here, class inclusion provides an illustration. Since children who fail class inclusion items do not respond randomly, but rather respond to the relationship between the two subordinate classes, cardinal number information is definitely being retained and processed. The computational procedures that are operating on this information, whatever they may be, are merely wrong.

This third locus of developmental change is where working-memory analysis makes closest contact with traditional theories of cognitive development. The "cognitive structures" that are so central in Piagetian theory seem to be special cases of the computational operations in working-memory models. Similarly, the notion of age-related changes in "rules"—which serves as the centerpiece of rule-based interpretations of concept development (Siegler, 1981; also, see Chapter 2 in this volume; Wilkinson, 1982), rule-sampling interpretations of children's concept learning (Brainerd, 1979a, 1982), and extensions of information integration theory to cognitive development (Anderson & Cuneo, 1978)—seem to be special cases of the notion of age-related changes in the software of working-memory systems.

4. *Retrieval failure.* If appropriate computational operations are stored in long-term memory, it does not necessarily follow that children will be able to retrieve them. As was the case for software failure, we may speak of two types of retrieval failure. First, children may be unable to find procedures in long-term memory that will operate on the stored information before that information has decayed, in which event guessing or some other irrelevant method must be used to respond. Second, children may retrieve procedures that will convert stored background facts into unique response alternatives, but their responses are wrong. In the class inclusion illustration, for example, the computational operations that are being retrieved obviously are not correct. If the subjects' long-term memories happen to contain the correct operations, class inclusion errors would be instances of retrieval failure rather than of software failure.

Less ambiguous examples of retrieval failure occur on tasks where short-term memory holds competing items of information, as it does on conservation problems. Remember here that the information stored in short-term memory presumably provides the retrieval cues that guide the search through long-term memory. When there is competing information, correct performance depends on the selection of those cues that will lead to retrieval of appropriate software. On conservation problems, the competition is between visual and quantitative information. Suppose that we administer a series of liquid quantity tests to 5- and 6-year-olds. Normative data show that children of this age almost always fail such items. The usual pattern is that one glass is judged to have more liquid "because it is taller." But when memory probes are administered to these subjects, the fact that the two quantities of water were equal at the outset still appears to be in storage (e.g., Brainerd, 1977). It seems, therefore, that the wrong traces may be being used to mediate retrieval.

If this interpretation is correct, we should be able to induce children to conserve by training them to use correct retrieval cues. Relevant findings are provided by feedback experiments, where nonconserving children are given a series of training trials on which they are informed about the correctness or incorrectness of their responses. Since this procedure does not teach any computational operations and does not alter the information available for encoding in any way, its apparent effect is to encourage children to switch to quantitative information as a basis for retrieval, thereby permitting them to bring their responses into conformity with the experimenter's feedback. That corrective feedback produces dramatic improvements in conservation among children who are in the first half of elementary school (e.g., Brainerd, 1972a, 1972b, 1976, 1979a, 1979b, 1982; Siegler & Liebert, 1972) is consistent with the view that retrieval failure is a major source of their conservation errors.

It should be added that this does not prove that conservation errors are always retrieval failures. It is conceivable, even likely, that there are gaps in younger children's long-term memories where the correct computational operations should be, and/or that younger children may not retain the critical information in short-term memory. On either hypothesis, one would anticipate that pure retrieval manipulations such as feedback would have less of an effect on the performance of preschoolers, a prediction that agrees with the data (Brainerd, 1974; Denney, Zeytinoglu, & Selzer, 1977). On the first hypothesis, one would also expect that instruction in a relevant computational operation would enhance the effectiveness of feedback with preschoolers, a prediction that also agrees with the data (Denney, Zeytinoglu, & Selzer, 1977).

5. *Work–space constraints.* Another possibility is that subjects who are capable of all the individual storing-processing operations demanded by a task nevertheless perform poorly because the combined load of these operations exceeds the chunk ceiling of short-term memory. It is not difficult to arrange such situations in adult reasoning and problem solving. For example, performance on elementary tests of language comprehension and arithmetic is known to deteriorate when adults must simultaneously hold a near-span set of irrelevant items (e.g., CVCs) for immediate recall. In mental arithmetic, it would be rare to find an undergraduate who could not perform perfectly on items such as 15 - 14 = 1 or 2? and 12 + 9 = 21 or 22? But it would be equally rare to find an undergraduate who

could perform perfectly on items such as $15 - 14 + 11 - 2 + 13 - 9 - 7 + 5 = 12$ or 13? Observe that the only alteration that has been made is to increase the number of numerals that must be stored and the number of calculations that must be executed. That problems with smaller numbers of numerals and calculations can be solved establishes that subjects can activate working-memory systems that contain all the necessary hardware and software for mental addition and subtraction. This point is also demonstrated by the fact that problems of the second type are readily solved when subjects are permitted to enlarge their working-memory system with some external work space (e.g., paper and pencil, a calculator).

For present purposes, the most interesting implication of performance failures due to space constraints is the possibility that working-memory capacity varies, in the sense of the combined storing-processing load that can be accommodated, with age. The reason that this possibility is interesting is that it would allow us to explain situations in which children perform poorly on certain tasks, although probes for the various hardware and software components all give positive readings.

Developmental increases in working-memory capacity might come about in at least three ways. First, it could be that the average number of short-term memory units increases with age—that is, the chunk ceiling rises (e.g., Biggs, 1971; McLaughlin, 1963). Second, it could be that the chunk ceiling is developmentally invariant but that the *efficiency* with which chunks are used for storing and processing improves with age (e.g., Case, 1975, 1978). The implication of this second hypothesis is that the average number of chunks that must be deployed to meet the demands of a target task decreases as individual storing-processing operations become more efficient. Third, it could be that both the chunk ceiling and storing-processing efficiency develop. At present, there is much dispute as to which of these alternatives is correct (cf. Dempster, 1981). However, they appear to have equivalent consequences for working-memory models of cognitive development. Each permits age changes in performance that are independent of the presence of specific storing and processing operations.

Suppose that children are confronted with some target task for which, on the one hand, all the essential hardware and software is available, but on the other hand, the combined storing-processing load exceeds available space constraints. At some point during processing, the capacity boundary will be reached. The working-memory system is now confronted with two options. First, like a computer that exceeds core, the system can simply shut down, with the subject selecting a response either by guessing or by considering irrelevant factors. Second and more interestingly, the system can opt to free up additional capacity by deleting stored information. This retroactive interference from processing will allow processing to continue. But it has the disadvantage that the deleted information will usually be critical to solution, and hence it will lead to incorrect response selections.

It is relatively easy to measure this second consequence of space constraints. About all that is required is to administer short-term memory probes for the essential background facts just before the experimenter's question (i.e., immediately after encoding and immediately before processing) and just after the subject's response to the experimenter's question (i.e., immediately after processing). Occasional probes of this sort are not difficult to incorporate into cognitive tasks that are commonly studied with children (e.g., Brainerd & Kaszor, 1974; Bryant & Trabasso, 1971; Lutkus & Trabasso, 1974). Obviously, performance on the prequestion probes should be better than performance on the postquestion probes if children are deleting stored information because of space constraints. Thus, depending on the sorts of scaling assumptions that one wishes to make, differential performance on short-term memory probes that are administered at different times provides a measure that should be at least monotonically related to space constraints on the working-memory system.

Note on the Structure of Hardware and Software Components. As we have seen, working-memory analysis seeks to explain age-related changes in cognitive performance by relying on age-related changes in five principal process variables, namely, encoding, short-term storage, retrieval from long-term memory, the contents of long-term memory (facts, rules, computational operations), and space constraints on working-memory systems. To avoid potential misinterpretation, it is worth emphasizing at this point that none of the first four variables is assumed to be a simple unitary process. On the contrary, available evidence is more consistent with the view that each is a complex multistage process, with one aim of research on working-memory models being to identify the component stages. Thus, "encoding," "storage in short-term memory," "retrieval from long-term memory," and "computation" are *categories* of memorial processes that one hopes to decompose through experimentation.

The multistage nature of these variables is clear enough in the case of retrieval and computation. Retrieval, as was discussed earlier, involves at least two substages —that is, the selection of search cues and the actual search process. If search involves the successive examination of the contents of different long-term memory loci, then these events are distinct components of retrieval. It may also be that cue selection and search have to be repeated several times before the subject manages to retrieve a set of computational operations to consciousness (or gives up and guesses). On a conservation problem, for example, suppose that a subject initially selects quantitative cues as the basis for retrieval but the search of long-term memory fails to turn up rules that will operate on such information. The subject may then select other cues (e.g., visual features of the stimulus array) and search for rules that will operate on the new information.

Insofar as computation is concerned, the iterative models discussed earlier are multistage theories of mental calculation (e.g., Groen & Parkman, 1972; Groen & Poll, 1973; Woods, Resnick, & Groen, 1975). According to these models, the computational phase of addition or subtraction consists of (a) stepping a counter by one, (b) storing the number of times the counter has been stepped in short-term memory, and (c) checking the number of times that the counter has been stepped. Moreover, the solution of individual problems typically requires several repetitions of the step-store-check sequence of stages.

Although previous examples make the complexity of retrieval and computation

more apparent than the complexity of encoding and storage, there is a large literature favoring the conclusion that the latter variables are also multistage processes (cf.
especially Chase, 1978). For this reason, modern theories of encoding and storage
(e.g., Craik & Lockhart, 1972; Flexer & Tulving, 1978) are all multistage models.

Illustrative Working-Memory Systems. Working-memory analyses of given phenomena in cognitive development normally involves three steps. First, a preliminary
working-memory system is constructed from task considerations and from available
data. Second, research is conducted with a view to localizing age-related variation in
performance on the target task within particular components of the working-
memory system and, where relevant, to discriminating different models of these
components. Third, the preliminary model is revised and articulated in light of
experimental findings.

It is the concern of this subsection to exemplify the first stage; the other two
stages will be considered presently. In particular, preliminary working-memory
systems for two tasks that show interesting age-related variation during childhood—
probability judgment and mental addition—are presented, and alternative models of
selected components are discussed.

1. *Probability Judgment.* The standard paradigm for assessing children's knowledge of probability concepts requires predictions about the results of random draws
from sets for which the relative frequencies of different types of elements are known.
This paradigm was introduced by Piaget and Inhelder (1951), and a review of the
subsequent literature on it can be found in a chapter by Hoemann and Ross (1982).

The usual materials for probability judgment consist of a set of tokens of different colors and an opaque container of some sort. The child is first asked to select a
certain number of tokens of a particular color (e.g., eight red ones) and place them
in the container. Next, the child is asked to select a different number of tokens of a
different color (e.g., three blue ones) and place them in the container also. (This
ensures that the child knows the relative frequencies of the two colors at the outset.) The experimenter then randomizes the contents of the container by shaking
it vigorously, and asks the child to predict which color is most likely to be obtained
on a random sample from the container, with "random sample" usually meaning
that the experimenter withdraws tokens without looking. As a rule, the child is
asked to predict the results of a series of random samples from the container. The
experimenter randomizes the contents of the container again after each draw.

There are two main informational variables that can be manipulated in this situation: (a) replacement versus nonreplacement of elements and (b) knowledge of
results. Regarding (a), the experimenter may either return each sampled element to
the container, or elements may be permanently removed as they are sampled. If
sampling is with replacement, then the relative frequencies of the two colors remain
invariant across a series of random samples and, naturally, the correct prediction is
always that the color that was more frequent at the outset is the one that is more
likely to be drawn. But if sampling is without replacement, predictive correctness
will depend on whether the child knows the results of each draw. When elements
are sampled without replacement, *but the subject has no knowledge of which elements were sampled on given draws*, the only information about the sampling space

that is relevant to probability judgment is the starting frequencies of the two colors. Hence, the correct prediction on all trials is that the color that was more frequent at the outset is the one that is more likely to be drawn. When elements are sampled without replacement and the child is also informed of the outcome of each draw, the correct prediction will depend on the starting frequencies of the two colors *and* on how many tokens of each color have been removed on previous draws. Regarding (b), the experimenter may or may not inform the child which elements are obtained on individual draws. The correct prediction as a function of knowledge of results will depend on whether or not sampling is with replacement. If sampling is with replacement, then it does not matter whether the subject knows the elements that are drawn. The color that was more frequent at the outset should be predicted on all trials because sampling probabilities remain invariant. But if sampling is without replacement, the correct prediction on each trial will depend on whether or not the child knows the outcome of previous draws.

Piaget and Inhelder (1951) reported three general findings about the relationship between age and performance on such tasks. First, below the age of 7 or 8 children rarely based their predictions on the relative frequencies of the elements. Second, between the ages of 7 or 8 and 11 or 12 children use relative frequency information on the first prediction in a sequence (when the cumulative information load is least) but not on later predictions. Last, after the age of 11 or 12, predictions usually agreed with relative frequency information on all trials in a sequence. Subsequent research has confirmed certain of these results and disconfirmed others. Contrary to Piaget and Inhelder, it has been found that the responses of even very young children (4- and 5-year-olds) are correct on the *first* trial in a predictive sequence more often than would be expected by chance (see Brainerd, 1981a). In agreement with Piaget and Inhelder, performance on later trials in a sequence appears to be relatively poor throughout most of the elementary school years (see Brainerd, 1981a; Ross, 1966).

The probability judgment paradigm poses a moderately complex problem in working-memory analysis because models with different amounts of internal structure are required in order to explain performance as a function of task variations. In all instances, the general problem is to devise a system that will deliver response decisions that agree with the relative frequencies of the event classes (in our example, colors) that constitute the sampling space. There are four preliminary models.

The simplest one is for the first prediction in a sequence, and it holds regardless of whether sampling is with or without replacement and with or without knowledge of results. The relevant working-memory system is shown in Figure 4-2. To make a frequency-based response on the first prediction in a sequence, the model assumes that the correct frequency differential must be encoded and retained in storage until processing has been completed, that the stored frequency information must be used to guide the search through long-term memory, and that computational rules must be retrieved that will convert the stored frequency information into correct response selections.

This model, although simple, provides considerable latitude, both with respect to possible loci of developmental change and with respect to the detailed structure of specific components. Concerning loci of development, all five degrees of freedom discussed earlier are available in this model. Concerning the structure of individual

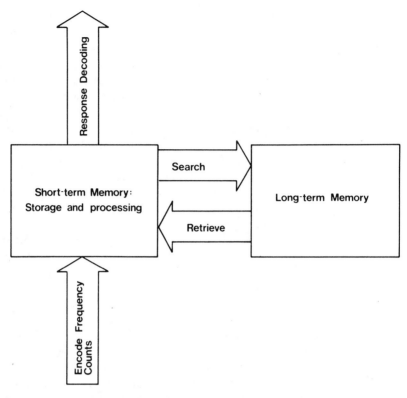

Figure 4-2. A simplified working-memory system for probabilistic predictions on the first trial of a probability judgment task.

components, there are a number of possibilities, for example, as to the nature of the the frequency traces that are actually stored and as to the nature of the computational operations that are brought to bear on them. Insofar as frequency traces are concerned, stored background facts such as "more reds than blues," "fewer blues than reds," and "eight reds and three blues" would all specify the frequency differential between the sets with sufficient precision for accurate probability judgment. Even certain types of incorrect information (e.g., "five reds and two blues") would be sufficient for correct responses on the first prediction. If the stored information takes the form of actual frequency counts (e.g., reds = 8 and blues = 3) rather than raw frequency differentials, then there would be several possible models of the configuration of the traces in short-term memory. To illustrate, Hintzman and his associates (Hintzman, 1969, 1976; Hintzman & Block, 1971, Hintzman, Block, & Summers, 1973; Hintzman & Stern, 1978; Hintzman, Summers, & Block, 1975; Hintzman & Waters, 1970) have reported a series of experiments designed to test three interpretations of how such counts are stored (as cumulative traces, as discrete traces, as propositions). Turning to processing, we find that many models of the computational operations are also conceivable. To a certain extent, what qualifies as an adequate package of computational software (i.e., operations that invariably deliver the response alternative that agrees with the stored frequency differential) will depend on the nature of the stored frequency information. If, for example, only the direction of the difference has been stored (e.g., "more reds than blues"), then a simple response rule of the form "Predict the class that has more" would be adequate. But if precise frequency counts have been stored, the subject may be able to apply the sorts of numerical comparison operations that have been identified in research on children's mental arithmetic (Ashcraft, 1982).

In our illustrative problem, which begins with eight reds and three blues in the container, suppose that after the first prediction children are asked to make a few additional predictions (say, four more) about this sampling space. Also, suppose that after each prediction, feedback is not provided about which element was obtained on the draw. That is, the only relevant frequency information that the children have is the starting counts. The second working-memory model applies to these subsequent no-feedback predictions, and it is applicable to both sampling with replacement and sampling without replacement.

The second model (Figure 4-3) differs from the first in only one respect: It assumes that children tend to encode and retain traces of the responses that they made on previous predictions. Relative to the first model, it is apparent that we expect poorer probability judgment performance in situations where the second model applies. First, the crucial information about the relative frequencies of the elements may fall out of short-term memory. As we saw in the earlier discussion of storage failure, encoding of subsequent information (in this case, response traces) may cause information that is currently in storage (in this case, frequency traces) to

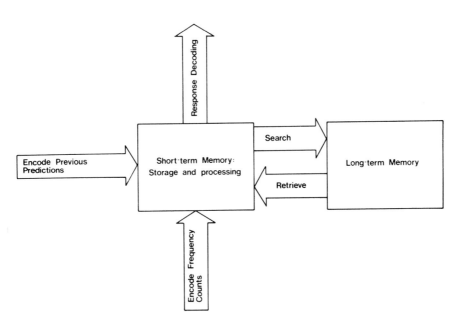

Figure 4-3. A simplified working-memory system for probabilistic predictions on later trials of a probability judgment task where outcome feedback is absent.

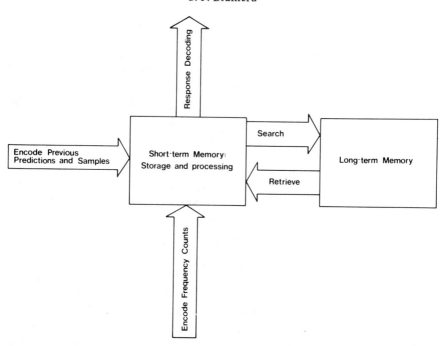

Figure 4-4. A simplified working-memory system for probabilistic predictions on later trials of a probability judgment task where outcome feedback is present.

be deleted. Second, even if the critical frequency information is retained, children may be less inclined to use it as a basis for retrieval. As we also saw earlier, when conflicting information is available in short-term memory, a decision is required as to which information should serve as the source of retrieval cues. If response information is available, it may sometimes be used as a basis for retrieval. Depending on the availability in long-term memory of software that will operate on such information, this should have one or both of two effects. [An example of such response-based rules would be one-trial response alternation (predict the color that was *not* predicted on the previous trial) and one-trial response perseveration (predict the color that was predicted on the previous trial).] If such rules are not usually present, the effect should be to increase the proportion of trials on which predictions are guesses. If such rules are present, the effect should be systematic deviations from correct performance that can be related in some way (e.g., alternation or perseveration) to the responses observed on previous predictions.

The first model covers all initial predictions in a sequence, regardless of whether sampling is with or without replacement or is with or without feedback, and the second model covers all subsequent predictions as long as sampling is without feedback. The remaining two models are concerned with subsequent predictions when there is feedback. The third model, which is shown in Figure 4-4, is the same as the second model except for one complication: Whereas both initial frequency information and subsequent response information are stored in the second model, stimulus information (i.e., the results of the experimenter's draw on each trial) is stored in the third model.

Like the second model, one anticipates that performance will be poorer in situations where the third model applies than in situations where the first model applies. To begin with, the previously discussed difficulties arising from the presence of response information in short-term memory also arise with the third model. In addition, there are parallel difficulties associated with the presence of stimulus information in short-term memory. The encoding of stimulus information, like the encoding of response information, may cause frequency information to fall out of storage. Even if frequency information is retained, stimulus information may interfere with retrieval. If stimulus information is used as a basis for retrieval and if stimulus-based software is available in long-term memory (e.g., "Choose the color that was drawn on the preceding trial" or "Choose the color that was not drawn on the preceding trial"), then systematic deviations from correct probability judgment that can be tied to previously sampled elements should be observed. But if stimulus information is used and such rules are not available in long-term memory, an increase in guessing should result.

Although accuracy clearly should be poorer with the second and third models than with the first, it is not immediately apparent whether performance should be worse with the second or third model. At first glance, it might seem as though the second model might produce better performance because it is less complex. If only response information competes with frequency information in the second model and both stimulus and response information compete with frequency information in the third model, it seems natural to assume that probability judgments will be less accurate in the latter case. Unfortunately, there are several complicating factors. For example, suppose that the capacity of short-term memory is so limited that the encoding of stimulus information tends to bump previously encoded response information out of storage. In this case, there is only one effective source of information at the time that children are asked to make judgments. Another complication is that stimulus information correlates with frequency information, but response information does not. The probability that the experimenter samples a given type of element on a random draw is always greater for the more frequent class in the sampling space. Hence, if subjects store stimulus information and retrieve stimulus perseveration rules (e.g., "Predict the element that was drawn on the preceding trial"), their predictions will tend to agree with the true frequency differentials in the sampling space more often than would be expected by chance. On the other hand, if subjects store stimulus information and retrieve stimulus avoidance rules (e.g., "Predict the element that was not drawn on the preceding trial"), their predictions will be much worse than if they had merely guessed.

The last model, which is shown in Figure 4-5, is the most complicated. Like the second and third models, it applies to subsequent predictions in a sequence. The situations covered by the second model (subsequent predictions without feedback) and the third model (subsequent predictions with feedback and replacement) have in common that the sampling probabilities of the classes remain invariant. Here, the basis for correct prediction is always the starting frequency counts. But if sampling is both with feedback and without replacement, the basis for correct pre-

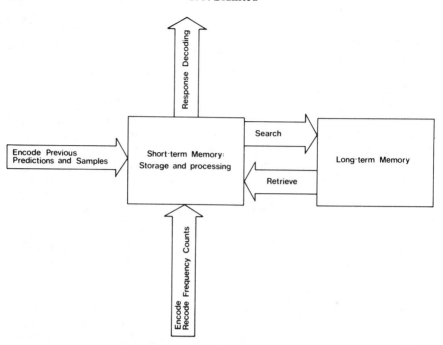

Figure 4-5. A simplified working-memory system for probabilistic predictions on later trials of a probability judgment task where outcome feedback is present and sampling is without replacement.

diction is the initial starting counts plus the elements drawn on previous trials. Thus, if the counts were reds = 5 and blues = 3 and if a red token were drawn on each of the first three trials, the correct predictions would be "red" on the first two trials, "either red or blue" on the third trial, and "blue" on the fourth trial. In short, correct prediction requires that information about previously sampled elements somehow be integrated with starting counts.

The fourth model, like the third, assumes the storage of both stimulus and response information. The key difference is that whereas the third model (and the two other models as well) assumes that stored frequency information is processed once, frequency information is processed twice in the fourth model. In addition to whatever operations are required in order to map relative frequency information into response alternatives, updating operations are required in order to find the true frequencies of the elements. Again, there are multiple possibilities. For example, the subject might retain traces of both the starting counts and the element drawn on each trial in short-term memory. Then, whenever a prediction is required, the numbers of elements of each type that have been previously sampled are subtracted from their respective starting counts to yield their current frequencies. This would clearly be an impractical procedure if the amount of work space were sharply constrained. Another possibility, one that would be more accommodating to capacity restrictions, involves updating the frequency counts after each draw and retaining only this information in short-term memory. In other words, the subject "recodes" the frequency information that was in storage at the start of a trial after each trial is completed.

To conclude, these models illustrate that all five loci of working-memory development (encoding, storage, retrieval, computation, space constraints) may be involved in age-related changes in probability judgment. Also, competing interpretations of what goes on at these loci (e.g., the configuration of stored frequency information, the nature of response-based computational operations) can be formulated. Consequently, probability judgment is an especially instructive phenomenon to study developmentally, at least insofar as working-memory analysis is concerned.

2. *Mental Arithmetic.* Children's performance on mental arithmetic items poses a more elementary problem in working-memory analysis than probability judgment does. This is not to say that children's mental arithmetic performance is better than their probability judgments. (Actually, the normative evidence shows that, say, second graders will normally perform more poorly on certain types of arithmetic items—multiplication and division—than on probability judgment tasks.) The statement simply means that the complexity of the models that are required to account for performance is less in the case of mental arithmetic.

In the standard mental arithmetic experiment with children, subjects are administered problems that involve "small-number facts" such as $5 + 2 = 7, 8 - 2 = 6$, and $9 + 1 = 10$. These problems are usually presented visually in arithmetical notation, either in the window of a memory drum or via a slide projector. Depending on the experiment, children respond in one of two ways. In one type of study (e.g., Groen & Parkman, 1972; Groen & Poll, 1973), children are given a response panel with numbered keys, and they respond by depressing the appropriate numbers. Visually, the problem is presented in the unsolved form "$m + n = ?$" In another type of study (e.g., Ashcraft, Hamann, & Fierman, 1981), children merely respond yes or no. Visually, these problems are presented in the solved form "$m + n = k?$" and the child's task is to decide whether or not the stated sum k is correct. Children usually work with a two-key response panel, depressing either the positive or the negative key accordingly as they think the stated sum is either correct or incorrect.

With the exception of some recent experiments by Ashcraft and his associates (Ashcraft, 1982; Ashcraft, Hamann, & Fierman, 1981), mental arithmetic research has not been much concerned to identify developmental changes in the working-memory structures that produce correct solutions. On the contrary, investigators have usually selected children who are old enough that their performance is virtually error free. In other words, whatever the encoding, storage, retrieval, and computational requirements of these tasks may be, the subjects are selected in such a way that they are capable of activating working-memory systems that meet these requirements. Since errors are uncommon occurrences in such experiments, the data of primary interest are response latencies.

From the perspective of working memory, solution of small-number problems requires that children be able to encode symbols such as "5" and "+" properly, that they be able to retain the encoded information in short-term memory, that there be procedures for arithmetical computation stored in long-term memory, and that the procedures be retrievable to consciousness. Since the children studied in most experiments evidently are capable of all these things, the focus of research has been on the fine-grain structure of the arithmetical software. Two theoretical interpretations, an iterative interpretation and a fact retrieval interpretation, have been extensively investigated.

The iterative interpretation, which was briefly discussed earlier, was originally proposed in a paper on mental addition by Groen and Parkman (1972). Groen and Parkman described a three-step algorithm for addition items: (a) Set a counter, (b) increment the counter in units of 1, and (c) keep track of how many times the counter has been incremented. There are at least five variations on this algorithm that would produce solutions to $m + n$ items. First, the counter is set to zero and is either incremented m times, then n times, or is incremented n times, then m times. Second, the counter is set to m (the leftmost numeral) and then incremented n (the rightmost numeral) times. Third, the counter is set to n (the rightmost numeral) and is then incremented m (the leftmost numeral) times. Fourth, the counter is set to the larger of the two numerals and is then incremented a number of times equal to the smaller numeral. Fifth, the counter is set to the smaller of the two numerals and is then incremented a number of times equal to the larger numeral.

What all five of these models have in common (and, therefore, what distinguishes them from other interpretations) is that children's response latencies on trials on which they solve the problem should be *linearly* related to problem variables. The main problem variables are the augend and the addend, m and n, and their sum, k. The models differ in their predictions about which of these three variables should account for the most variance in the latency data. In the first model, the counter is always incremented k times, so latency should be linearly related to the sum. In the second model, the counter is always incremented m times, so latency should be linearly related to the value of the leftmost numeral. In the third model, the counter is always incremented n times, so latency should be linearly related to the value of the rightmost numeral. In the fourth model, the counter is always incremented a number of times equal to the minimum, so latency should be linearly related to the value of the smaller numeral. In the fifth model, the counter is always incremented a number of times equal to the maximum, so latency should be linearly related to the value of the larger numeral.

Groen and Parkman (1972) found that the fourth model, which they called the "max-min" interpretation, gave the best account of their data. They reported an experiment of the first type mentioned above in which 37 first-grade children solved 55 addition problems, all of whose sums were less than 10. In general, correct-response latencies were a linearly increasing function of the value of the smaller numeral. The slope of the best fitting line was 410 msec, indicating that passes through the cycle of incrementing the counter by one and storing the result require 410 msec on the average. The sole exception to this relationship occurred with "tie" items—that is, items for which the values of m and n were the same. Correct-response latencies on ties were unrelated to any of the problem variables, and they were much faster than on untied items.

The fact retrieval interpretation was originally formulated in an article on adults' mental addition by Ashcraft and Battaglia (1978), although it is closely related to some suggestions in an earlier paper on multiplication by Parkman (1972). Ashcraft and Battaglia assumed that adults have tables of number facts stored in long-term memory that resemble the table shown in Figure 4-6. (Although it is mental addition that we are concerned with, analogous tables supposedly are available for subtraction, multiplication, and division.) To solve a mental addition item, the subject retrieves the appropriate fact table to consciousness and scans it to find the solution. Because of the structure of the table, the search process is presumed to be an intersection operation. Note that the table in Figure 4-6 is constructed in such a way that the columns correspond to values of m in $m + n$ problems, and the rows correspond to values of n. The cells of the table contain the correct sum for the row and column

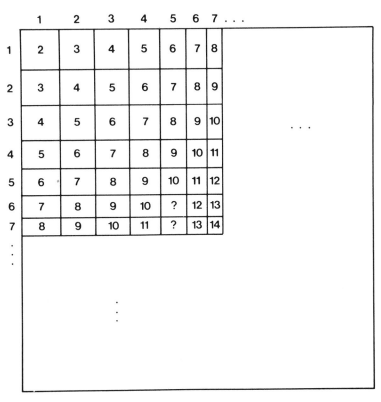

Figure 4-6. A table of arithmetic facts for mental addition problems solved by the fact retrieval method. If the problem is of the form $m + n = ?$ the subject simultaneously enters the table at the column corresponding to m and the row corresponding to n, or conversely. The problem is solved by scanning down the column and across the row until the two operations intersect at a given cell. The value in the cell is then read out as the solution. If the cell is empty, the problem is solved by iteration or the subject guesses.

values. Thus, the subject enters the table at row n and column m, simultaneously scanning across the row and down the column until the two operations intersect at a particular cell. At this point, the solution can be read out.

There are two other features of the fact table in Figure 4-6 that should be borne in mind. First, the "distance" between successive row values and successive column values shrinks as the numbers become larger. Second, a few of the cells are empty. The first feature is motivated by the results of numerical comparison studies of adults (e.g., Moyer & Landauer, 1967) and children (Sekuler & Mierkiewicz, 1977). The task in such experiments is to identify the larger (or the smaller) of a pair of numerals, usually in the 1-100 range, as rapidly as possible. Latencies are again the response measure. Two general relationships hold in such studies: (a) The time that it takes to identify the larger (or the smaller) member decreases as the distance between the numerals increases (e.g., latencies on 2 vs. 7 items are shorter than latencies on 7 vs. 9 items), and (b) this "distance effect" decreases as the members of a numeral pair become larger (2 vs. 7 is faster than 7 vs. 9 and 32 vs 37 is faster than 37 vs. 39, but the latter difference is smaller than the former). The second relationship suggests that the representation of the number line in long-term memory is foreshortened at the high end, which is reflected in the foreshortenings of the rows and columns of Figure 4-6. The second feature of Figure 4-6, occasional empty cells, is motivated by the obvious possibility that some subjects may not have values for all the simple number facts stored in long-term memory. Here, the assumption is that whenever the intersection operator terminates at an empty cell, the subject falls back on some sort of rote computation (e.g., the iteration procedure in the Groen-Parkman models).

The fact retrieval model leads to two predictions that serve to distinguish it from the max-min model. To begin with, latencies on $m + n$ items should be more closely related to the value of the sum, k, than to the value of either numeral. If these items are solved by scanning a fact table like the one in Figure 4-6, solution time will depend on how long it takes for the row and column operators to intersect. It is easy to see that, other things being equal, total time to intersection increases whenever the value of m or the value of n increases. In itself, the prediction that latency varies chiefly as a function of k does not differentiate iterative and fact retrieval models, because the first iterative model (set to zero and increment k times) also anticipates this result. However, the second prediction does. According to this prediction, the relationship between response latency and k will not be linear, but will be some negatively accelerated function (e.g., latency will increase as k increase, but the increase will be smaller for larger values of k than for smaller values of k). A negatively accelerated relationship between latency and k is a direct consequence of the fact that the distances between cells decrease as the row and column values increase.

In two experiments of the second type (yes-no) mentioned above, Ashcraft and Battaglia (1978) found that adult addition latencies were more strongly related to the value of the sum than to the value of either numeral and that this relationship was negatively accelerated. If L is latency in msec, the actual function that gave the best fit to Ashcraft and Battaglia's data was

$$L = a + b(k)^2, \tag{4-1}$$

a finding that was subsequently replicated by Ashcraft et al. (1981).

The question now becomes whether Ashcraft's results hold only for adults or whether there is a developmental trend away from iteration and toward fact retrieval. Ashcraft et al. (1981) reported an experiment that was designed to provide relevant data. They administered $m + n$ items to college students and to elementary schoolers. They found that Equation 4-1 once again gave the best account of the adult data. It also gave the best account of the data of older elementary schoolers. However, this was not true at younger age levels. With first graders, Groen and Parkman's (1972) max-min model delivered the best fit (i.e., the latencies of first graders were linearly related to the value of the minimum numeral). With second graders, the max-min model and Equation 4-1 gave equally good accounts of the data. Ashcraft (1982) has interpreted these data as showing, first, that there is a developmental trend from iteration to retrieval; second, that third grade is the youngest level at which most children are using fact retrieval on most items; and third, that second grade is a transition level where neither fact retrieval nor iteration clearly predominates.

Illustrative Experiments: The Qualitative Sieve

Now that the nuts and bolts of working-memory analysis have been considered, it is time to take up research that seeks to tie age-related changes in cognition to the development of aspects of working memory. Throughout this section, it may be useful to bear in mind that the objective of any working-memory analysis is to explain all the age-related variation in performance on the target tasks, at least within permissible limits of statistical error. Although this idealized goal has not yet been achieved for any task, we shall see that some close approximations are possible.

It has already been noted that research on working-memory models of children's cognition has been of two general types—namely, studies designed to localize age-related variation within particular components of working memory and studies designed to test competing models of particular components. Both forms of research are important, and their findings are complementary. However, research of the former sort has logical priority because the formulation of alternative models of a specific working-memory component will usually be motivated by evidence that it is a major source of age-related variation on the target task. For this reason, the present section deals exclusively with localization research.

We saw that working-memory models suggest five general sources of age-related variation on cognitive tasks (encoding, short-term storage, retrieval from long-term memory, computational rules, and space constraints), with further differentiation being possible within each category. Given some task of interest, the problem becomes how to decide which loci are important and how to determine whether the factors that produce age-related variation are different for different age ranges. The decision strategy exemplified in this section consists essentially of putting the working-memory factors through an empirical strainer, with the idea being that those factors which fall through are the important ones.

The strainer itself is a sequence of experimental manipulations, each designed to embody one or more working-memory factors. For example, if one suspected that the premise information in a transitivity problem tended to be deleted from young children's short-term memories, one might refresh their memories with prompts (Roodin & Gruen, 1970) or transfer all the premises to long-term memory (Bryant & Trabasso, 1971) or merely encourage the children to rehearse. This "qualitative sieve" is a common procedure in adult cognitive research. Insofar as working-memory analyses of cognitive development are concerned, the strategy has proved to be productive because experience has shown that it tends to localize age variation within a few, not all, of the working-memory factors. That is, when manipulations designed to affect encoding, short-term storage, retrieval, computational rules, and space constraints are studied, one typically finds that only the manipulations in one or two categories give positive signals.

In this section the qualitative sieve is illustrated in action by means of a series of experiments on probability judgment. Because working-memory systems for probability judgment have already been examined (Figures 4-2 to 4-5), we can proceed directly to the research. Full details of these experiments have been published elsewhere (Brainerd, 1981a). In what follows, I summarize only those results that bear on potential working-memory loci of children's probability judgment. A brief synopsis of pertinent methodological points is presented before the data are taken up.

General Methodology

In all of the experiments, a random-draws paradigm of the sort introduced by Piaget and Inhelder (1951) was used. The apparatus was a small opaque container with a tight-fitting cover. At the start of each problem, a small number of same-size plastic tokens was placed in the container by the child. The tokens bore pictures of familiar animals (horse, bird, rabbit, etc.). Depending on the problem, the tokens in the container contained either pictures of two types of animals (two-class problems) or pictures of three types of animals (three-class problems). The different animal classes were always represented with unequal frequencies. Thus, there was always a High class and a Low class on two-class problems, and a High class, a Medium class, and a Low class on three-class problems. On two-class problems, the frequencies were usually High = 7 and Low = 3. On three-class problems, the frequencies were usually High = 8, Medium = 5, and Low = 2.

The subjects in most experiments were administered a series of five probability judgment problems, a warm-up task followed by four main problems. On each problem, the subjects' task was to predict a sequence of five one-element draws from the container. Before Trial 1 of a problem, the subject was asked to deposit in the container the appropriate numbers of animal tokens for that problem (e.g., "Put seven turtles and three rabbits in here"). The experimenter then placed the cover on the container and shook it vigorously to randomize its contents. On Trial 1, the subject was asked to predict which of the two (or three) types of animals would be more likely to be obtained on a random draw (e.g., "If I take a picture without looking, will I get a turtle or a rabbit?"). After a prediction had been made, the experimenter made a random draw. After the draw, the experimenter either did or did not display the picture to the subject (feedback vs. no feedback) and either did or did not replace the token in the container before the next draw (replacement vs. nonreplacement). Last, the experimenter shook the container vigorously again and proceeded to Trial 2. This procedure was repeated until the subject had made five predictions.

Experiment 1

Piaget and Inhelder (1951) reported that young children's performance on probability judgment items was poor (i.e., they did not consistently predict the High class). But if working-memory analysis is to explain young children's performance, we need a more fine-grained picture of their actual predictions; we require benchmark data. The aim of this study was to generate such data.

A mixed sample of 50 children 4 and 5 years of age (mean age = 5 years, 5 months) was administered five two-class problems—one warm-up task followed by four main problems—of the sort just described. On the four main problems, the experimenter did not provide feedback as to the element sampled on each random draw. Hence, the only correct basis for predictions was the initial frequencies of the two animal classes. Sampling was with replacement on two of the main problems and without replacement on the other two.

The principal findings can be summarized by referring to performance on the first prediction for a problem (Trial 1) versus performance on all subsequent predictions (Trials 2-5). On Trial 1, subjects' predictions were imperfect, but they nevertheless predicted the High class more often than would be expected by chance. Summing across the four main problems and across subjects, the High class was predicted 66% of the time on Trial 1. Since a correct prediction could occur 50% of the time by chance, the 66% figure suggests that about one-third of the Trial 1 predictions were based on the actual frequency differential between the High and Low classes.

A different pattern was observed on Trials 2-5. Summing across problems and subjects, the High class was predicted slightly *less* than half the time. The reason for this surprising result can be seen when the subjects' predictions on each trial are conditionalized on the predictions on the immediately preceding trial. The results can be conveniently summarized in a transition matrix:

	High ($n+1$)	Low ($n+1$)
High (n)	.28	.72
Low (n)	.67	.33

This matrix is to be read as follows. The rows give the subjects' predictions (High class or Low class) on each trial in the sequence, and the columns give the subjects' predictions (High class or Low class) on the next trial. Hence, each number in the matrix is the proportion of times that a certain column class was predicted, given that the indicated row class was predicted on the immediately preceding trial. What emerges in this matrix is that, by and large, the predictions on Trails 2-5 conformed to a simple response alternation rule: When a given class was predicted on Trial n (whether High or Low), the other class was usually predicted on Trial $n + 1$.

To sum up, Experiment 1 produced three qualitative findings that will now serve as reference points for later experiments. First, the predictions on Trial 1 preserved the ordering of the relative frequencies of the elements in the sampling space, which suggests that young children are capable of activating the simplest of the three working-memory systems for probability judgment (Figure 4-2) at least some of the time. Second, the frequency of correct predictions on Trial 1, although higher than chance expectation, was far from perfect, with the indication being that there were failures somewhere in the working-memory system about two-thirds of the time. Third, predictions after Trial 1 did not preserve the sampling probabilities and appeared to be primarily under the control of response information.

Experiment 2

The purpose of this experiment was to evaluate an explanation of the pattern of results in Experiment 1 that is weighted toward the encoding-storage end of working memory. The concepts of encoding failure and storage failure could bring order to both the Trial 1 results and Trials 2-5 results as follows. Suppose that the children are sometimes incapable of encoding some or all of the information about the relative frequencies of the classes that is provided at the outset. Also, suppose that when such information is encoded into short-term memory it tends to decay rapidly, and in addition, it is rarely present on Trials 2-5 because of retroactive interference from response traces. According to this explanation, the necessary frequency information is present some of the time on Trial 1. When it is, it serves as a basis for retrieval, and subjects manage to retrieve appropriate computational rules (i.e., retrieval failure and software failure are not problematical). This accounts for the fact that High predictions are significantly more frequent on Trial 1 than Low predictions. But thanks to encoding failure, it is often the case that frequency information is absent, which is why Trial 1 performance is not perfect. As regards Trials 2-5, the fact that frequency information is no longer in storage means that it cannot be used as a source of retrieval cues—hence, poorer performance on Trials 2-5 than on Trial 1. The additional fact that it has been supplanted by response information means that response traces can be used as a basis for retrieval—hence, the strong control of subsequent predictions by previous predictions.

If the encoding-storage interpretation is correct, then any manipulation that makes it easier to encode frequency information and/or to retain it in short-term memory should increase the correlation between subjects' predictions and the relative frequencies of the classes that constitute the sampling space. The obvious manipulation is to provide children with an external frequency store. Since the frequency counts are now displayed externally, they cannot be lost as the problem proceeds, thereby reducing the probability of storage failure. The external availability of the counts means that there are now increased opportunities for encoding, thereby reducing the incidence of encoding failure.

A minor modification in the design of Experiment 1 was all that was required. Recall that at the start of each problem the subject was asked to deposit the appropriate numbers of animal tokens in the container. In Experiment 2, the subject was also asked to place the same numbers of tokens in a row in front of the container. Thus, if there were seven dogs and three birds in the container on a given problem, there was a row of seven dogs and row of three birds displayed in front of the container on all predictions. Apart from the external frequency store, Experiment 2 was the same as Experiment 1. The 50 subjects were a mixed sample of 4- and 5-year-olds (mean age 5 years, 3 months).

Contrary to the encoding-storage explanation, the manipulation did not affect performance relative to Experiment 1. Summing across problems and children, the High class accounted for 72% of the Trial 1 predictions. On Trials 2-5 the results were as follows.

	High ($n+1$)	Low ($n+1$)
High (n)	.24	.76
Low (n)	.80	.20

This failure to find support for an encoding-storage interpretation is surprising from the standpoint of one of the most influential views of cognitive development, attentional theory. According to attentional theorists (e.g., Gelman, 1969; Odom, 1978), young children's errors on thinking and reasoning tasks are rooted in their failure to pay attention to (i.e., to encode and store) the relevant information. On the other hand, the results of Experiment 2 are in agreement with earlier research on human frequency memory per se. The ability of subjects to retain frequency information has been extensively investigated in both adults (for a review, see Hintzman, 1976) and children (for a review, see Ghatala & Levin, 1976). The results of these experiments favor the conclusion that frequency encoding is an automatic and obligatory process in humans (Hintzman & Stern, 1978). Even incidental-memory experiments, in which subjects are not informed that memory for frequency will be tested, have shown good retention. Some especially interesting results were obtained in an experiment with elementary schoolers by Ghatala, Levin, and Truman (1978). During the study phase of the experiment, the children read a prose passage. One day later, during the test phase, they were given a surprise frequency-memory test, which consisted of presenting pairs of words and asking the children to select the pair member that had appeared more often in the prose passage. Performance was generally quite accurate.

Experiment 3

Since the results of Experiment 2 argued against encoding and storage failures as sources of young children's probability judgment errors, explanations from the processing side will now be considered. I begin by discussing two hypotheses, one based on the notion of software failure and the other on the notion of retrieval failure, that are capable of explaining the general pattern of predictions observed in Experiments 1 and 2. It turns out that these hypotheses lead to different predictions about how responses in three-class problems (High, Medium, Low) will differ from those in the two-class problems. Consequently, an experiment of this sort is reported.

Software Failure. In line with the results of the first two experiments, this hypothesis assumes that the pertinent frequency counts have been encoded and the traces are still in storage on most trials. The hypothesis also assumes that subjects use the stored frequency traces as a basis for their initial atte..ipts at retrieval. However, the hypothesis continues, there often are holes in long-term memory where frequency-based computational operations should be; although children search their long-term memories using fequency cues as a guide, they often are unable to find computational rules that will operate on stored frequency traces. When this happens, the subject must either guess or recycle the retrieval operation in order to make use of other cues in short-term memory. This software-failure hypothesis explains the principal results of the first two experiments as follows.

Combining the data of the two experiments, we find that the children's Trial 1 predictions were correct 69% of the time. When the 50% guessing probability is taken into account, the suggestion is that children's predictions were based on the correct frequency differential about 38% of the time on Trial 1. According to the software-failure hypothesis, the latter value is roughly the percentage of children who possess appropriate frequency software in long-term memory. On Trial 1, the other 62% of the children either guess or they generate predictions by processing other information in short-term memory. Since frequency is the only type of information that correlates with correctness and incorrectness, non-frequency-based predictions are correct with probability ½. As regards Trials 2-5, the software-failure hypothesis assumes that although frequency processing operations are absent in the preponderance of young children, response processing operations are readily available. (Incidentally, there is considerable support for such an assumption in the literature on children's discriminating learning. In such experiments, high incidences of response alternation and response perseveration are observed in young children—e.g., Phillips & Levine, 1975.) Thus, when the retrieval operation is recycled after failure to locate frequency processing operations, recently encoded response information (i.e., the subject's prediction on the immediately preceding trial) is the most salient source of retrieval cues, and hence response processing operations are usually retrieved. The latter events would, of course, lead to the marked response dependencies on Trials 2-5 observed in the first two experiments.

Retrieval Failure. The second hypothesis is simpler. Like the first hypothesis, it assumes that frequency counts are properly encoded and that they are available in short-term memory on most trials. Unlike the first hypothesis, it assumes that young children have frequency processing operations stored in long-term memory and that these operations will normally be retrieved if the appropriate retrieval cues are used. The problem is that the retrieval cues are often something other than the stored frequency traces. The second hypothesis explains the data of the first two experiments as follows.

On Trial 1, the 69% correct figure, together with the 50% guessing probability, is interpreted as showing that retrieval is guided by frequency cues on about 38% of the predictions. The rest of the time other information stored in short-term memory (e.g., contextual features of the experiment) provides the retrieval cues. On subsequent trials, a new and highly salient form of information, the subjects' previous responses, is also available in short-term memory. Therefore, response traces are routinely used as retrieval cues on Trials 2-5, hence the strong response dependency of predictions after Trial 1. If retrieval failure is the main problem, it is likely that the presence of recently encoded response information would also decrease, relative to Trial 1, the incidence of frequency retrieval. However, this assumption is not necessary in order to produce response-dependent predictions on Trials 2-5; it is sufficient to assume that response cues are frequently used to guide retrieval.

Procedure and Results. Suppose that an experiment were conducted that was identical to the first two experiments, save that the sampling spaces for all problems consisted of three classes of unequal frequency rather than two classes. The software-failure and retrieval-failure hypotheses lead to some straightforward predictions about how responses in such an experiment should differ from those previously reported.

On Trial 1, both hypotheses anticipate that the frequency with which the High class is predicted should decline, and more important, it should decline by a specific amount. Recall that both hypotheses assume, albeit for different reasons, that about 62% of the Trial 1 predictions in the first two experiments were based on irrelevant information that is uncorrelated with frequency differentials. Thus, the lower guessing probability on three-class items should cause the rate at which the High class is predicted on Trial 1 to decline. Moreover, the assumption that 38% of the Trial 1 predictions were frequency based, together with the one-third guessing probability in a three-class experiment, implies that the High class prediction rate will decline to somewhere in the neighborhood of 59%.

On Trials 2-5, the software-failure hypothesis expects that evidence of frequency-based responding will be observed under certain conditions, but the retreival-failure hypothesis does not. To see why, recall first that software failure assumes that children use frequency cues for retrieval and that when they manage to locate frequency processing operations (roughly one-third of the cases), they use them to generate predictions. However, these frequency-based predictions are swamped in the two-class percentages by the much larger proportion of trials on which the retrieval operation is recycled to use response cues. But the three-class percentages should reveal a different picture. First, consider those trials in a sequence for which the correct (High) prediction was made on the preceding trial. According to the software-failure hypothesis, some of these High predictions resulted from the correct processing of frequency information and others resulted from other forms of processing (e.g., response alternation). Second, consider those trials in a sequence for which an incorrect prediction (Medium or Low) was made on the preceding trial. Since they are all incorrect, none of these predictions resulted from correct processing of frequency information. Thus, consideration of whether or not a High prediction occurred on a given trial tends to divide subjects into groups with higher and lower probabilities of possessing frequency processing operations. The obvious prediction, therefore, is that the response alternation tendency in three-class experiments should be *less* pronounced for those $n/n+1$ pairs for which the Trial n response is High. In contrast, the retrieval-failure hypothesis does not forecast this this result: If young children are relying on response cues and ignoring frequency cues when they retrieve, there is no reason to suppose that this tendency should be more or less pronounced following a High prediction than following a Medium or a Low prediction.

The experiment whose results I now report was identical to Experiment 1, except that the opaque container held three animal classes (High = 8, Medium = 5, Low = 2) on all problems. Forty-six 4- and 5-year-olds served as subjects (mean age = 5 years, 6 months). As in Experiment 1, there were four main problems, two with replacement and two without replacement, and the experimenter did not provide feedback as to the element sampled on any prediction.

The Trial 1 responses were consistent with what the two hypotheses predict. The Trial 1 High prediction rate declined to 60%, a value that did not differ significantly from the predicted value of 59% but was significantly smaller than the 68% prediction rate obtained in the first two experiments. It should be noted here that these Trial 1 results provide further evidence against the encoding-storage explanations considered in Experiment 2. If children have trouble encoding frequency counts and/or retaining them in storage, these problems should be compounded by the addition of a third class to the sampling space. Hence, the decline in the High prediction rate should be more pronounced than the amount anticipated by the two processing hypotheses.

The Trials 2-5 responses were more in line with the retrieval-failure interpretation than the software-failure interpretation. The matrix of transition probabilities indicates that response alternation was still occurring:

	High (n+1)	Medium (n+1)	Low (n+1)
High (n)	.16	.45	.39
Medium (n)	.42	.16	.42
Low (n)	.43	.44	.13

Contrary to the software-failure hypothesis, the estimated probabilities of two consecutive High predictions, two consecutive Medium predictions, and two consecutive Low predictions were .16, .16, and .13, respectively. Once the response on the immediately preceding trial is held constant, the matrix shows that the prediction rates for the remaining two responses do not differ. Thus, the picture that emerges for Trials 2-5 is that on most trials the subject eliminated the preceding prediction and then selected between the remaining two alternatives either by guessing or by processing information that is unrelated to frequency or response information.

Experiment 4

So far, the results are consistent with the following explanation. On Trial 1, children often (over half the time) fail to use stored frequency traces as a basis for retrieval. When they do, however, they usually find frequency-based processing operations in long-term memory. On Trials 2-5, interference from highly salient response information virtually eliminates frequency-based retrieval, and response cues are predominately used for retrieval. The next two experiments were designed to provide more direct evidence on this interpretation.

In Experiment 4, the same five problems administered in Experiment 1 were administered again, with the slight change that they were administered *simultaneously* rather than successively. In Experiment 1, the subject began by constructing the sampling space for the warm-up problem, and then five predictions were made about that space. The procedure was then repeated for the first experimental problem, and so on until the four experimental problems had been completed. In Experiment 4, however, the subject began by constructing the sampling spaces for *all five* problems. The subject then made a total of 25 predictions, 5 for each sampling space, organized in blocks of 5 predictions containing 1 prediction for each sampling space.

After the subject had constructed the five sampling spaces, there were five opaque containers arranged in front of him or her. At the start of the first block of five predictions, the experimenter requested a prediction about the warm-up container. After the prediction had been made and an element had been sampled, the experimenter requested one prediction about each of the other four containers. When these predictions had been made and elements had been drawn, the experimenter rerandomized the contents of the five containers and proceeded to the next block of five predictions. Sampling was always with replacement and without feedback. To avoid any possibility of storage failure due to the large numbers of classes involved, there was an external store for all five containers.

The retrieval-failure hypothesis implies that there should be some dramatic differences in performance, relative to Experiment 1, under conditions of simultaneous presentation. The hypothesis assumes that children often fail to rely on stored frequency traces for retrieval cues because of interference from other stored information, especially recently encoded response information. On this interpretation, we expect that Trial 1 performance should be much poorer in this experiment than in previous experiments, but that the response alternation tendency should more or less disappear. The first prediction follows from the fact that under simultaneous presentation, information about previous responses is present on Trial 1 for each of the four main problems. Recall here that in the first block of five predictions (i.e., Trial 1 for each sampling space), each prediction for a given container was preceded by a prediction about some other container (either the warm-up container or one of the other three containers for the main experimental problems). Hence, the presence of such information should have the same deflating effect on Trial 1 performance that it had on Trials 2-5 in the first three experiments. As regards Trials 2-5, the retrieval-failure hypothesis assumes that the response alternation tendency observed in the first three experiments results from using stored information about the preceding prediction as a retrieval cue. But note that the preceding prediction under conditions of simultaneous presentation is always about some container other than the one for which a prediction is currently being made. Thus, if this information is used as a basis for retrieval, there is no computational operation that will work, and the subject is confined to guessing, with the obvious prediction being that all the entries in the transition matrix for Trials 2-5 should be ½.

The 48 subjects in Experiment 4 were a mixed sample of 4- and 5-year-olds (mean age = 5 years, 8 months). The results for Trial 1 and for Trials 2-5 were consistent with what retrieval failure anticipates. On Trial 1, the High class was predicted only 53% of the time, a value that is significantly lower than the 68% rate observed in the first two experiments and that does not differ significantly from ½. The matrix for Trials 2-5 reveals the expected decline in response alternation:

	High $(n+1)$	Low $(n+1)$
High (n)	.44	.56
Low (n)	.51	.49

None of the four values differs significantly from ½. These results also provide rather striking support for the view that salient intertrial information blocks the use of frequency cues for retrieval. Since information about the previous prediction is complately irrelevant in simultaneous presentation, it might be supposed that after a few retrieval failures, the children would shift to frequency-based retrieval. Apparently this does not happen.

Experiment 5

The purpose of this experiment was to broaden our understanding of the limits of retrieval failure. The suggested interpretation of the data reported up to this point is that other stored information interferes with the use of frequency traces and that this interference is more or less total on Trials 2-5 but not on Trial 1. A question arises as to whether the degree of interference depends on the type of information in storage or whether it depends only on relative recency. Either interpretation is possible on the basis of the response alternation evidence from the first three experiments. On the one hand, it might be that there is something especially salient about stored response information. On the other hand, it might be that the fact that response information has been more recently encoded than frequency information is what makes it so salient.

These possibilities were explored in the fifth experiment. The 50 subjects were a mixed sample of 4- and 5-year-olds (mean age = 5 years, 7 months). Each subject was administered five two-class problems (a warm-up plus four experimental problems) like those in Experiment 1. However, there were two differences between these problems and those in Experiment 1. First, sampling was always with replacement. Second and more important, sampling was with feedback—after each prediction, the experimenter withdrew an element and displayed it to the subject.

The retrieval-failure hypothesis expects different effects from the feedback manipulation, accordingly as one assumes that the response-dependent predictions observed earlier are a consequence of the special properties of response information or that such predictions are a consequence of the recency of response information. Note that whereas the sequence of events in earlier experiments was randomization → prediction → sampling, the sequence of events on each trial in this experiment is randomization → prediction → sampling → feedback. Thus, feedback information is interposed between response information and the next prediction. If response-dependent retrieval is due to the special properties of stored response traces, then one would not expect that this change would have much of an effect on performance (i.e., strong response dependencies would still be apparent). But if response-dependent retrieval is due to the recency of response information, one would expect a new form of interference, namely, stimulus-based retrieval. This suggests the possibility of stimulus-dependent predictions on Trials 2-5, with stimulus alternation (predicting whatever class was not obtained on the preceding draw) and stimulus perseveration (predicting the same class that was obtained on the preceding draw) being likely candidates.

In the event, the data of Experiment 5 were consistent with the view that recency of encoding is the critical variable in retrieval failure. On Trial 1, performance was analogous to that in Experiments 1 and 2. The High class was predicted on 66% of the trials. Since subjects did not receive feedback until *after* the first prediction, the Trial 1 data should be the same as in Experiments 1 and 2. But the results for Trials 2-5 were quite different. These data can be displayed to best advantage in a matrix that expresses subjects' predictions on each trial as a function of both their response on the previous trial and the stimulus that was drawn after that response:

	$H_r H_s (n+1)$	$H_r L_s (n+1)$	$L_r H_s (n+1)$	$L_r L_s (n+1)$
$H_r H_s (n)$	.52	.21	.19	.08
$H_r L_s (n)$	.20	.03	.49	.28
$L_r H_s (n)$	.57	.16	.21	.06
$L_r L_s (n)$	.24	.05	.53	.18

The notation is read as follows: $H_r H_s$ denotes trials on which the subject predicted High and the experimenter drew High; $H_r L_s$ denotes trials on which the subject predicted High and the experimenter drew Low; $L_r H_s$ denotes trials on which the subject predicted Low and the experimenter drew High; $L_r L_s$ denotes trials on which the subject predicted Low and the experimenter drew Low.

It can be seen from the matrix that predictions in Trials 2-5 were heavily weighted toward the outcome of the experimenter's draw. Summing across different feedback events on the preceding trial, we find that 68% of the Trial $n + 1$ predictions were High when High was sampled on Trial n, and 74% of the Trial $n + 1$ predictions were Low when Low was sampled on Trial n. In short, there was now a strong stimulus perseveration bias where there had previously been a response alternation bias. Summing across different prediction events (High or Low), we find that 43% of the Trial $n + 1$ predictions were High when High was the Trial n prediction, and 44% of the Trial $n + 1$ predictions were Low when Low was the Trial n prediction.

Experiment 6

The purposes of Experiment 6 were to provide more direct data on the retrieval-failure hypothesis and to provide further data on storage failure. Concerning the first aim, although the findings up to this point implicate retrieval failures as the proximal causes of young children's probability judgment errors, more direct evidence is desirable. Specifically, one anticipates on the basis of this hypothesis that the accuracy of probability judgments should improve dramatically on items where subjects are constrained to use the relevant frequency differential in retrieval. Concerning the second aim, the fact that an external frequency store does not improve probability judgment (Experiments 1 and 4), together with other results (Ghatala & Levin, 1976), suggests that young children have little difficulty encoding frequency information. However, it can be argued that this manipulation does not provide the best evidence as to the possibility of storage failure. Storage failure (i.e., the absence of the relevant frequency traces at the time the subject is asked to make a prediction) can occur in two basic ways. First, information may not be encoded into short-term memory in the first place, with performance in the presence of an external frequency store arguing against this interpretation in the case of frequency information. Second, previously encoded information may decay from short-term memory. Since the elapsed time during a sequence of predictions for the forgoing tasks is always less than 2 minutes, the likely reasons for such decay would be retroactive interference from subsequently encoded information and retroactive interference from processing (space constraints). Although the negative results from the external store manipulation make it doubtful that frequency decay is a major problem, they still leave open the possibility that the relevant frequency differential is absent from short-term memory on a proportion of the trials.

The first problem is to find a manipulation that serves to ensure that children use frequency information as a basis for retrieval. The strong stimulus and response dependencies observed earlier, plus the ineffectiveness of the external store manipulation, point to a simple procedure. The results of Experiment 2 suggest that, for the most part, the frequency counts are still in short-term memory. The results of Experiments 4 and 5 suggest that children are prone to use the most recently encoded information in short-term memory as the source of retrieval cues. The manipulation suggested by these results is to ask subjects to recall the relevant frequency differential just before they are asked to make a prediction. If the frequency counts are still in storage, then young children should be able to reproduce them on demand. (In theoretical interpretations of short-term memory—e.g., Greeno, 1967—it is normally assumed that whereas information stored in long-term memory cannot always be retrieved, information stored in short-term memory is retrievable.) In addition, if young children rely on recently encoded information as a basis for retrieval, they should now use frequency cues because the response to the frequency probe immediately precedes the experimenter's request for a prediction.

Hence, the introduction of probes for frequency information appears to yield a fairly unambiguous test of the retrieval-failure hypothesis. If the hypothesis is sound, then young children should be able to answer frequency probes correctly and their predictive accuracy should increase. One also expects that the conditional probability of a correct prediction given a correct answer to a frequency probe should be close to unity. Frequency probes provide additional evidence as to whether there are some residual storage failures due to space constraints on working memory. If it is assumed that the guessing probability on the frequency probes is known, estimates can be made about the proportion of trials on which the relevant frequency differential was absent from short-term memory.

The subjects were a mixed sample of 54 children 4 and 5 years old (mean age = 5 years, 8 months). The procedure was the same as that of Experiment 1 (i.e., a warm-up problem followed by four main problems), except for two changes. First, sampling was with replacement on all five problems (and without feedback). Second, a forced-choice frequency probe was administered just before each prediction. These probes consisted of posing questions such as: "Did we have more _____ (name of animal class) or more _____ (name of animal class) when we started?" "Do you think that there are more _____ or more _____ in here now?" "Did we put more _____ than _____ in here at the start?"

As anticipated by the retrieval-failure hypothesis, the subjects' frequency memories were quite good and there was a considerable improvement in their probability judgments. On Trial 1, 89% of the retrieval probes were answered correctly, and the High class was correctly predicted 94% of the time on Trial 1. The conditional probability of a correct prediction on Trial 1 given a correct response to the frequency-memory probe was unity. The results for Trials 2-5 are best displayed in another matrix:

	$H_pH_r\,(n+1)$	$H_pL_r\,(n+1)$	$L_pH_r\,(n+1)$	$L_pL_r\,(n+1)$
$H_pH_r\,(n)$	.81	.01	.06	.12
$H_pL_r\,(n)$	.91	.02	.04	.03
$L_pH_r\,(n)$	.88	.05	.00	.07
$L_pL_r\,(n)$	.86	.03	.07	.04

The notation is read as follows: H_pH_r denoes trials on which High was the response on both the frequency probe and the prediction; H_pL_r denotes trials on which High was the probe response and Low was the prediction; L_pH_r denotes trials on which Low was the probe response and High was the prediction; and L_pL_r denotes trials on which Low was the response on both the frequency probe and the prediction.

According to the data in the matrix, performance on Trials 2-5 was, for the first time, analogous to performance on Trial 1. Summing across subjects and trials shows that roughly 86% of the frequency-memory probes were answered correctly on Trials 2-5, a value that does not differ significantly from the 89% success rate observed on Trial 1. Also, the subjects almost always predicted that an element from the High class would be sampled when they had responded High to the probe.

The conditional probability of a High prediction given a High probe response was .95, which does not differ significantly from the value of .94 observed on Trial 1. Finally, the unconditional probability of predicting High on Trials 2-5 was .86. This value is significantly smaller than unity and significantly smaller than the .94 unconditional probability on Trial 1, whereas the latter value does not differ significantly from unity.

Thus, young children were able to identify the more frequent class on the great preponderance of the probes, which shows that the relevant frequency differential was still in storage on most problems, and answering frequency-memory problems dramatically improved probability judgments, which is consistent with the view that the principal locus of working-memory failures in these children is a tendency to use the most recently encoded information in short-term memory as a basis for retrieval. Despite these findings, it should be noted that there is some residual variance that is not accounted for by the retrieval-failure hypothesis. Whereas the hypothesis predicts perfect performance on the frequency-memory probes and on the prediction trials, neither result was obtained. The probability of a High probe response, although large in absolute terms, was significantly smaller than unity. The observed values were .89 on Trial 1 and .86 on Trials 2-5. The probability of a High prediction on Trials 2-5 was .86. If it is assumed that responses to probes that were not based on frequency information were either guesses or based on information that is uncorrelated with frequency, the 10-15% error rate and the ½ guessing probability suggest that frequency information was still in storage on about 70-80% of the items. Since external frequency stores do not appear to enhance the probability judgments of 4- and 5-year-olds, it seems more likely that retroactive interference (rather than encoding failure) is responsible for the absence of frequency information on 20-30% of the trials. If one accepts the view that such interference is most likely to occur when work space is limited, the suggestion is that although most 4- and 5-year-olds' working memories are adequate for the storing-processing load imposed by probability judgment, the load exceeds the capacity ceilings of some of these children.

Remarks on Experiments 1-6

The first six experiments illustrate that it is possible to implicate working-memory variables in young children's errors on cognitive tasks in reasonably direct ways and that it is sometimes possible to attribute nearly all the variation for a given age level to a single working-memory locus. It will be remembered that the original retrieval-failure hypothesis in Experiment 3 assumed that 4- and 5-year-olds (a) have no appreciable difficulty encoding frequency information into short-term memory, (b) have no appreciable difficulty retaining frequency traces in storage across a short sequence of predictions, (c) have the necessary frequency processing operations stored in long-term memory, but (d) habitually use the wrong cues to guide their search through long-term memory for computational operations. Generally speaking, this hypothesis covers the facts that have been reported. The only major exception occurred in Experiment 6, where frequency counts appeared to have fallen out of storage on a small but significant proportion of the problems.

However, this finding can be accommodated by a revised retrieval-failure hypothesis in which Assumption (c) is weakened somewhat. According to the revision, 4- and 5-year-olds' probability judgment errors are normally retrieval failures, but in a small percentage of cases the frequency counts have fallen out of storage, presumably as a result of retroactive interference prompted by space constraints on working memory. In these cases, probability judgment errors are storage failures.

Given that working-memory analysis has enjoyed some success in explaining the probability judgments of a particular age level, the next question is whether it does a comparable job with development. Extant data on probability judgment (e.g., see Hoemann & Ross's 1982 review) show that predictive accuracy improves substantially between the ages of 4 and 5 and the ages of 7 and 8. Why? On the basis of the evidence considered so far, one would expect that these improvements are not chiefly a consequence of increased ability to encode frequency information or increased availability of the frequency processing software in long-term memory, because neither of these variables appeared to be influential with 4- and 5-year-olds. Instead, age improvements in probability judgment should result primarily from an increased reliance on frequency-based retrieval cues, with some additional contribution from a decline in the storage-failure rate due to increased working-memory capacity. The experiments that I now summarize were designed to determine whether or not such predictions could be confirmed in data.

Experiment 7

Except for the age of the subjects, this study was identical to Experiment 1 in both methodology and purpose. A sample of second-grade children ($N = 53$, mean age = 8 years, 4 months) was administered a sequence of five two-class problems (a warm-up task plus four experimental problems) identical to those described in Experiment 1.

The pattern of predictions indicated that second graders were different than preschoolers in some respects and similar in others. Concerning differences, predictive accuracy was better on Trial 1 and the response alternation tendency on Trials 2-5 varied as a function of whether the immediately preceding prediction was correct or incorrect. Concerning similarities, the rate at which the High class was predicted on Trial 1 was still less than unity, and the response alternation tendency was still apparent on Trials 2-5.

Turning to the detailed findings, the High class was predicted 87% of the time on Trial 1. This is about 20% better than the level of Trial 1 accuracy observed in 4- and 5-year-olds. However, although this value is beginning to approach unity, significance tests showed that it was still smaller than 100%. The detailed findings for Trials 2-5 were as follows.

	High ($n+1$)	Low ($n+1$)
High (n)	.41	.59
Low (n)	.84	.16

As can be seen, second graders, like preschoolers, were inclined to predict whichever class had not been predicted on the immediately preceding trial. However, there is a new finding. If the transition matrices for Experiments 1 and 2 are examined, it will be noted that the tendency to alternate after a High prediction (i.e., to predict Low on the next trial) and the tendency to alternate after a Low prediction (i.e., to predict High on the next trial) are roughly equal. With second graders, however, Low → High alternation is much more pronounced than High → Low alternation.

A possible interpretation of the discrepancy between the High→Low and Low→ High alternation rates is that whereas preschoolers almost never use frequency cues for retrieval after Trial 1, second graders use such cues a significant proportion of the time on Trials 2-5. I shall return to this possibility to seek support for it in Experiment 9. For the present, however, I consider questions of encoding and storage failure for second graders.

Experiment 8

That external frequency stores did not affect the probability judgments of 4- and 5-year-olds (Experiments 2 and 4) was interpreted as showing that encoding operations for frequency information are present during early childhood and that most young children can hold frequency traces in short-term memory across a short sequence of predictions. If this view is correct, then encoding-storage manipulations should not have much of an effect on the probability judgments of second graders. An obvious test of the interpretation is to replicate Experiment 2 with second graders. If encoding and storage of frequency information are essentially perfect in early childhood, manipulations designed to enhance encoding and storage of such information should not be any more successful with second graders than they were with preschoolers.

In this experiment, the same tasks described in Experiment 2 were administered to a mixed sample of 7- and 8-year-olds ($N = 42$, mean age = 8 years, 6 months). On Trial 1, the High class was predicted 91% of the time, a value that did not differ significantly from the 89% rate obtained in Experiment 7. On Trials 2-5, the results were as follows.

	High ($n+1$)	Low ($n+1$)
High (n)	.38	.62
Low (n)	.89	.11

Significance tests revealed that none of the four values in this matrix differed from the corresponding value obtained in Experiment 7. Hence, the availability of an external source of frequency information had no measurable effect, relative to Experiment 7, on the probability judgments of second graders.

Experiment 9

In Experiment 3, three-class problems were used to tease apart the retrieval-failure and software-failure hypotheses, with the latter predicting that the response alternation tendency should vary as a function of the correctness or incorrectness of the immediately preceding prediction and the former predicting that it should not. In Experiments 7 and 8, it was found that High → Low alternation was less pronounced than Low → High alternation, and it was suggested that second graders are using frequency retrieval cues at least some of the time on Trials 2-5. Suppose that this interpretation is correct. If so, it leads to two predictions about three-class experiments. To begin with, of course, the High → Medium and High → Low alternation rates should be lower than the Medium → High and Low → High alternation rates. Second and more interesting is that increased reliance on frequency retrieval cues suggests that even on alternation trials (i.e., when the prediction is not the same as on the immediately preceding trial), the choice between the remaining two classes should favor their relative frequency. The rationale for this prediction is as follows. Suppose that on a given trial the subject uses response cues as a basis for retrieval and retrieves a response alternation rule. This eliminates whichever class was predicted on the immediately preceding trial. But it does not provide a basis for choosing between the remaining classes. The three-class data for young children (Experiment 3) suggested that once the class predicted on the preceding trial is eliminated, the choice between the remaining classes is either a guess or based on information that is uncorrelated with frequency. But if older children spontaneously use frequency cues for retrieval on Trials 2-5, a logical strategy would be for them to recycle the retrieval operation by using the frequency information for the two classes that are not eliminated by the response alternation rule. Consequently, we would be likely to find (a) that the Medium prediction rate should be higher than the Low prediction rate on trials where High was the immediately preceding prediction, (b) that the High prediction rate should be higher than the Medium prediction rate on trials where Low was the immediately preceding prediction.

This experiment was a replication of the three-class experiment reported for 4- and 5-year-olds, except for the subjects ($N = 58$, mean age = 8 years, 9 months). On Trial 1, the prediction rates were High = 74%, Medium = 23%, and Low = 3%. The 74% rate for High was significantly less than unity, but it was significantly larger than the 60% value for younger children. The data for Trials 2-5 were as follows.

	High ($n+1$)	Medium ($n+1$)	Low ($n+1$)
High (n)	.08	.64	.28
Medium (n)	.71	.06	.23
Low (n)	.76	.24	.00

Obviously, the response alternation tendency is still in evidence. Unlike Experiments 7 and 8 (and contrary to prediction), there was no tendency for the alternation rate following High predictions to be smaller than the alternation rates following Medium and Low predictions. This datum is inconsistent with the view that the lower High → Low alternation rates in Experiments 7 and 8 reflect increased frequency retrieval among second graders on Trials 2-5. In contrast, the other three predictions that follow from this interpretation were confirmed: There were 36% more Medium predictions than Low predictions when High was the previous response, 48% more High than Low predictions when Medium was the preceding response, and 52% more High than Medium predictions when Low was the preceding response.

The latter findings indicate that older children are processing frequency information of some sort on Trials 2-5. The discrepancy between the two-class transition matrices and the three-class matrix can be eliminated by assuming that older children behave somewhat differently on the two types of items. On two-class problems, they use *either* response information or frequency information on a given trial —hence, the difference between the High → Low and Low → High transition rates. But in three-class problems they normally use both response and frequency information, relying first on response cues to eliminate the class predicted on the preceding trial and then relying on frequency cues to decide between the remaining classes. A plausible reason why younger children may not use this two-step strategy on three-class problems is that space constraints on working memory simply will not permit it, a notion that is consistent with the occasional loss of frequency information from storage in such subjects.

Experiments 10 and 11

If we accept for the moment, pending more direct evidence, the suggestion that older children are more apt to use frequency retrieval cues on all trials of a five-prediction sequence, the next question is, Why? In Experiments 4 and 5, it appeared that young children are disinclined to use frequency cues because retrieval is dominated by recency of encoding. Explicitly, it appeared that retrieval was guided by relative frequency when that was the most recently encoded information (Trial 1 in Experiments 1-3 and 5), by response information when that was the most recently encoded information (Trials 2-5 in Experiments 1-4 and Trial 1 in Experiment 4), and by stimulus information when that was the most recently encoded information (Trials 2-5 in Experiment 5). A reasonable hypothesis for older children, therefore, is that the increased incidence of frequency-guided retrieval is a consequence of an increasing tendency to select retrieval cues on the basis of content rather than recency.

A second explanation of developmental improvements in retrieval relies on the notion of space constraints. To begin with, recall that working-memory models assume that the sheer capacity of short-term memory (measured in chunks) and the efficiency with which this capacity is used may vary with age. The results of Experiment 6 suggested that young children's working-memory capacity is usually adequate for the storing-processing load imposed by probability judgment. On the other hand, the number of trials on which frequency information had apparently fallen out of storage (about one-quarter) was sufficiently large that it can be argued that the load may have come close to exceeding available capacity in most subjects. In such circumstances, it is likely that working memory would be strongly inclined to favor information that can be more efficiently processed and that, therefore, reduces the possibility that space constraints will be exceeded. According to this argument, reliance on recently encoded information as a source of retrieval cues stems from the fact that, for whatever reasons, such information can be more efficiently processed than information that was stored in short-term memory some time ago.

Essentially, the first hypothesis views the increased incidence of frequency-based retrieval as a consequence of older children's more discriminating use of the traces in short-term memory (presumably accruing from their greater experience with quantitative reasoning situations), whereas the second hypothesis says that it is an automatic consequence of greater working-memory capacity. A third hypothesis, which is a variation on the second, is also possible. It states that the second explanation is correct up to the point where it assumes that there are age changes in efficiency of processing such that less frequently encoded information can be more efficiently processed by older children. This would, of course, eliminate the motivation for using response and stimulus information on Trials 2-5.

The next two experiments provide a differential test of these three explanations. What all three have in common is the prediction that concurrent processing manipulations of the sort studied in Experiment 4 (simultaneous presentation of problems) and Experiment 5 (standard presentation with feedback) should have less of an effect on second graders than they did on 4- and 5-year-olds. But they diverge on other, more detailed predictions. To see what the differences are, suppose that Experiments 4 and 5 are replicated with both younger and older children. Suppose also that the procedure is modified to incorporate occasional short-term memory probes for response information (the immediately preceding prediction) in Experiment 4 and occasional short-term memory probes for stimulus information (the immediately preceding feedback event) in Experiment 5. What would the three hypotheses lead us to expect about the data?

The most interesting results are those concerned with potential age differences in subjects' retention of irrelevant stimulus and response information. The first and third hypotheses do not assume that working-memory capacity is increasing with age. Increased use of frequency retrieval cues is attributed either to better knowledge of their relevance or to greater ease of processing, relative to more recently encoded information. It seems clear that neither of these hypotheses would expect that children's memory for irrelevant information should increase with age. Since working-memory capacity, relative to the demands of probability judgment tasks, evidently is limited, the most plausible scenario is that older children would be less inclined to retain irrelevant task information, either because they are more likely to recognize its irrelevance or because frequency information is becoming easier to process. In contrast, the second hypothesis clearly anticipates that memory for irrelevant information should improve with age, even though such information has a smaller effect on probability judgments in older children. If working-memory capacity is increasing, then there is more space available to older subjects for storing and processing irrelevant information as well as relevant information.

The subjects in Experiment 10 were 30 kindergarteners (mean age = 5 years, 8 months) and 30 third graders (mean age = 8 years, 9 months). The subjects in Experiment 11 were also 30 kindergarteners (mean age = 5 years, 5 months) and

30 third graders (mean age = 8 years, 10 months). The procedure was the same as in Experiment 1, except that the four experimental problems were presented in two pairs and that outcome feedback was provided. In Experiment 10, after the warm-up task had been administered, the subject was asked to construct the sampling spaces for the first two problems (e.g., "Put seven horses and three cats in this container" and then "Put seven turtles and three cows in this other container"). To avoid possible storage failures arising from the use of four different classes, the same numbers of animals of each type deposited in the containers were also displayed in rows in front of the appropriate container. Next, the subject made a sequence of 10 predictions, 5 for each container. The sequence began with the random selection of one of the two containers, with predictions alternating between containers thereafter. After each prediction, the experimenter sampled an element from the container about which the prediction had just been made, displayed it to the subject, and then returned the element to its container. Hence, on each prediction in a 10-trial sequence save the first, a prediction about a given container was preceded by a stimulus information about the *other container.* Probes for this stimulus information were administered immediately after some predictions. Specifically, following four (randomly selected) of the predictions, two for each container, the subject was asked, "The last time I took a picture from here, did I get a ____ or a ____ ?" When the 10-prediction sequence with four probes had been completed for the first pair of experimental problems, it was repeated for the other pair of experimental problems, yielding a total of 20 probability judgments and eight probe responses for each subject.

Experiment 11 was similar to Experiment 10, with the only important change being the nature of the feedback event. Immediately before requesting a prediction about a given container, the experimenter sampled an element from that container, displayed it to the subject, and then returned it to the container. On each prediction in a 10-trial sequence, therefore, a prediction about a given container was preceded by stimulus information about *that same container.*

The question of principal interest is whether or not there were age trends in memory for the feedback information, and if so, whether the direction was positive or negative. In the event, the probe data favored the second hypothesis (developmental improvements in working-memory capacity) because memory for irrelevant stimulus information was better in third graders in both experiments. In Experiment 10, kindergarteners selected the element that had been drawn from the other container at the start of the trial 76% of the time, whereas 95% of the probes were correctly answered by the third graders. In Experiment 11, the corresponding figures were 74% correct for kindergarteners and 94% correct for third graders.

Experiment 12

The last experiment was an attempt to implicate age improvements in frequency retrieval more directly in the age improvements in probability judgment discussed earlier. In Experiment 6, it will be recalled that 4- and 5-year-olds appeared to have access to the correct frequency counts on about three-quarters of the trials and that being constrained to remember these counts on a memory probe greatly enhanced performance. In fact, the conditional probability of predicting High given a High response to the frequency probe did not differ significantly from 1. What does one expect for older children? To begin with, the conditional probability of predicting High given a High response to the frequency probe should be as great in older children as in young children. In addition, if age-related increases in the use of frequency cues are attributable to age-related increases in the capacity of working memory, then the absolute level of accuracy on the frequency probes should be greater in older children. This prediction follows from the fact that decay of stored frequency traces due to retroactive interference from recently encoded information should be less severe if working-memory capacity is greater (cf. Experiment 6).

A replication of the frequency probe study with older children produced data that were generally consistent with these predictions. Apart from the subjects ($N = 64$, mean age = 8 years, 9 months), the design was the same as that of Experiment 6. On Trial 1, the High class was correctly predicted 97% of the time and the frequency probe was correctly answered 99% of the time. The results for Trials 2-5 were as follows.

	$H_p H_r$ $(n+1)$	$H_p L_r$ $(n+1)$	$L_p H_r$ $(n+1)$	$L_p L_r$ $(n+1)$
$H_p H_r$ (n)	.96	.00	.02	.02
$H_p H_r$ (n)	.57	.14	.29	.00
$L_p H_r$ (n)	.00	.25	.75	.00
$L_p L_r$ (n)	.00	1.00	.00	.00

The notation for this matrix is the same as for the matrix in Experiment 6. The only values that are meaningful are those in the first row of the matrix. The fact that 97% of the Trial 1 responses were $H_p H_r$, together with the fact that 96% of $H_p H_r$ transitions were to another $H_p H_r$ trial, means that virtually all of the responses for Trials 2-5 are in the first row.

For purposes of developmental comparison, it will be recalled that 82% of the frequency probes were correctly answered in Experiment 6, a datum that was interpreted as showing that the relevant frequency differential was still available in short-term memory on about two-thirds of the trials. The present subjects answered 97% of the Trial 1 frequency probes correctly and 96% of the Trials 2-5 frequency probes correctly. Both values are significantly larger than the corresponding percentages in Experiment 6 and neither differs significantly from 100%, with the latter result suggesting that frequency counts were in storage on nearly all trials with these subjects. The absolute level of accuracy of probability judgment was also higher with these subjects. On Trial 1, 99% of the predictions were High, compared to 94% in Experiment 6. These two values do not differ significantly from each other. On Trials 2-5, however, 95% of the predictions were High, compared to 86% in Experiment 6. The former value is reliably larger than the latter but not reliably smaller than unity.

Remarks on Experiments 7-12

The results of the experiments with older children converge on two conclusions about the working-memory loci of age-related changes in predictive accuracy on these tasks. First, the proximal cause of these changes seems to be age-related changes in subjects' tendency to use frequency cues as a basis for retrieval. Although it is quite possible that other working-memory loci are contributing small slices of the age variation, it is difficult to escape the conclusion that retrieval development is the key factor, especially when one compares the large differences in accuracy with and without frequency probes. The other conclusion is that retrieval development is more the result of age-related changes in the capacity of working memory than of age-related changes in specific knowledge about the pertinence of frequency information or age-related changes in the efficiency with which frequency information is processed. This second conclusion is frankly speculative and rests primarily on the fact that memory for irrelevant stimulus events improves with age (Experiments 10 and 11) and the fact that the rate of storage failure for frequency information declines with age (Experiment 12).

Random Notes on Metatheory

Throughout this chapter, I have been concerned to argue, more by example than by statement, that the litmus test for any theory of cognitive development is explanation. It should permit us to formulate sensible hypotheses about the sources of age-related variation in performance on tasks of the sort that were considered in the first two sections of this chapter, and these hypotheses should lend themselves to straightforward experimental tests such as those presented above.

This is not to say that the explanatory emphasis of working-memory analysis is commonly accepted as the chief aim of cognitive-developmental theorizing. Many investigators, perhaps a majority, are of the opinion that theories should be primarily heuristic or, in plain language, inspirational (e.g., Feldman, 1980, 1981). Inspirational theories differ from explanatory theories in that the former are judged by aesthetic criteria, whereas the latter are judged by the pragmatic yardstick of whether or not they deliver the goods when it comes to accounting for specific types of age variation. While I agree that inspirational theories have a role to play in most areas of psychology, principally during early phases of research (cf. Brainerd, 1981c), I also maintain that there is a strong case to be made that our highest priority at present should be explanation.

In part, this case rests on the current situation in the literature. The revival of Piagetian theory during the early 1960s was followed by two decades of intensive study of cognitive development. This research has put us into possession of many important facts about children's concepts, children's reasoning, children's learning, children's reading, children's memories, and so forth. The literature on cognitive development has grown to the point that, for example, an entire volume of the most recent revision of *Carmichael's Manual of Child Psychology* has been devoted to reviewing it. But by consensus, this same research has dealt body blows to the theory that inspired much of it in the first place. Thus, although we know far more about the basic facts of cognitive development than we did 20 years ago, our theoretical understanding of what these facts mean has diminished—hence, the need for concerted and comprehensive attempts at explanation.

Although the need for explanation seems clear enough, most students of cognitive development are also interested in conceptual questions that are broader than how to account for data points. Such questions are properly called "metatheoretical issues" because they are not directly connected to whether or not a theory delivers the explanatory goods for specific data. Assuming that some theory enjoys modest explanatory success, it is natural to inquire whether or not it provides us with any leverage on traditional metatheoretical concerns.

In the case of working-memory analysis, the answer appears to be yes, and consequently I conclude this chapter with a brief overview of three metatheoretical issues from the perspective of working memory. It should be stressed, however, that this is not intended to be a systematic treatment of the metatheoretical implications of working memory. My only purposes are to suggest that working-memory distinctions are not entirely devoid of such implications and to give some textbook illustrations of metatheoretical issues that these distinctions may serve to clarify.

Origins of Cognitive Development

Perhaps the oldest dilemma in cognitive-developmental theory concerns the causes of the age-related changes that we observe in the process variables that seem to be implicated in children's performance on cognitive tasks. Are these changes the result of learning experiences that are relatively specific to the tasks in question, or do they originate in more global developmental events, such as maturational changes and experiences that are not task specific (e.g., play, acquisition of language)? As things now stand, theories of cognitive development that aspire to some level of generality either focus on task-specific experiences and say little about nonspecific factors or they focus on nonspecific factors and say little about task-specific experiences. This is equally true of theories that seek to explain the development of particular concepts. A classic illustration is provided by the numerous theories of conservation development, which can be classified (see Brainerd, 1979a) either as stressing the role of particular conservation-related skills (e.g., the knowledge of a certain rule, paying attention to a certain type of stimulus information) or as stressing global prerequisites (e.g., cognitive structures, language development).

I think we can safely conclude that task-specific experience and nonspecific developmental changes must both be invoked, and hence that a successful theoretical framework will have to take both into account. If motivation is required to accept this view, it can be found in profusion in the literature on children's concept learning. On the one hand, experiments have firmly established that young children's performance on a long list of tasks that ostensibly measure various logical, mathematical, physical, and social concepts can be improved by training task-specific skills (e.g., see reviews by Beilin, 1971, 1978). These improvements are typically quite durable, and they transfer well (Brainerd, 1978a). On the other hand, the size of these learning effects appears to be limited by general variables such as social class, psychometric intelligence, and creativity.

Another motivation for incorporating general and specific factors in a theory of cognitive development is that their relative contributions are likely to vary as a function of the type of cognitive task that is being studied and the age level being considered. It is not unreasonable to suppose that task-specific experiences will be more influential with paradigms that measure things which are purely matters of social consensus (e.g., concepts such as animism or subjective morality) than with paradigms that measure information that is more objective (e.g., concepts such as number or length or weight). Concerning age, it has often been speculated (e.g., Flavell & Wohlwill, 1969) that the influence of general factors is more pronounced during the initial phases of age-related changes on a task, with specific factors becoming more influential during later phases.

A key advantage of working-memory analysis is that the five degrees of freedom that one manipulates (encoding, short-term storage, retrieval from long-term memory, computational operations stored in long-term memory, and space constraints) include variables that (a) presumably are affected primarily by task-specific experiences, (b) presumably are affected primarily by general developmental factors, and (c) presumably are affected by both. Using a computer metaphor, one can divide the five degrees of freedom into "hardware" variables and "software" variables, with computational procedures stored in long-term memory being the software variables and encoding, storage, retrieval, and space constraints being the hardware variables. The software plus retrieval would seem to fall naturally into Category (a) in that knowledge of what sorts of information to use as a basis for retrieval and the presence of algorithms for processing particular types of information should both depend on experiences that are rather closely connected to the task. Thus, the counting algorithm posited in iterative theories of mental addition (Groen & Parkman, 1972) evidently requires counting experience, and the intersection search algorithm posited in fact retrieval theories evidently requires experience with number facts.

In contrast, general developmental factors appear to be major contributors to the rest of the working-memory hardware. Concerning space constraints, this variable falls naturally into Category (b) because it is presumed to be independent of the storing-processing operations that constitute the working-memory system for any given task. Whether the general factors that control the development of working-memory capacity are experiential or maturational or both depends on the sorts of assumptions that one makes about how capacity develops. We saw earlier that some investigators assume that the sheer number of chunks available in short-term memory increases with age, others assume that the number of chunks is fixed but processing efficiency increases, and still others assume that both processing efficiency and chunk number are increasing. Under the chunk increase hypothesis, neurological development is probably the most promising explanation of age-related trends in capacity. (In this connection, it is interesting to note that the largest changes in the length of short-term memory span occur during the same age range as myelination of the corpus collosum.) Under the processing-efficiency increase hypothesis, the acquisition of general mnemonic strategies (grouping, chunking, rehearsal, image formation, etc.) may explain age-related trends in capacity. If the number of chunks and the efficiency with which they are used both change with age, then neurological developmental and nonspecific memory experience leading to the acquisition of general mnemonics can probably both be implicated in capacity development.

Last, the encoding and storage variables seem to belong in Category (c). With respect to encoding, it is possible to affect the information that children will encode by training them on the specific aspects of the language that is used on a target task (e.g., relational terminology) or by training them to pay attention to certain types of perceptual information. Such task-specific encoding manipulations are known to improve performance on certain problems that measure Piagetian concrete-operational concepts. On the other hand, the encoding skills that children bring with them to an experiment, which are mostly under the control of experiences that are not directly connected to the task at hand, also contribute to performance. Concerning storage, children can also be trained to retain the relevant background information on a task in preference to irrelevant information, with the large literature on so-called "dimensional sensitivity" training in children's concept identification (for a review, see Esposito, 1975) being a case in point. The information that children choose to retain in storage is also affected by various preferences that they have at the outset of the experiments, with the literature on how preexperimental dimensional preferences affect discrimination transfer being a case in point (e.g., Caron, 1969; Seitz & Weir, 1971; Smiley, 1973; Smiley & Weir, 1966). Like encoding tendencies, these preexperimental storage preferences are under the control of experiential variables that presumably are not directly connected to the target task.

Qualitative Change and Quantitative Change

Another ancient dilemma, which is usually called the continuity-discontinuity problem, concerns whether cognitive development should be viewed as a morphogenic process involving changes in type or as a nonmorphogenic process involving smooth, continuous change. Historically, answers have tended to vary as a function of what sorts of data are emphasized. On the one hand, there are many aspects of cognitive performance that remain developmentally invariant, a fact that is suggestive of continuity. Perhaps the most obvious illustration is that the *direction* of effects of task-difficulty manipulations is almost always developmentally invariant. That is, a manipulation (e.g., concreteness, familiarity, organization, meaningfulness) that enhances or inhibits the performance of younger subjects normally has the same effect on the performance of older subjects. In short, Age × Treatment interactions involving "crossovers" are rare in comparison with other types of Age × Treatment interactions (e.g., converging and diverging fans). There is also considerable evidence of very basic developmental invariances at the level of the mathematical structure of the data generated by specific paradigms. The age-related changes in performance that are observed on such tasks seem to exclude the possibility of a transformation of the underlying model of the data. To date, developmental invariance in the underlying mathematical model of the data has been observed for age-related changes in recognition memorizing (Brainerd, 1983; Brainerd & Howe, 1980), age-related changes in recall memorizing (Brainerd, 1983; Brainerd & Howe, 1978, 1982; Brainerd et al., 1982), age-related changes in discrimination learning (Brainerd, 1983; Brainerd & Howe, 1979; Greenberg, 1981), age-related changes in discrimination transfer (Brainerd, 1981; Greenberg, 1981), and age-related changes in certain forms of socialized language (Sedlak & Walton, 1982). In all of these areas, the numerical values of the parameters of the best fitting model may change with age, but the model itself evidently does not. Obviously, such results are suggestive of deep underlying continuity.

On the other hand, performance on cognitive tasks routinely shows dramatic age-related variation, often within remarkably narrow age ranges, a datum that is usually taken as evidence of qualitative change. Between the ages of 5 and 7, for example, performance on a wide assortment of measures (discrimination learning, classification, mental arithmetic, conservation, etc.) improves markedly. Similarly, although the underlying mathematical model of the data appears to be invariant with tasks such as those mentioned above, there are other tasks for which mathematical models are not developmentally invariant. An example has already been encountered in latency models of children's mental addition. If L is latency to solve an $m + n = k$ item, where $m > n$, $L = a + bn$ is the best fitting model for young children, but $L = a + b(k)^2$ is the best fitting model for older children. Results such as these are as suggestive of fundamental changes in underlying processes as the results in the preceding paragraph are suggestive of fundamental continuity.

As a rule, cognitive-developmental theorists have been more impressed by evidence of discontinuity than by evidence of continuity. Hence, qualitative-change theories have tended to predominate. Since Freud's time, the hallmark of such theories has been that development is described in terms of sequences of stages, with stage transitions implying qualitative changes in process. Of course, Piaget's stages and those of neo-Piagetian theorists, such as Kohlberg's stages of moral development, are the standard examples. However, stage typologies have also been popular in areas such as the development of learning, with Kendler and Kendler's (1962) mediational and nonmediational stages and Hebb's (1949) set-influenced and nonset-influenced stages being the best known illustrations.

The problem with stage theories is that they resolve the continuity-discontinuity dilemma largely by ignoring it. Although it is true that some attention is given to continuous factors (e.g., the functional invariants in Piaget's theory), it is stages that are the centerpieces of such theories, and it is stages that are most directly tied to age variation. It has never been clear how stage changes are linked to continuous-change variables, a difficulty that is usually called the "transition problem." Because of the transition problem, plus a long list of other difficulties with stages (see commentaries by various writers in Brainerd, 1978b, 1979c), proposing stage sequences does not appear to be a satisfactory method of dealing with the continuity-discontinuity issue.

Although the continuity-discontinuity issue has hitherto proved intractable, the dimensions of a satisfactory solution are fairly clear, at least in the abstract. What is apparently called for is a mechanism whereby qualitative perturbations can be introduced into a theory while enough overall continuity is preserved to account for developmental invariances. If this method of introducing qualitative perturbations while preserving overall continuity is to be maximally useful as a theoretical tool, it should be readily adaptable to most cognitive tasks. This brings us back to working-memory analysis.

Working-memory models permit the imposition of qualitative perturbations by allowing for the possibility of alterations in the basic structure of individual storing and processing operations. For example, we have seen that the computational operations that are activated on a mental addition item may change from one-step iterations (Groen & Parkman, 1972) to intersection search of a fact table (Ashcraft, 1982). Similarly, the configuration of the background information that is stored on a given task may change with age. Here, consider the transitivity paradigm again. On a three-term problem of the form $A > B > C$, the critical background information consists of the premises $A > B$ and $B > C$. Research on children's understanding of such information indicates that very young children tend to encode and store traces that carry absolute rather than comparative information. That is, the premises $A > B$ and $B > C$ may be stored as propositions of the form "A is long," "B is short," "B is long," and "C is short." In contrast, older children appear to encode and store traces that carry comparative information, which means that the premises $A > B$ and $B > C$ may be stored in a single serial structure.

In sum, working-memory models accommodate both discontinuity and continuity within the same framework. Discontinuity is accommodated by allowing the structure of encoding operations, stored traces, retrieval operations, and computational operations to be qualitatively different for different age levels. Continuity is accommodated by preserving the macrostructure of a working-memory system. The fine-grain structure of encoding, storing, retrieving, and computing aside, a given task always demands the activation of a working-memory system that will encode and store certain types of information, that will use this information to guide retrieval, and that will bring to bear computational operations that are capable of processing this information. Roughly, then, the basic diagram of information flow (Figure 4-1) is developmentally invariant, and the sequence in which the principal components of a working-memory system are activated is invariant in the face of qualitative changes in the architecture of the components themselves.

Sensitivity, Invariant Sequences, and Measurement Error

The final metatheoretical question, a question of more recent origin than the other two, is closely connected to stage theories of cognitive development. It concerns which procedures are "best" for measuring children's understanding of certain concepts. Following a paper by Flavell (1971), this has usually been called "the sensitivity problem." There are two contexts in which this problem most often arises in the literature, namely, with reference to evidence of conceptual precocity and with reference to invariant sequence studies. I discuss these two contexts separately and then consider what light working-memory analysis may shed on the sensitivity problem.

Conceptual Precocity. A standard type of experiment in concept-development research consists of presenting data which seem to show that children understand some logical, mathematical, physical, or social concept much earlier than Piagetian theory supposes. Research of this sort may properly be said to have begun with Braine's (1959) doctoral thesis on transitivity. Braine argued that for any given concept, Piaget's clinical method measures many abilities other than the concept itself, a criticism that has been echoed in any number of subsequent methodological commentaries (e.g., Braine, 1962; Brainerd, 1973a; Bryant & Trabasso, 1971; Gelman, 1972; Siegel, 1978; Trabasso, 1977). If Braine's reasoning were to be translated into working-memory language, the essence of a concept would be the processing operations (rules, strategies, etc.) whereby background information is converted into responses. Thus, tasks that do not take into account the possibilities of encoding failure, storage failure, retrieval failure, and space constructs are not the best measures because they are prone to high levels of false negative error. Piaget's clinical method, in particular, was criticized as being overly conservative because it places excessive demand on children's verbal sophistication and on their memories.

To deal with this possibility, Braine suggested that concept assessment procedures be simplified by reducing their demands on ancillary skills. He applied this strategy to the transitive inference paradigm, using a nonverbal discrimination-learning task that resembled the well-known intermediate size transposition paradigm (e.g., see Stevenson, 1970, 1972). Whereas Piaget (1952; Piaget, Inhelder, & Szeminska, 1960) had reported that few children make transitive inferences before 7 or 8 years of age, Braine found that most 5-year-olds passed the new test. During the intervening two decades, this same sequence of criticizing Piagetian measurements for false negative bias, followed by the construction of new and simplified dependent variables, followed by data showing precocious knowledge of concepts has been repeated for all of the principal concepts from Piaget's stages. For example, extensive literatures of this sort exist for ordering concepts (e.g., Siegel, 1971), classification concepts (e.g., Siegel, McCabe, Brand, & Matthews, 1978), transitive inference (e.g., Trabasso, 1977), probability concepts (e.g., Yost, Siegel, & Andrews, 1962), cardinal number concepts (e.g., Gelman, 1972), various magnitude concepts (e.g., Siegel, 1978), various perspective-taking concepts (e.g., Borke, 1978), object permanence (e.g., Bower, 1974), and causal inference (e.g., Hood, & Bloom, 1979). The evidence of conceptual precocity using the "simplification strategy" is so vast that many investigators have concluded that hereditary programming must play a much more direct role in concept development than has been previously supposed.

Unfortunately, there is an automatic counterargument to such data that is based on the idea of false positive error, a point that was first elucidated in some commentaries by Smedslund (1963, 1969) on Braine's papers. It may be true, as adherents of the simplification strategy maintain, that the revised measures simply reduce the incidence of false negative error. But it could also be true that performance is better on simplified tasks because they inflate the incidence of false positive error. (In the language of working-memory analysis, performance is not better because encoding, storage, and retrieval failures are less likely to occur, but because children can now activate other processing operations that are more primitive than those that define the concept that we actually seek to measure.) In line with this argument, it has been possible to identify sources of false positive error on simplified tests of concepts such as transitivity (e.g., Murray & Youniss, 1968), cardinal number (e.g., Brainerd & Siegel, 1978), perspective taking (e.g., Chandler & Greenspan, 1972), and class inclusion (e.g., Brainerd & Kaszor, 1974). Although specific false positive errors can normally be controlled once they have been identified, the more serious problem is that there may be numerous other sources of false positive error operating on any given task of which we are completely unaware.

It has proved to be impossible, in principle, to decide between the false negative and false positive interpretations of precocity data at our present level of theoretical sophistication. As is often the case with metatheoretical issues, the underlying reason for the dilemma becomes clear when some equations are considered. Suppose that we perform an elementary experiment in which we measure some concept A by using two tests i and j. Suppose further that j is a simplified version of i. For the sake of argument, let us assume that i and j are both valid measures of Concept A— that is, subjects who have this concept will perform better on either test than subjects who do not. The only empirical information that these tests produce when they are administered to children is level of performance.

Let $p(i)$ be an appropriate performance measure for Test i (e.g., the average probability of a correct response for the population being studied) and let $p(j)$ be the same measure for Test j. Since Test i is assumed to be a valid measure of Concept A, the performance level can be expressed as

$$p(i) = P_A(1 - \beta_i) + (1 - P_A)\alpha_i, \tag{4-2}$$

where P_A is the proportion of subjects who have Concept A, β_i is the characteristic false negative error rate for Test i, and α_i is the characteristic false positive error rate for Test i. The performance level for Test j can be expressed as

$$p(j) = P_A(1 - \beta_j) + (1 - P_A)\alpha_j, \tag{4-3}$$

where P_A is defined as before, but β_j and α_j are the characteristic false negative and false positive error rates, respectively, for Test j.

Insofar as differential performance on these tests is concerned, Equations 4-2 and 4-3 pose what is usually called a parameter identifiability problem. Since j is a simplified version of i, we naturally expect that performance will be better on j— that is, $p(j) > p(i)$ in data. Given that the same competence or "knowledge of the concept" parameter appears in both expressions, the different performance levels must be attributable to a higher false positive rate on Test j or a lower false negative rate on Test j or both. But it is impossible to decide between these interpretations because although we have only one empirical degree of freedom—the performance level—for each test, we have three theoretical degrees of freedom to contend with.

This interpretative impasse stems from the fact that, generally speaking, we do not know what it means to "have Concept A." Without such knowledge, we cannot devise independent procedures for measuring conceptual competence, false positive error, and false negative error. And unless such procedures are available, it is painfully evident from Equations 4-2 and 4-3 that we shall not be able to decide between the false negative and false positive interpretations of conceptual precocity data.

Although I have stressed the theoretical ramifications of whether one sees performance on simplified tests as evidence of conceptual understanding or as evidence of false positive error, this matter also has implications for the psychology of instruction. For some years now, recommendations about when to introduce certain components of elementary school mathematics and science curricula have been influenced by normative findings on certain concrete-operational skills (cf. Brainerd,

1978c, 1978d). Under the first interpretation of performance on simplified tests, most of the basic concepts of arithmetic and the physical sciences are in children's repertoires by the time they enter kindergarten, and therefore we need not be overly concerned about the precise timing of the introduction of these concepts in the classroom. But if the false positive interpretation is accepted, instruction in most of these concepts should probably not begin before the middle of elementary school (see also Sigel, 1969).

Invariant Sequences. At one time, studies designed to determine whether or not the concepts associated with Piaget's stages develop in fixed sequences were a dominant theme of concept-development research (for reviews of the early literature, see Flavell, 1970; Hooper, Goldman, Storck, & Burke, 1971). Since Piagetian theory anticipates many such sequences, it was originally thought that such studies afford direct tests of the theory's claim that there are culturally universal stages of cognitive development. Eventually, substantial literatures accumulated on sequences in the acquisition of various conservation concepts (e.g., Brainerd & Brainerd, 1972; Uzgiris, 1964), sequences in the acquisition of object search skills (e.g., Gratch & Landers, 1972; Miller, Cohen, & Hill, 1970), sequences in the understanding of identity and equivalence (e.g., Brainerd & Hooper, 1975, 1978), sequences in the understanding of compensation and conservation (e.g., Gelman & Weinberg, 1972; Larsen & Flavell, 1970), sequences in the understanding of ordinal and cardinal number (e.g., Brainerd, 1973b; Seigel, 1974), sequences in the understanding of class inclusion and transitivity (e.g., Brainerd, 1974; Hooper, Swinton, & Sipple, 1979b), and sequences in the understanding of seriation and transitivity (e.g., Murray & Youniss, 1968; Youniss & Murray, 1970).

Although these so-called invariant sequence studies continue to be reported, measurement error problems analogous to those just discussed have made them far less popular than heretofore. Along the way in such research, it was discovered that "universal sequences" were in fact highly unstable and that seemingly trivial procedural variations produced different sequences for the same concepts. More particularly, it was found that (a) sequences originally obtained in Geneva with the clinical method were not necessarily obtained outside Geneva with more objective tests and that (b) different sequences were often observed for the same concepts with slightly different versions of objective tests. For example, although Piaget (e.g., 1968) concluded that identity and equivalence are concurrent achievements, early evidence from North America (e.g., Hooper, 1969) seemed to show that identity precedes equivalence. But later North American studies, using objective tests that differed in details such as the presence or absence of explanations, showed in some cases that identity preceded equivalence (e.g., Rybash, Roodin, & Sullivan, 1975) and in other cases that equivalence preceded identity (e.g., Silverstein, Pearson, Aguinaldo, Friedman, Takayama, & Weiss, 1982); in still other cases, however, these studies produced data in agreement with Piaget's (e.g., Koshinsky & Hall, 1973).

However, the most extensive evidence on the instability of an ostensible invariant sequence concerns transitivity and conservation. Piaget (1952) originally reported that children conserve before they make transitive inferences. He went on to argue, largely on theoretical grounds, that conservation of quantitative invariants is an inescapable prerequisite for transitivity. Some years later, Lovell and Ogilvie (1961) conducted an experiment in which children's understanding of weight conservation and their ability to make transitive inferences about weight were compared. Their tests of conservation and transitivity, although similar to Piaget's, were simplified and objective. Their subjects made transitive inferences and understood conservation at about the same time. Subsequently, Smedslund (1963) and McManis (1969) both found that conservation preceded transitivity, as Piaget had originally reported. Their tests were also objective, simplified versions of the Genevan clinical interview, although these tests differed somewhat from Lovell and Ogilvie's. Next, during the early 1970s, several investigators (e.g., Brainerd, 1973c; Toniolo & Hooper, 1975) found that transitivity preceded conservation. Again, their tests were objective, simplified versions of the Genevan measures, and they differed in small ways from the tests of Lovell and Ogilvie, Smedslund, and McManis. The coda, so to speak, to research on transitivity-conservation sequences was an experiment by Keller and Hunter (1973). They studied conservation of length and transitivity of length, and more important, they manipulated a task-difficulty variable (visual illusions) that affects children's length judgments across conservation and transitivity items. In some conservation-transitivity comparisons, conservation performance was better; in others, transitivity performance was better; and in still others there was no difference. Which result is to be believed?

The answer is not clear, and the reason becomes apparent if we again consider some simple equations. Suppose that we are interested in investigating possible developmental sequences in two concepts, A and B. Assume that we have two tests for Concept A, T_{A1} and T_{A2}, which differ in minor procedural details. Assume that we also have two tests for Concept B, T_{B1} and T_{B2}, which differ in minor procedural details. Let $p(T_{A1})$, $p(T_{A2})$, $p(T_{B1})$, and $p(T_{B2})$ be the appropriate empirical measures of performance (e.g., correct response probability) on the respective tests. The relevant expressions for these performance measures are

$$p(T_{A1}) = P_A(1 - \beta_{A1}) + (1 - P_A)\alpha_{A1}, \tag{4-4}$$

$$p(T_{A2}) = P_A(1 - \beta_{A2}) + (1 - P_A)\alpha_{A2}, \tag{4-5}$$

$$p(T_{B1}) = P_B(1 - \beta_{B1}) + (1 - P_B)\alpha_{B1}, \tag{4-6}$$

and

$$p(T_{B2}) = P_B(1 - \beta_{B2}) + (1 - P_B)\alpha_{B2}, \tag{4-7}$$

where P_A is the relevant competence parameter for Concept A, P_B is the relevant competence parameter for Concept B, the α's are the characteristic false positive rates for the tests, and the β's are the characteristic false negative rates for the tests.

Now suppose that these tests are administered to a large sample of subjects and that the results are as follows: $\hat{p}(T_{A1}) = .5$, $\hat{p}(T_{A2}) = .25$, $\hat{p}(T_{B1}) = .5$, $\hat{p}(T_{B2}) = .25$. Note that the apparent developmental relationship between A and B depends on which tests we compare, just as in the literature on identity-equivalence, the literature on conservation-transitivity, and so on. Concept A seems to precede Concept B if T_{A1} and T_{B2} are compared, Concept B seems to precede Concept A if

T_{A2} and T_{B1} are compared, and there seems to be no sequence if the comparison is either T_{A1} versus T_{B1} or T_{A2} versus T_{B2}. Because the same competence parameter appears in the expressions for the A tests and the same competence parameter appears in the expressions for the B tests, this variation in results must be due to variations in the false positive and/or the false negative rates. But since we have no methods for assessing measurement error rates independently, we cannot say which of the test-performance comparisons provides the more accurate picture of the relationship between P_A and P_B, the two parameters that we actually wish to make inferences about.

The problem of invariant sequences, like the problem of conceptual precocity, has practical as well as theoretical implications. One of the oldest issues in elementary education is that of sequencing—that is, the order in which the building blocks of reading, arithmetic, science, writing, and the like should be introduced in the classroom. Because many of the concepts associated with Piaget's concrete-operational stage also appear in elementary mathematics and science curricula, it has often been suggested that decisions about sequencing can be based on the data of invariant sequence studies. But because the data of such studies have a way of conflicting with each other, instructional programmers are confronted with the dilemma of either making no recommendations about sequencing or making recommendations that agree with some results but disagree with others.

Working Memory and Measurement Error. It is obvious from Equations 4-2 to 4-7 that both the precocity problem and the sequence problem are rooted in a deeper question about the nature of measurement error on concept tests. On the one hand, we seek, for practical as well as theoretical reasons, to discover when the average child grasps certain concepts and what the normal acquisition sequence is for certain groups of concepts. On the other hand, we do not have much more than a vague, intuitive idea of what it means to "have a concept." Without more precise definitions, we cannot say which aspects of performance are indicative of conceptual understanding and which aspects of performance are indicative of measurement error. (Or, in the language of the 1960s, we do not know what is competence and what is performance.) Unless progress can be made in this area, we can forget about trying to answer age-of-acquisition and sequence-of-acquisition questions.

How does working memory provide leverage on the nature of measurement error? It does so primarily by allowing investigators to draw a distinction between the short-term memory hardware and the long-term memory software. Encoding operations, short-term storage operations, and retrieval operations constitute the short-term memory hardware, whereas the facts, rules, and transformational procedures in long-term memory, which have been discussed under the collective heading "computational operations," constitute the software. The definition of "having a concept" that comes closest to the spirit of the cognitive-developmental literature, especially the Piagetian area of the literature, is one that relies on software. In other words, when a child is described as having a certain type of conceptual competence, one usually means that he or she possesses some rule, operation, strategy, fact, or the like in long-term memory. But one does not usually mean that he or she is capable of encoding a certain type of information, or of holding certain information in short-term storage, or of using certain types of traces as retrieval cues. Such variables are almost universally regarded as "performance factors" (e.g., cf. Flavell & Wohlwill, 1969), and consequently as sources of measurement error.

The hardware-software distinction provides a conceptually simple definition of what it means to commit a false positive or a false negative error. If a target concept is defined in terms of a certain software package, then concept test errors attributable to hardware failure (encoding failure, storage failure, retrieval failure, space constraints) that occur *when the appropriate software is present in long-term memory* are automatically false negative errors. Concept test errors caused by hardware failures when the appropriate software is absent are not false negatives, however. Turning to false positives, suppose that it is sometimes possible to make a correct response on a certain test without using the software that defines the concept (e.g., by guessing or by retrieving other types of computational operations). Correct responses of this sort that occur in the absence of the relevant software are automatically false positive errors.

Although the hardware-software distinction is an appealing way of dealing with the measurement error problem, it would not be of much use if it were impossible to implicate hardware failures and software failures, respectively, in concept test performance. But as the earlier experiments on probability judgment were intended to illustrate, it is possible to generate convergent evidence on hypotheses about encoding failure, storage failure, retrieval failure, software failure, and space constraints with reasonably uncomplicated experiments. Ultimately, of course, we shall wish to devise general mathematical models whose parameters will provide numerical estimates of the failure rates of the various loci of working-memory systems. Some small progress has lately been made in this direction, but much more remains to be done. The main point is that the hardware-software distinction provides some grounds for optimism about being able to find data-based answers to age-of-acquisition and sequence-of-acquisition questions.

Acknowledgment. The research reported in this chapter was supported by Grant No. A0668 from the Natural Sciences and Engineering Research Council. Computer funds were provided by a grant from the Faculty of Social Science, University of Western Ontario. [I would like to thank Alan Pauro, Michael Pressley, and James Turnure for their comments on an earlier draft of this chapter.]

References

Anderson, N. H., & Cuneo, D. O. The height + width rule in children's judgments of quantity. *Journal of Experimental Psychology: General*, 1978, *107*, 335-378.

Ashcraft, M. H. The development of mental arithmetic: A chronometric approach. *Developmental Review*, 1982, *2*, in press.

Ashcraft, M. H., & Battaglia, J. Cognitive arithmetic: Evidence for retrieval and decision processes in mental addition. *Journal of Experimental Psychology: Human Learning and Memory*, 1978, *4*, 527-528.

Ashcraft, M. H., Hamann, M. S., & Fierman, B. A. *The development of mental addition.* Paper presented at Society for Research in Child Development, Boston, April 1981.

Atkinson, R. C., & Shiffrin, R. M. Human memory: A proposed system and its control processes. In K. W. Spence & J. T. Spence (Eds.), *The psychology of learning and motivation* (Vol. 2). New York: Academic Press, 1968.

Baddeley, A. D., & Hitch, G. Working memory. In G. H. Bower (Ed.), *The psychology of learning and motivation* (Vol. 8). New York: Academic Press, 1974.

Baddeley, A. D., Scott, D., Drynan, R., & Smith, J. C. Short-term memory and the limited-capacity hypothesis. *British Journal of Psychology*, 1969, *60*, 51-55.

Beilin, H. The training and acquisition of logical operations. In M. F. Rosskopf, L. P. Steffe, & S. Taback (Eds.), *Piagetian cognitive-developmental research and mathematics education*. Washington, D.C.: National Council of Teachers of Mathematics, 1971.

Beilin, H. Inducing conservation through training. In G. Steiner (Ed.), *Psychology of the twentieth century* (Vol. 7). Munich, Federal Republic of Germany: Kindler, 1978.

Biggs, J. B. *Information and human learning*. Glenview, Ill.: Scott, Foresman, 1971.

Binet, A., & Henri, V. La psychologie individuells. *L'Année Psychologique*, 1895, *2*, 411-465.

Boersma, F., & Wilton, K. M. Eye movement and conservation acceleration. *Journal of Experimental Child Psychology*, 1974, *17*, 49-60.

Borke, H. Piaget's view of social interaction and the theoretical construct of empathy. In L. S. Siegel & C. J. Brainerd (Eds.), *Alternatives to Piaget: Critical essays on the theory*. New York: Academic Press, 1978.

Bower, T. G. R. The development of object permanence: Some studies of existence constancy. *Perception and Psychophysics*, 1967, *2*, 411-418.

Bower, T. G. R. *Development in infancy*. San Francisco: W. H. Freeman, 1974.

Braine, M. D. S. The ontogeny of certain logical operations: Piaget's formulation examined by nonverbal methods. *Psychological Monographs*, 1959, *73*(5, Whole No. 475).

Braine, M. D. S. Piaget on reasoning: A methodological critique and alternative proposals. In W. Kessen & C. Kuhlman (Eds.), Thought in the young child. *Monographs of the Society for Research in Child Development*, 1962, *27*(2, Whole No. 83).

Brainerd, C. J. Reinforcement and reversibility in quantity conservation acquisition. *Psychonomic Science*, 1972, *27*, 114-116. (a)

Brainerd, C. J. The age-stage issue in conservation acquisition. *Psychonomic Science*, 1972, *29*, 115-117. (b)

Brainerd, C. J. Judgments and explanations as criteria for the presence of cognitive structures. *Psychological Bulletin*, 1973, *79*, 172-179. (a)

Brainerd, C. J. Mathematical and behavioral foundations of number. *Journal of General Psychology*, 1973, *88*, 221-281. (b)

Brainerd, C. J. Order of acquisition of transitivity, conservation, and class inclusion of length and weight. *Developmental Psychology*, 1973, *8*, 105-116. (c)

Brainerd, C. J. Training and transfer of transitivity, conservation, and class inclusion of length. *Child Development*, 1974, *45*, 324-334.

Brainerd, C. J. Does prior knowledge of the compensation rule increase susceptibility to conservation training? *Developmental Psychology*, 1976, *12*, 1-5.

Brainerd, C. J. Feedback, rule knowledge, and conservation learning. *Child Development*, 1977, *48*, 404-411.

Brainerd, C. J. Learning research and Piagetian theory. In L. S. Siegel & C. J.

Brainerd (Eds.), *Alternatives to Piaget: Critical essays on the theory.* New York: Academic Press, 1978. (a)

Brainerd, C. J. The stage question in cognitive-developmental theory. *The Behavioral and Brain Sciences,* 1978, *1,* 173-213. (b)

Brainerd, C. J. *Piaget's theory of intelligence.* Englewood Cliffs, N.J.: Prentice-Hall, 1978. (c)

Brainerd, C. J. Cognitive development and instructional theory. *Contemporary Educational Psychology,* 1978, *3,* 37-50. (d)

Brainerd, C. J. Markovian interpretations of conservation learning. *Psychological Review,* 1979, *86,* 181-213. (a)

Brainerd, C. J. Concept learning and developmental stage. In H. J. Klausmeier et al. (Eds.), *Cognitive learning and development: Piagetian and information processing perspectives.* Cambridge, Mass.: Ballinger, 1979. (b)

Brainerd, C. J. Continuing commentary. *The Behavioral and Brain Sciences,* 1979, *2,* 137-154.

Brainerd, C. J. Working memory and the developmental analysis of probability judgment. *Psychological Review,* 1981, *88,* 463-502. (a)

Brainerd, C. J. *Young children's mental arithmetic errors: A working-memory analysis.* Research Bulletin No. 547, Department of Psychology, University of Western Ontario, 1981. (b)

Brainerd, C. J. Stages II. *Developmental Review,* 1981, *1,* 63-81. (c)

Brainerd, C. J. Children's concept learning as rule-sampling systems with Markovian properties. In C. J. Brainerd (Ed.), *Children's logical and mathematical cognition: Progress in cognitive development research.* New York: Springer-Verlag, 1982.

Brainerd, C. J. Structural invariance in the developmental analysis of learning. In J. Bisanz, G. Bisanz, & R. V. Kail (Eds.), *Learning in children: Progress in cognitive development research.* New York: Springer-Verlag, 1983.

Brainerd, C. J., & Brainerd, S. H. Order of acquisition of number and quantity conservation. *Child Development,* 1972, *43,* 1401-1406.

Brainerd, C. J., & Hooper, F. H. A methodological analysis of developmental studies of identity conservation and equivalence conservation. *Psychological Bulletin,* 1975, *82,* 725-737.

Brainerd, C. J., & Hooper, F. H. More on the identity → equivalence sequence: An update and some replies to Miller. *Psychological Bulletin,* 1978, *85,* 70-75.

Brainerd, C. J., & Howe, M. The origins of all-or-none learning. *Child Development,* 1978, *48,* 1028-1034.

Brainerd, C. J., & Howe, M. L. An attentional analysis of small cardinal number concepts in five-year-olds. *Canadian Journal of Behavioural Science,* 1979, *11,* 112-123.

Brainerd, C. J., & Howe, M. L. Developmental invariance in a mathematical model of associative learning. *Child Development,* 1980, *50,* 349-363.

Brainerd, C. J., & Howe, M. L. Stages-of-learning analysis of developmental interactions in memory, with illustrations from developmental interactions in picture-word effects. *Developmental Review,* 1982, *2,* in press.

Brainerd, C. J., Howe, M. L., & Desrochers, A. The general theory of two-stage learning: A mathematical review with illustrations from memory development. *Psychological Bulletin,* 1982, *90,* 634-665.

Brainerd, C. J., & Kaszor, P. An analysis of two proposed sources of children's class inclusion errors. *Developmental Psychology,* 1974, *10,* 633-643.

Brainerd, C. J., & Siegel, L. S. *How do we know that two things have the same number?* Research Bulletin No. 469, Department of Psychology, University of Western Ontario, 1978.

Brown, R., & Fraser, C. The acquisition of syntax. In C. N. Cofer & B. S. Musgrave (Eds.), *Verbal behavior and learning: Problems and processes*. New York: McGraw-Hill, 1963.

Bryant, P. E., & Trabasso, T. Transitive inference and memory in young children. *Nature*, 1971, *232*, 456-458.

Caron, A. J. Discrimination shifts in three-year-olds as a function of dimensional salience. *Developmental Psychology*, 1969, *1*, 333-339.

Case, R. Gearing the demands of instruction to the developmental capacities of the learner. *Review of Educational Research*, 1975, *45*, 59-87.

Case, R. Intellectual development from birth to adulthood: A neo-Piagetian interpretation. In R. S. Siegler (Ed.), *Children's thinking: What develops?* Hillsdale, N.J.: Erlbaum, 1978.

Chandler, M. J., & Greenspan, S. Ersatz egocentrism: A reply to H. Borke. *Developmental Psychology*, 1972, *7*, 104-106.

Chase, W. G. Elementary information processes. In W. K. Estes (Ed.), *Handbook of learning and cognitive processes* (Vol. 5). Hillsdale, N.J.: Erlbaum, 1978.

Coltheart, V. The effects of acoustic and semantic similarity on concept identification. *Quarterly Journal of Experimental Psychology*, 1972, *24*, 55-65.

Cornell, E. H. The effects of cue distinctiveness on infant's manual search. *Journal of Experimental Child Psychology*, 1981, *32*, 330-342.

Craik, F. I. M., & Lockhart, R. S. Levels of processing: A framework for memory research. *Journal of Verbal Learning and Verbal Behavior*, 1972, *11*, 671-684.

Daneman, M, & Carpenter, P. A. Individual differences in working memory and reading. *Journal of Verbal Learning and Verbal Behavior*, 1980, *19*, 450-466.

Dempster, F. N. Memory span: Sources of individual and developmental differences. *Psychological Bulletin*, 1981, *89*, 63-100.

Denney, N. W., Zeytinoglu, S., & Selzer, C. Conservation training in four-year-old children. *Journal of Experimental Child Psychology*, 1977, *24*, 129-146.

Emmerich, H. J., & Ackerman, B. P. Developmental differences in recall: Encoding or retrieval? *Journal of Experimental Child Psychology*, 1978, *25*, 514-525.

Erdelyi, M. H., Finkelstein, S., Herrell, N., Miller, B., & Thomas, J. Coding modality vs. input modality in hypermnesia: Is a rose a rose a rose? *Cognition*, 1976, *4*, 311-319.

Erdelyi, M. H. & Kleinbard, J. Has Ebbinghaus decayed with time?: The growth of recall (Hypermnesia) over days. *Journal of Experimental Psychology: Human Learning and Memory*, 1978, *4*, 275-289.

Esposito, N. J. Review of discrimination shift learning in young children. *Psychological Bulletin*, 1975, *82*, 432-455.

Feldman, D. H. *Beyond universals in cognitive development*. Norwood, N.J.: Ablex, 1980.

Feldman, D. H. The role of theory in cognitive developmental research: A reply to Brainerd. *Developmental Review*, 1981, *1*, 82-89.

Flavell, J. H. Concept development. In P. H. Mussen (Ed.), *Carmichael's manual of child psychology* (Vol. 1). New York: Wiley, 1970.

Flavell, J. H. Stage-related properties of cognitive development. *Cognitive Psychology*, 1971, *2*, 421-453.

Flavell, J. H., & Wohlwill, J. F. Formal and functional aspects of cognitive development. In D. Elkind & J. H. Flavell (Eds.), *Studies in cognitive development*. New York: Oxford University Press, 1969.

Flexer, A. J., & Tulving, E. Retrieval independence in recognition and recall. *Psychological Review*, 1978, *85*, 153-171.

Galton, F. Notes on prehension in idiots. *Mind*, 1887, *12*, 79-82.

Gelman, R. Conservation acquisition: A problem of learning to attend to relevant attributes. *Journal of Experimental Child Psychology*, 1969, *7*, 167-187.

Gelman, R. The nature and development of early number concepts. In H. W. Reese (Ed.), *Advances in child development and behavior* (Vol. 7). New York: Academic Press, 1972.

Gelman, R., & Weinberg, D. H. The relationship between liquid compensation and conservation. *Child Development*, 1972, *43*, 371-383.

Ghatala, E. S., & Levin, J. R. Children's recognition memory processes. In J. R. Levin & V. L. Allen (Eds.), *Cognitive learning in children: Theories and strategies*. New York: Academic Press, 1976.

Ghatala, E. S., Levin, J. R., & Truman, D. L. Varieties of frequency interference in children's recognition of sentence information. *Journal of Experimental Child Psychology*, 1978, *25*, 354-365.

Gratch, G., Appel, K. J., Evans, W. F., LeCompte, G. K., & Wright, N. A. Piaget's stage IV object concept error: Evidence of forgetting or object conception? *Child Development*, 1974, *45*, 71-77.

Gratch, G., & Landers, W. F. Stage IV of Piaget's theory of infant's object concepts: A longitudinal study. *Child Development*, 1971, *42*, 359-372.

Greenberg, N. A. *Young children's perceptual judgments of nonredundant cardinal number equivalence*. Unpublished doctoral dissertation, University of Western Ontario, 1981.

Greeno, J. G. Paired-associate learning with short-term retention: Mathematical analysis and data regarding identification of parameters. *Journal of Mathematical Psychology*, 1967, *4*, 430-472.

Groen, G. J., & Parkman, J. M. A chronometric analysis of simple addition. *Psychological Review*, 1972, *79*, 329-343.

Groen, G. J., & Poll, M. Subtraction and the solution of open sentence problems. *Journal of Experimental Child Psychology*, 1973, *16*, 292-302.

Harris, P. L. Development of object search and object permanence during infancy. *Psychological Bulletin*, 1975, *82*, 332-344.

Hebb, D. O. *The organization of behavior*. New York: Wiley, 1949.

Heisel, B. E. *Children's use and transfer of a retrieval strategy*. Unpublished doctoral dissertation, University of Western Ontario, 1981.

Hintzman, D. L. Apparent frequency as a function of frequency and the spacing of repetitions. *Journal of Experimental Psychology*, 1969, *80*, 139-145.

Hintzman, D. L. Repetition and memory. In G. H. Bower (Ed.), *The psychology of learning and motivation* (Vol. 10). New York: Academic Press, 1976.

Hintzman, D. L., & Block, R. A. Repetition and memory: Evidence for a multiple-trace hypothesis. *Journal of Experimental Psychology*, 1971, *88*, 297-306.

Hintzman, D. L., Block, R. A., & Summers, J. J. Modality tags and memory for repetitions: Locus of the spacing effect. *Journal of Verbal Learning and Verbal Behavior*, 1973, *12*, 229-239.

Hintzman, D. L., & Stern, L. D. Contextual variability and memory for frequency. *Journal of Experimental Psychology: Human Learning and Memory*, 1978, *4*, 539-549.

Hintzman, D. L., Summers, J. J., & Block, R. A. Spacing judgments as an index of study-phase retrieval. *Journal of Experimental Psychology: Human Learning and Memory*, 1975, *1*, 31-40.

Hintzman, D. L., & Waters, R. M. Recency and frequency as factors in list discrimination. *Journal of Verbal Learning and Verbal Behavior*, 1970, 9, 218-221.

Hitch, G. J. The role of short-term working memory in mental arithmetic. *Cognitive Psychology*, 1978, *10*, 302-332. (a)

Hitch, G. J. Mental arithmetic: Short-term storage and information processing in a cognitive skill. In A. M. Lesgold, J. W. Pelligrino, J. W. Fokkema, & R. Glaser (Eds.), *Cognitive psychology and instruction*. New York: Plenum, 1978. (b)

Hoemann, H. W., & Ross, B. M. Children's concepts of chance and probability. In C. J. Brainerd (Ed.), *Children's logical and mathematical cognition: Progress in cognitive development research*. New York: Springer-Verlag, 1982.

Hood, L., & Bloom, L. What, when, and how about why: A longitudinal study of early expressions of causality. *Monographs of the Society for Research in Child Development*, 1979, *44*(6, Whole No. 181).

Hooper, F. H. Piaget's conservation tasks: The logical and developmental priority of identity conservation. *Journal of Experimental Child Psychology*, 1969, *8*, 234-249.

Hooper, F. H., Goldman, J. A., Storck, P. A., & Burke, A. M. Stage sequence and correspondence in Piagetian theory: A review of the middle-childhood period. *Research relating to children*. (Bulletin No. 28.) Washington, D.C.: U.S. Government Printing Office, 1971.

Hooper, F. H., Swinton, S. S., & Sipple, T. W. *An initial analysis of concrete operations task performances and memory variables for children aged 5 to 13 years.* Technical Report No. 371, Research and Development Center for Cognitive Learning, University of Wisconsin, 1976.

Hooper, F. H., Swinton, S. S., & Sipple, T. W. Logical reasoning in middle childhood: A study of the Piagetian concrete operations stage. In H. J. Klausmeier and associates. *Cognitive learning and development: Piagetian and information-processing perspectives*. Cambridge, Mass.: Ballinger, 1979.

Hooper, F. H., Toniolo, T. A., & Sipple, T. S. A longitudinal analysis of logical reasoning relationships: Conservation and transitive inference. *Developmental Psychology*, 1978, *14*, 674-682.

Huttenlocher, J., & Burke, D. Why does memory span increase with age? *Cognitive Psychology*, 1976, *8*, 1-31.

Inhelder, B. Memory and intelligence in the child. In D. Elkind & J. H. Flavell (Eds.), *Studies in cognitive development*. New York: Oxford University Press, 1969.

Inhelder, B., Sinclair, H., & Bovet, M. *Learning and the development of cognition*. Cambridge, Mass.: Harvard University Press, 1974.

Jacobs, J. Experiments on prehension. *Mind*, 1887, *121*, 75-79.

Jensen, A. R. *Individual differences in learning: Interference factor*. (Final Report, Cooperative Research Project No. 1897.) Washington, D.C.: U.S. Department of Health, Education and Welfare, 1964.

Keller, H. R., & Hunter, M. L. Task differences on conservation and transitivity problems. *Journal of Experimental Child Psychology*, 1973, *15*, 287-301.

Kendler, H. H., & Kendler, T. S. Vertical and horizontal processes in problem solving. *Psychological Review*, 1962, *69*, 1-16.

Koppitz, E. M. *The visual aural digit span test*. New York: Grune & Stratton, 1977.

Koshinsky, C., & Hall, A. E. The developmental relationship between identity and equivalence conservation. *Journal of Experimental Child Psychology*, 1973, *15*, 419-424.

Larsen, G. Y., & Flavell, J. H. Verbal factors in compensation performance and the relationship between conservation and compensation. *Child Development*, 1970, *41*, 965-977.

Liben, L. S. Memory in the context of cognitive development: The Piagetian approach. In R. V. Kail, Jr., & J. W. Hagen (Eds.), *Perspectives on the development of memory and cognition*. Hillsdale, N.J.: Erlbaum, 1977.

Lovell, K., & Ogilvie, E. A study of the conservation of weight in the junior school child. *British Journal of Educational Psychology*, 1961, *31*, 138-144.

Lutkus, A., & Trabasso, T. Transitive inferences by preoperational retarded adolescents. *American Journal of Mental Deficiency*, 1974, *78*, 599-606.

McLaughlin, G. H. Psycho-logic: A possible alternative to Piaget's formulation. *British Journal of Psychology*, 1963, *33*, 61-67.

McManis, D. L. Conservation and transitivity of weight and length by normals and retardates. *Developmental Psychology*, 1969, *1*, 373-382.

Miller, G. A. The magical number seven, plus or minus two: Some limits on our capacity for processing information. *Psychological Review*, 1956, *63*, 81-87.

Miller, D., Cohen, L., & Hill, K. A methodological investigation of Piaget's theory of object concept development in the sensory-motor period. *Journal of Experimental Child Psychology*, 1970, *9*, 58-85.

Morrison, F. J., & Manis, F. R. Cognitive processes and reading disability: A critique and proposal. In C. J. Brainerd & M. Pressley (Eds.), *Verbal processes in children: Progress in cognitive development research*. New York: Springer-Verlag, 1982.

Moyer, R. S., & Landauer, T. K. Time required for judgments of numerical inequality. *Nature* (London), 1967, *215*, 1519-1520.

Murdock, B. B., Jr. Item and order information in short-term serial memory. *Journal of Experimental Psychology: General*, 1976, *105*, 191-215.

Murray, J. P., & Youniss, J. Achievement of inferential transitivity and its relation to serial ordering. *Child Development*, 1968, *39*, 1259-1268.

Odom, R. D. A perceptual-salience account of decalage relations and developmental change. In L. S. Siegel & C. J. Brainerd (Eds.), *Alternatives to Piaget: Critical essays on the theory*. New York: Academic Press, 1978.

Palermo, D. Still more about the comprehension of "less." *Developmental Psychology*, 1974, *10*, 827-829.

Parkman, J. M. Temporal apsects of simple multiplication and comparison. *Journal of Experimental Psychology*, 1972, *95*, 437-444.

Patterson, K. A. *Limitations on retrieval from long-term memory*. Unpublished doctoral dissertation, University of California, San Diego, 1971.

Phillips, S., & Levine, M. Probing for hypotheses with adults and children: Blank trials and introtacts. *Journal of Experimental Psychology: General*, 1975, *104*, 327-354.

Piaget, J. *Classes, relations et nombres: Essai sur les "groupements" de la logistique et la réversibilité de la pensée*. Paris: Vrin, 1942.

Piaget, J. *The child's conception of number*. New York: Humanities, 1952.

Piaget, J. *The construction of reality in the child*. New York: Basic Books, 1954.

Piaget, J. *The mechanisms of perception*. New York: Basic Books, 1967.

Piaget, J. *On the development of memory and identity*. Worcester, Mass.: Clark University Press, 1968.

Piaget, J., & Inhelder, B. *La genèse de l'idée de hasard chez l'enfant*. Paris: Presses Universitaires de France, 1951.

Piaget, J., & Inhelder, B. *Mental imagery in the child*. New York: Basic Books, 1971.

Piaget, J., & Inhelder, B. *Memory and intelligence*. New York: Basic Books, 1973.

Piaget, J., Inhelder, B., & Szeminska, A. *The child's conception of geometry*. New York: Harper, 1960.

Pressley, M. Imagery and children's learning: Putting the picture in developmental perspective. *Review of Educational Research*, 1977, *47*, 585-622.

Rabbitt, P. B. Channel-capacity, intelligibility, and immediate memory. *Quarterly Journal of Experimental Psychology*, 1968, *20*, 241-248.

Reese, H. W. Imagery and associative memory. In R. V. Kail, Jr., & J. W. Hagen (Eds.), *Perspectives on the development of memory and cognition*. Hillsdale, N.J.: Erlbaum, 1977.

Riley, C. A., & Trabasso, T. Comparatives, logical structures, and encoding in a transitive inference task. *Journal of Experimental Child Psychology*, 1974, *17*, 187-203.

Roodin, P. A., & Gruen, G. E. The role of memory in making transitive judgments. *Journal of Experimental Child Psychology*, 1970, *10*, 264-275.

Ross, B. M. Probability concepts in deaf and hearing children. *Child Development*, 1966, *37*, 917-927.

Rothkopf, E. Z. Copying span as a measure of the information burden in written language. *Journal of Verbal Learning and Verbal Behavior*, 1980, *19*, 562-572.

Rybash, J. M., Roodin, P. A., & Sullivan, L. F. The effects of a memory aid on three types of conservation judgments. *Journal of Experimental Child Psychology*, 1975, *19*, 358-370.

Sedlack, A., & Walton, M. D. The discourse of making amends: A demonstration of an approach for the creation and use of a finite-state grammar of children's discourse. *Developmental Review*, 1982, *2*, in press.

Seitz, V., & Weir, M. W. Strength of dimensional preferences as a predictor of nurseryschool children's performance on a concept-shift task. *Journal of Experimental Child Psychology*, 1971, *12*, 370-386.

Sekuler, R., & Mierkiewicz, D. Children's judgments of numerical inequality. *Child Development*, 1977, *48*, 630-633.

Shallice, T., & Warrington, F. K. Independent functioning of verbal memory stores: A neuropsychological study. *Quarterly Journal of Experimental Psychology*, 1970, *22*, 261-273.

Siegel, L. S. The sequence of development of certain number concepts. *Developmental Psychology*, 1971, *5*, 357-361.

Siegel, L. S. The development of number concepts: Ordering and correspondence operations and the role of length cues. *Developmental Psychology*, 1974, *10*, 907-912.

Siegel, L. S. The relationship of language and thought in the preoperational child: A reconsideration of nonverbal alternatives to Piagetian tasks. In L. S. Siegel & C. J. Brainerd (Eds.), *Alternatives to Piaget: Critical essays on the theory*. New York: Academic Press, 1978.

Siegel, L. S. The development of quantity concepts: Perceptual and linguistic factors. In C. J. Brainerd (Ed.), *Children's logical and mathematical cognition: Progress in cognitive development research*. New York: Springer-Verlag, 1982.

Siegel, L. S., McCabe, A. E., Brand, J., & Matthews, J. Evidence for the understanding of class inclusion in preschool children: Linguistic factors and training effects. *Child Development*, 1978, *49*, 688-693.

Siegler, R. S. Developmental sequences within and between concepts. *Monographs of the Society for Research in Child Development*, 1981, *46* (2, Whole No. 189).

Siegler, R. S., & Liebert, R. M. Effects of presenting relevant rules and complete feedback on the conservation of liquid quantity task. *Developmental Psychology*, 1972, *7*, 133-138.

Sigel, I. E. The Piagetian system and the world of education. In D. Elkind & J. H. Flavell (Eds.), *Studies in cognitive development*. New York: Oxford University Press, 1969.

Silverstein, A. B., Pearson, L. B., Aguinaldo, N. E., Friedman, S. L., Takayama, D. L., & Weiss, Z. I. Identity conservation and equivalence conservation: A question of developmental priority. *Child Development, 1982, 53,* 819-821.

Smedslund, J. Development of concrete transitivity of length in children. *Child Development*, 1963, *34*, 389-405.

Smedslund, J. Psychological diagnostics. *Psychological Bulletin*, 1969, *71*, 237-248.

Smiley, S. S. Optional shift behavior as a function of age and dimensional dominance. *Journal of Experimental Child Psychology*, 1973, *16*, 451-458.

Smiley, S. S., & Weir, M. W. Role of dimensional dominance in reversal and non-reversal shift behavior. *Journal of Experimental Child Psychology*, 1966, *4*, 296-307.

Stevenson, H. W. Learning in children. In P. H. Mussen (Ed.), *Carmichael's manual of child psychology* (Vol. 1). New York: Wiley, 1970.

Stevenson, H. W. *Children's learning*. New York: Appleton-Century-Crofts, 1972.

Taylor, D. A. Stage analysis of reaction time. *Psychological Bulletin*, 1976, *83*, 161-191.

Toniolo, T. A., & Hooper, F. H. *Micro-analysis of logical reasoning relationships: Conservation and transitivity*. Technical Report No. 326, Research and Development Center for Cognitive Learning, University of Wisconsin, 1975.

Trabasso, T. Representation, memory and reasoning: How do we make transitive inferences? In A. D. Pick (Ed.), *Minnesota symposia on child psychology* (Vol. 9). University of Minnesota Press, 1975.

Trabasso, T. The role of memory as a system in making transitive inferences. In R. V. Kail, Jr., & J. W. Hagen (Eds.), *Perspectives on the development of memory and cognition*. Hillsdale, N.J.: Erlbaum, 1977.

Trabasso, T., & Riley, C. A. The construction and use of representations involving linear order. In R. L. Soslo (Ed.), *Information processing and cognition: The Loyola symposium*. Hillsdale, N.J.: Erlbaum, 1975.

Trabasso, T., Riley, C. A., & Wilson, E. G. The representation of linear order and spatial strategies in reasoning: A developmental study. In R. Falmagne (Ed.), *Reasoning: Representation and process in children and adults*. Hillsdale, N.J.: Erlbaum, 1975.

Uzgiris, I. C. Situational generality of conservation. *Child Development*, 1964, *35*, 831-841.

Vellutino, F. R., & Scanlon, D. M. Verbal processing in poor and normal readers. In C. J. Brainerd & M. Pressley (Eds.), *Verbal processes in children: Progress in cognitive development research*. New York: Springer-Verlag, 1982.

Wanner, E., & Shiner, S. Measuring transient memory load. *Journal of Verbal Learning and Verbal Behavior*, 1976, *15*, 159-167.

Warrington, E. K., Logue, V., & Pratt, T. C. The anatomical localization of selective impairment of auditory and verbal short-term memory. *Neuropsychologia*, 1971, *9*, 377-387.

Warrington, E. K., & Shallice, T. The selective impairment of auditory short-term memory. *Brain,* 1969, *92,* 885-896.

Warrington, E. K., & Weiskrantz, L. An analysis of short-term and long-term memory defects in man. In J. A. Deutsch (Ed.), *The psychological basis of memory.* New York: Academic Press, 1973.

Wilkinson, A. C. Theoretical and methodological analysis of partial knowledge. *Developmental Review,* 1982, *2,* in press.

Wohlwill, J. F. Responses to class-inclusion questions for verbally and pictorially presented items. *Child Development,* 1968, *39,* 449-465.

Woods, S. S., Resnick, L. B., & Groen, G. J. An experimental test of five process models for subtraction. *Journal of Educational Psychology,* 1975, *67,* 17-21.

Yost, P. A., Siegel, A. E., & Andrews, J. M. Non-verbal probability judgments by young children. *Child Development,* 1962, *33,* 796-780.

Youniss, J., & Murray, J. P. Transitive inference with nontransitive solutions controlled. *Developmental Psychology,* 1970, *2,* 169-175.

5. An Ethological Approach to Cognitive Development

William R. Charlesworth

The title of this chapter needs an explanation. *Cognitive* refers here to brain processes that organize relatively complex behaviors. Examples of such processes are storing, retrieving, and transforming information picked up from the environment by perceptual mechanisms. It is assumed that these processes are functions of the brain, just as contractions are functions of heart muscle. Further, it is assumed that the neurophysiological mechanisms that enable these processes to perform these functions are products of evolutionary history. The content on which these processes operate—the images, rules, and other forms of information represented in the brain—are viewed here as products of ontogeny, that is, the stored cumulations of the individual's everyday experiences. *Development* is employed here as referring to the sequence of progressive, non-repetitive changes undergone by an organism over its lifespan.

The term *approach* is used here in the dictionary sense of preliminary steps taken toward something. In the present context it refers specifically to a means of access to fuller knowledge of cognitively mediated behavior and its function. This definition is important to keep in mind because what is being offered here is not a theory. What is offered is a way, rather, of viewing and dealing with cognitive phenomena from a particular point of view labeled here as ethological.

Ethology is now generally understood to refer to the biological study of naturally occurring behavior with emphasis on its proximate causal mechanisms, adaptive function, ontogenesis, and general evolutionary or phylogenetic significance (Lorenz, 1981; Thorpe, 1979; Tinbergen, 1963). Labeling the present approach as ethological, though, may cause some confusion. In 1976 Griffen encouraged ethologists to study the mental experiences of animals; two years later, he proposed a new discipline called "cognitive ethology" (Griffen, 1978). In reviewing Griffen's book, Mason (1976), however, pointed out that "cognitive ethology is not a new or emerging discipline" (p. 930). According to Mason, Griffen's proposal was anticipated years ago by Yerkes, Köhler, Lashley, Tolman, Hebb, and Harlow, all of whom "have attempted to deal with the complexities of the animal mind in a disciplined manner" (pp. 930-931).

The approach being presented here has nothing to say about animal or human awareness and is therefore in a different category than Griffen's. Also, it is not an extension of the Yerkes, Köhler, et al. approach, for important conceptual and methodological reasons. In a number of earlier papers (Charlesworth, 1976, 1978), I presented the thesis that by the end of the 19th century, research in psychology had split into two quite different camps—the psychometric and the naturalistic. Members of the former engaged in testing and experimenting with subjects under conditions arranged by the investigator; members of the latter engaged in observing and describing the subjects (usually animals) in their natural habitat with little or no intervention by the investigator. The two approaches differed significantly in terms of the questions asked as well as in terms of the operations used to answer the questions. For various reasons the psychometric approach to studying cognitive processes came to dominate the field. Animal researchers, most of whom were labeled comparative psychologists, were part of this approach. Those representing the naturalistic approach, in contrast, worked with animals under a greater range of conditions—in the field, field stations, barnyards, zoos, vivaria—observing, describing, writing ethograms, and conducting field experiments with various degrees of rigor. For the most part, these researchers, most of whom were labeled ethologists, studied animal social behavior. With the exception of Konrad Lorenz (1971), who concerned himself with problems of perceptions, cognition, and intelligence, none of the ethologists studied cognition in any significant way.

The present approach, then, is *ethological* for the following reasons: It proposes field research on cognitively mediated behavior, and it argues that this research can best be organized around the notion of adaptation as viewed from an evolutionary perspective. Cognitive abilities are viewed here as evolved adaptations that aid animals in their interactions with complex, variable, and hazardous features of their environments. The goal of this approach is twofold: to contribute to a unified body of knowledge on cognitive behaviors and their relationship to environmental demands, and to connect this knowledge to various indices of adaptation.

Forerunners of the Ethological Approach

An account of the forerunners of the ethological approach to human cognition and the historical conditions surrounding them has been provided elsewhere (Charlesworth, 1978); hence these researchers will only be mentioned here. While viewed as essential for developing an evolutionary view of intelligence, naturalistic observation of intelligent behavior in animals consisted for the most part during Darwin's time of anecdotal accounts and nonsystematic observation by untrained observers (Romanes,

1884, 1889). An exception to this was Wesley Mills (1898), who argued strongly for naturalistic observation as the first step toward laying a foundation for psychology. Mills, however, had little impact on psychology. Even though William James (1910) and other members of the functionalist school, such as Hall, Angell, Judd, and Thorndike, postulated a connection between intelligent behavior and adaptation, no significant field research to test their arguments was undertaken. Most behavioral research continued to be conducted in test and experimental settings. There were some exceptions to this, however. William Stern (1920), for example, attempted to evaluate intelligence in other ways than by using paper and pencil tests. Stern made a distinction between theoretical intelligence and practical intelligence, and suggested that parents, teachers, and other caretakers of children be trained to observe and describe how the latter dealt with everyday problems. As far as can be determined, this suggestion was not followed up systematically. Other forerunners of the ethological approach as it would apply to human behavior included Mason (1966), who provided anthropological accounts of how pre-industrial peoples mastered their physical and social environments by employing cognitive skills in daily problem solving situations; Tolman (1932), who viewed cognitive maps as important adaptations that animals acquired in order to guide themselves in their physical environments; Brunswick (1956), who developed the concept of molar and purposive behavior as a means of dealing adaptively with a probabilistic environment; and Heider (1958), who developed the theory that humans regulate their social behavior by means of a "naive theory" of human behavior and social interactions.

In short, a number of researchers and writers during and since Darwin's time have emphasized the need to study cognition under natural conditions, but they have had no significant effect on research. Ethologists, for the most part, had focused their attention on social behavior and the mechanisms controlling it. Psychologists, in contrast, were intent upon establishing rigorous control over cognitive subject matter, which meant refining tests and experimental methods. Field work was viewed by most psychologists as productive of anecdote and description rather than scientific fact and explanation.

Today, the intellectual climate has changed somewhat. Precision and rigor are not considered the only marks of significant research; generalizability and practical applicability of findings have also become important. Furthermore, divisions between disciplines are breaking down, especially between the biological, behavioral, and social sciences. Connections between ethology and social psychology have already been established and current conditions are favorable for forging connections between ethology and the cognitive sciences.

Conditions Favoring the Ethological Approach

There are at least three current conditions that favor the ethological approach to cognition. These conditions have their origins in three areas—evolutionary biology, which is now in the position of providing a theoretical rationale for an ethological approach to cognition; traditional psychology, which because of various methodological overcommitments has produced an empirical vacuum that needs to be filled; and current educational and therapeutic practice, which provides a strong practical need for the kinds of data the ethological approach can produce.

Evolutionary Biology

The strongest rationale for studying the adaptive value of cognitive processes in animals can be found in evolutionary biology. Evolutionary changes in behavioral adaptation (in animals in general and mammals in particular) can now be linked to brain size (Jerison, 1973). It also appears that there has been a strong trend in primate evolution toward the associating of large brains with behavioral despecialization, man being the most despecialized species in the primate order (Wilson, 1980). Such despecialization is characterized by greater coordination and flexibility of responses to variations in environmental conditions, both characteristics made possible by the brain's ability to acquire, store, and appropriately use information acquired during ontogeny. The term *intelligence* has come to epitomize the collective operations of these characteristics. Concept learning, symbol formation, insight, analytical thinking, and other cognitive skills are also subsumed under intelligence.

The evolution of such cognitive abilities is usually accounted for in terms of natural selection. The genes for large brain size (which make these abilities possible) spread rapidly throughout small, isolated populations of primates by conferring more sophisticated and flexible responses to environmental challenges. In other words, there is reason to believe that modern man's intellectual status relative to that of other animals is a consequence of a particular evolutionary history. It seems reasonable, as Reed (1965) points out, that genes supporting higher intellectual functioning and learning spread rapidly through small isolated population units. The consequences of this spread put other hominids not having the genes at a disadvantage, either in direct competition for insufficient resources or in dealing with harsh climate and terrain conditions. That such selection may still be operating today is suggested by Higgins, Reed, and Reed (1962), who show that the average number of offspring of individuals with IQs below 70 is less than that of those with higher IQs.

Genotype and corresponding brain abilities are necessary but not sufficient conditions for the emergence of adaptive behavior. Social and physical environments that provide the young animal with learning experiences from which to develop the abilities are also necessary. Individuals having the genes necessary for the development of higher cognitive functioning, but not having proper environments in which to express themselves, are just as disadvantaged as those not having the genes. The kinds of environments that conceivably could have stimulated and supported cognitive development during evolution have not been extensively investigated. This omission has left a great empirical lacuna in the theory.

A prominent feature of higher cognitive functioning is the relatively long period early in ontogeny during which it becomes operative. An extended period of learning appears necessary both for the development of normal functions and for the programming of specific information on social and physical environments necessary for independent action. The prolonged period of immaturity is characterized in most primates by playfulness, heightened curiosity, and exploratory and manipulative behavior. In human children imaginative play enters the behavioral repertoire quite early. All these activities make possible great strides in learning, and as a consequence, contribute to the individual's ability to adjust to traditional cultural tasks as well as to new situations and the particular features of the environment.

The most salient characteristic of man as a cultural animal is the rapid change induced in cultural patterns from generation to generation. Every new invention made in response to an environmental challenge requires a series of new adaptations in order to deal with its direct and indirect consequences. These adaptations have to be made *de novo* by each new generation. No genetic change could possibly keep up with them, nor could response systems less flexible than those made possible by current human brain capacities. Therefore, it is very important that cultures constantly update educational content and objectives as well as methods for transmitting them.

What is important in the evolutionary approach to the study of cognition is that environmental demands be studied along with their relationship to cognitive behavior. This requires developing methods for observing, identifying, describing, and evaluating such demands. To date, those working in the area of animal intelligence have for the most part not done this. Bindra (1976), Bitterman (1965), and Razran (1971), for example, all touch on the biological utility or evolutionary significance of intelligent behavior, but the question of the actual survival value of intelligent behavior vis-à-vis known environmental requirements is not answered. We still do not know what factors specifically caused the evolution of cognitive functioning and what features of such functioning currently contribute to survival and reproduction. It is easy to speculate about the environmental demands that may have put pressure on early man's cognitive abilities—the extremes of Pleistocene weather (Klein, 1973), the need for cooperation in a hunter-gatherer society (Humphrey, 1976). But it is not easy to document such demands empirically, and evolutionary theory requires their documentation in order to include them as a major factor in the basic equation of adaptation.

For this reason, then, evolutionary research on intelligence requires us to go beyond tests and experiments and to engage in extensive field observations of cognitive behavior and the environmental conditions that release, reinforce, and extinguish such behavior. These observations obviously will have to take place in the animal's natural habitat where adaptational demands are made; otherwise we will never know what environmental conditions are implicated in the occurrence of cognitive behavior and its development. As already noted, ethologists have made such observations on animals' social behavior. More recently, other modes of adaptation, such as foraging, navigating, hunting, and food caching have become foci of attention. Many of the behaviors involved in these activities could be classified as cognitively guided and organized.

Further impetus to the study of cognitive behavior from an evolutionary viewpoint also comes from biologists who recognize the role that culture and mind play in the process of animal and human adaptation. Bonner (1980), for example, views the capacity for culture as a trait evolved by natural selection that allows animals to acquire information about their habitats, food sources, and predator behavior that could not possibly be encoded in the genome. Lumsden and Wilson (1981) maintain that individual mental and behavioral development are the crucial processes linking genetic and cultural evolution and require the study of developmental or epigenetic rules and processes that make the formation of culture possible.

Traditional Psychology

Within certain areas of psychology, great emphasis has traditionally been placed on the role of the environment in shaping behavior. The mechanism of shaping has been broadly conceived of in associative learning terms, and since the turn of the century a great deal of psychological research has been directed toward studying such learning. The environment, as manifested in the home and community and in the culture itself, has been viewed as the primary socializing agent of the child. When we turn to research, however, we discover that virtually none of it was directed toward studying environments per se. The few investigators (see Wright, 1960; and Barker, 1968) who studied environments usually made no attempt to connect environmental factors to individual differences in short- or long-term adaptation. Only relatively recently have serious moves been made to connect environmental research to problems of human adaptation (e.g., Willems & Rausch, 1969; Bronfenbrenner, 1979).

Most researchers who maintained the prepotency of environmental determination either studied individual abilities and processes in test and laboratory settings or interviewed individuals about their backgrounds and child-rearing practices. For example, in comparative psychology, laboratory research was the dominant approach to studying problems in learning. This was true even for those who subscribed to evolutionary theory and recognized the significant role environmental factors played in natural selection. Thorndike (1898), Maier and Schneirla (1935), and Bitterman (1965), for example, recognized the importance of evolutionary theory but nevertheless did their best work with laboratory preparations. They produced much data on the learning and cognitive potentialities of their subjects, but they did not examine the extent to which such potentialities were actually useful to the species under natural conditions. The results of their efforts were mixed. As Lockhard (1971) points out, comparative psychology, as a consequence of its preoccupation with laboratory work, became a "confused scatter of views of nature, problems, and methods" (p. 168). There was nothing outside the laboratory with which to make validating connections. The question whether learning, as learning researchers perceived it, was the animal's major mode of adapting to its environment was never directly answered. Today, most learning research has not changed substantially. As Johnston (1981) indicates, only very recently have there been attempts to bring learning and ecology together, and these attempts have so far not been met with any great support.

In social psychology, especially that which focuses on the development of social behavior during early development, great emphasis was placed on the environment as determinative of behavior, but individual-environment interaction was rarely studied. Environmental conditions were usually inferred from interviews, measures of parents' socioeconomic status, or other indices, or from cursory observations of neighborhood and family conditions (Sears, Maccoby, & Levin, 1957). With few exceptions, the observation of everyday child-environment interaction required to make valid and reliable statements about the origins of socialization was usually not carried out.

In cognition research, things were not substantially different. Piaget's work was welcomed because he recognized child-environment interactions as indispensable for cognitive growth. The child's biological predispositions and prior experience were considered crucial in the adaptational act, as were the immediate environmental conditions surrounding the act. Understanding child-environment interaction required observational data on the child and the environment. In his infancy research, Piaget (1952, 1954) fulfilled this requirement. The three infants he studied were his own; hence he was sufficiently in their presence to obtain a good picture of the kind and frequency of environmental challenges that presumably were implicated in their development. Although his observations do not appear to have been preplanned and systematic, he was on much firmer ground in discussing environmental factors than infancy researchers who assessed infants' cognitive abilities in test settings.

In his later research, Piaget conducted no field work, but still engaged in extensive speculation on an environment-subject interaction and its role in cognitive development. Such speculation gradually became well established in the literature, but without an empirical foundation. As Brainerd (1981) points out, Piaget proposed "a free floating set of assumptions that is not motivated by prior empirical findings and whose connections to the children's behavior are vague" (p. 64). Not only the world of the child's everyday behavior but also the actual functions of such behavior are vague in Piaget's formulations. Many key questions relative to Piaget's theory are still not answered. For example, we could ask in what circumstances a child encounters instances where the cognitive ability to conserve substance is required; how often, on the average, these circumstances occur; and what happens when the child responds to them. Such questions ultimately have to be answered if the theory of child-environment interaction as implicated in cognitive development is to be scientifically useful. It should also be noted here that Piaget (1978) has acknowledged the significance of behavior in evolution because of its adaptive value. However, Piaget falls short of being convincing because he does not seem to recognize that field observation is the only method that can be used to test such a notion.

In short, by arguing that environmental factors are the major causal agent in shaping human behavior, but failing to conduct the necessary research, psychologists have inadvertently produced a vacuum waiting to be filled by empirical findings. Whether this vacuum will be filled in the near future remains to be seen. There is no doubt, however, that traditional psychology will have to undergo a major paradigm shift from the relatively restrictive, reductionistic approach that has characterized much of its research so far to a more holistic, functional approach that requires systematic sampling of everyday life situations.

Education and Therapy

In the world of applied psychology and psychiatry there is a continuing need for more information on how individuals learn and develop adaptive and maladaptive behaviors. The possible contributions of ethology to education and psychiatry have been discussed by several writers (White, 1974; Tinbergen, 1974; Charlesworth & Spiker, 1975; Charlesworth & Bart, 1976). They range from providing general theoretical support for adopting the concept of adaptation to giving more specific support in the form of the concepts of sign stimuli, behavioral stereotypies, and observational procedures. However, the most important current contribution ethology can make to education and therapy is to provide a convincing rationale for studying adaptation in everyday circumstances. There is no longer any question that observational research is needed in educational psychology (Weinberg & Wood, 1975). This holds true for remedial work with retarded children as well. Observational research in the area of mental retardation has already been addressed on a number of occasions (Sackett, 1978; Charlesworth, in press). In behavioral therapy, students of behavior modification have stressed the necessity of establishing behavioral base rates *and* the stimulus contexts in which the behaviors occur. The success of the work of Patterson, Littman, and Bricker (1967) and Patterson and Cobb (1971) is a case in point. Behavior modifiers recognized early that there was no substitute for directly observing the life situation and recording targeted features of it.

Summary

These, then, are the background conditions viewed here as favoring the ethological approach to the human behavioral sciences in general and to the study of cognition in particular. Why cognition is singled out for special attention should be clear: Cognitively mediated behavior appears to be a significant form of human adaptation to environmental conditions; it mediates the actions of all individuals—children and adults, normal and retarded, the mentally disturbed, and those in preliterate and industrialized societies. Its pervasiveness almost makes cognitive behavior invisible, and the ubiquitousness of the conditions that elicit, reinforce, maintain, and extinguish it are often so familiar that they hardly attract our attention. Therefore, a special effort is necessary in order to convince researchers to study it. What cognitive science needs now is a method to study such behavior and the conditions surrounding it. The following is a step toward developing such a method.

Problem-Behavior Analysis

There are undoubtedly numerous ways to conceptualize and identify behavioral events occurring in everyday life that we would agree are cognitively mediated. In the present scheme (referred to hereafter as **PROBA**, problem-behavior analysis) the concept of problem is given primary status.[1] A *problem* is defined

[1] After PROBA was developed, it was discovered that Ragle (1957) had already developed a scheme for identifying problem episodes in the lives of children observed in the classic study of children in the Midwest by Barker and Wright (1955). Ragle's schema shares clear similarities with PROBA. As a test of the latter, two coders examined a number of Ragle's observational protocols by using the PROBA scheme. They identified 72 of the 74 problems identified by Ragle as well as an additional 142 problems that fit minor features of the PROBA definition. In short, PROBA agreed with Ragle and also proved sensitive to detecting other, less salient problems in the child's everyday life.

here as a block to ongoing behavior that elicits a response that an observer has reason to believe is mediated by some form of cognitive process (Charlesworth, 1978). The choice of the concept of problem has a number of advantages: Problems have been a standard means in research of assessing cognitive abilities; they play a major role in theorizing on the evolution of intelligence; and they have, for the most part, an effect that can be detected by an outside observer.

On the basis of approximately 50 hours of field observation of young children, a great variety of blocks to ongoing behavior were observed and recorded; a sample of blocks was also obtained from self-reports by young adults. In the case of young children, behavior was interrupted, for example, by such things as falling, being challenged by another child, being asked questions by parents and teachers, doors that refused to open, an object or food that was unobtainable, and situations that aroused curiosity. In the case of the young adults, ongoing behavior was interrupted or blocked by, for example, demands made by friends, bad weather conditions, difficult test items, missing library materials, the forgetting of daily tasks, and the car getting stuck on a slippery hill. Such events obviously vary in the extent to which they implicate complex cognitive mediation. Many of them would traditionally be excluded by cognition researchers. Our first response to this variation was the feeling that the definition of problems as blocks or disruptions may have been too broad. Although the definition had the advantage of allowing us to identify problematic behavioral events, many of the events extended far beyond traditional definitions of problems in the research literature: The vast majority of the problems did not resemble, for example, the tower of Hanoi or missionary-cannibal problems. Furthermore, a wide range of responses were employed to remove these blocks, responses that could have been accounted for in terms ranging from simple recall to deductive reasoning. To make matters more difficult, validly inferring what cognitive processes mediated the response to the problem was a virtually impossible task.

In spite of these shortcomings, we kept the definition of a problem as an observable block to ongoing behavior. The net we would cast with our observational method would catch problems traditionally defined in research along with a disproportionately larger number of other situations that individuals have to cope with every day. All problems could be evaluated after we recorded them. Not recording them while in the field, it was felt, would be a greater loss than the time spent processing and evaluating those ultimately found useless for one reason or other. As long as the observer had reason to believe that a block had occurred, the block and the response to it were noted in the observational protocol.

It was at this point in the project that the decision was made to rely solely on commonsense notions about cognitive processes and to forgo any attempt to explore the nature of the cognitive processes that mediated problem solving behavior. Inferences about processes could be made, but with no control over the stimulus situation involved, they would be primitive at best. For example, if a child whose ball rolls under the sofa immediately gets a yardstick and retrieves it, we can assume prior experience with such a situation (long-term memory), the recognition that the present situation shares similarities with prior experiences, and the ability to generalize from them. If the child reaches in vain for the ball, gives up, walks around aimlessly, picks up the yardstick, handles it, and then suddenly goes to the sofa and retrieves the ball, we could assume that something akin to insight ocucrred. This would be the best we could do by the PROBA method. As Bindra (1979) points out in a critique of this aspect of PROBA, a method that relies on observations of spontaneous behavior will not lead "to the isolation and definition of the cognitive processes that contribute to the production of different types of intelligent actions" (p. 575). Such information on cognitive processes can only be achieved by experimental control through task selection, repeated manipulations of known stimuli, and control over response variation. The field method obviously lacks these controls. But such controls do not help us answer questions regarding the nature and frequency of cognitive challenges that an individual experiences on a day-to-day basis and how the results of these experiences are implicated in short- and long-term adaptation. These questions can only be answered by field work.

A second reason to forgo explicating cognitive processes was the feeling, based on observing children, that problem solving, learning, and habit were closely related developmentally and that all three involved some form of cognitive processing. For example, what is a problem for a child at time T and involves much struggle and trial and error to solve becomes somewhat easier to deal with at time $T + 1$ and even easier at time $T + 2$. At each of the three times, nevertheless, the problem may block the child's ongoing behavior and have to be dealt with one way or another. An individual child's ability to deal with the problem would therefore vary over developmental time. For example, a child who at time T cries in response to a scraped knee until help comes, may at time $T + 1$ rub his scraped knee and call his mother. At time $T + 2$, he may cry briefly, look at his knee, and tie his handkerchief around it; and at time $T + 3$, he may quickly hold his knee tightly, assess the damage, put on a Band-Aid, and eventually call his mother. At all four times, the problem is the same, but the response to it shows an increase in complexity and cognitive involvement. To document such developmental changes appears worthwhile, especially from an adaptational point of view, where individual differences are clearly observable. Children move at variable rates through cycles of problem solving, learning (or retention of prior successful problem solving behavior), and habit (immediate employment of the successful response). The degree of cognitive mediation may vary considerably between children and over the cycle: This we will not know for certain, but we will know what behaviors the child engages in when facing problems, as well as whether or not the problem diminishes in frequency over time. It should be noted here that problem episodes which elicit rapid responses suggest that the individual has had experience with such problems. In PROBA these episodes are labeled "bit problems" and analyzed separately from those episodes that require slower and usually more complex responses. An episode involving a bit problem, for example, would be a child's immediately taking back a toy another child had pulled out of his hand. A problem episode, in contrast, would involve the child's crying, attempting to take back the toy, and claiming that it is his. A response to a bit problem need not be successful, as in the case of a child who has acquired the habit of complying immediately with her mother's commands.

A number of elements are posited here as essential to the PROBA scheme. The observer, focusing on one individual, records, along with general contextual information (time, place, activity engaged in, etc.), five basic elements: (1) ongoing behavior the individual is engaged in that is interrupted by the block; (2) the block itself (i.e., the stimulus conditions the observer judges to be responsible for the interruption); (3) the individual's response to the block; (4) whether the block is removed or not by the response; and (5) whether the ongoing behavior is renewed or not. All five elements constitute a problem or problem episode.

Ongoing behavior is usually categorized on the basis of pilot observations. For example, in the home setting study with preschool children, ongoing behavior was categorized as playing, socially interacting, caring for the body, dressing, eating, self-stimulating, toileting, locomoting toward a goal, looking intently at something (casual looking excluded, attempting to acquire an object, and doing nothing. These categories were checked every 60 seconds until a block occurred. The block was recorded in narrative form, along with the response to it. After the block was recorded, ongoing behavior was checked again, or a new category was checked if the ongoing behavior was not renewed.

The block, as already noted, can consist of a wide range of events produced by different sources. As will be seen in more detail later, blocks can consist of such events as others' making demands on the individual, another person's asking the individual a question or requesting the individual to do things, the blocking of the individual's physical movements by objects or the absence of needed objects; blocks can also be situations that demand information from the individual or situations that elicit curiosity and questioning.

The reaction to the block can consist of any response the individual engages in to remove it. For example, responses can include attempting verbally or physically to compel another person to do something, using physical force, complying with the wishes or demands of another, asking questions, searching for a desired object, refusing to comply with another's impositions, or going through many related and unrelated verbal steps. Whatever the observer judges to be the individual's response (there may be more than one response) is recorded in narrative form, or with one word when the response is a relatively simple, high-frequency response such as "ignores," "refuses," "complies" (with a command), or "cries."

Whether the response to the block removes it or not is also recorded. If a block is repeated after an interval, it is also noted. Finally, as already mentioned, a note is made after the episode with the block indicating whether the original ongoing behavior was renewed or not.

On the basis of approximately 1,000 problem episodes, a classificatory scheme was developed in order to organize problems or blocks into a taxonomy. Two major dimensions were posited. One dimension consisted of the content of the problem in terms of the substantive nature of its source; the other dimension consisted of the determinants of the block. The content was divided into three categories—social, physical, and informational. Social blocks were defined as involving other persons; physical blocks as involving objects or object-related phenomena such as having accidents; and informational blocks as involving information or knowledge. All three categories of blocks were assumed to be cognized by the individual and all three were assumed to elicit some form of cognitively mediated responses. A response to a social block, for example, might involve a careful mental weighing of many alternatives (a problem), whereas a response to an informational block, such as a request for information, might involve a quick, one-word answer (a bit problem).

The second dimension for organizing blocks dealt with the determination of the block. Determinants were broken down into two classes—impositions and needs. An observable interruption of ongoing behavior was labeled an *imposition*: A person might interrupt another's conversation and demand an explanation that the latter is forced to provide; a window might not immediately open, and the individual might struggle with it; a novel sound might startle the individual and elicit an orienting response followed by a search for the source of the sound. In the case of needs, the individual was observed to be in such a state of need that searching or seeking behavior resulted. The individual would seek social contact, look for a drinking fountain, consult research literature for certain information. In all instances the responses reflect the individual's need regarding the object of search and the lack of anything immediately present to satisfy this need. (If the object is immediately present, there is no problem.)

The PROBA scheme, as developed here, has a number of advantages from the ethologist's point of view. First, it contains observational units that are objective and still general enough to document environment-behavior events at different developmental levels as well as across different cultures. Such a feature makes comparative analysis possible. Second, the scheme includes elements that allow predictions of blocks as well as prediction of responses to them and the outcomes of such responses. This feature makes possible functional analyses as well as identification of learned modifications of adaptive behavior over time. Third, the scheme provides data on how individuals cope under everyday conditions. These data can be related to standard indices of cultural adaptation—for example, performance on developmental tests in early childhood, achievement tests in school-age children, job performance and social and personal adjustment in adults, and more "biological" adaptation, having to do with health, reproductive success, and longevity.

Empirical Findings

To date, research involving PROBA has concentrated mainly on developing procedures for carrying out field observations with different subject populations and constructing a method for coding and classifying the observations. Work on this procedure is continuing. In the process of establishing the PROBA method, it was possible, however, to obtain reliable data of general interest to those working on substantive issues of problem solving. Reliability consists of interobserver agreements on the identifying and recording of the various elements of the problem episode of 80% or more and intercoder agreements of 90% or more in coding and classifying the narrative portions of the observational protocols. Summary findings from six projects are presented next as illustrations of the application of PROBA to a variety of subject populations—toddlers, preschoolers, physically handicapped schoolchildren, and undergraduate honors students. Analysis of the findings to date have been limited, for the most part, to establishing frequencies of the five problem elements (ongoing behavior, block, response to block, efficacy of response, and outcome) and relationships of the elements to contextual and subject variables. No attempt has been made to examine the possible functional value of problem solving episodes, developmental changes in blocks and block removal behavior, or the connection between problem solving behavior and various measures of adaptation. This work still has to be completed.

Project I

A 2-year longitudinal observational study was done of problem solving behavior in response to problems encountered by four toddlers (1½ to 3½ years old) in their homes and surrounding neighborhoods. Total observation time was 180 hours.

This study was carried out in order to develop the PROBA scheme for observing and coding narrative recordings made during field observation. Toddlers were chosen as the first sample for at least two reasons—the relative simplicity of their behavior and life situations compared to those of older children, and the fact that earlier field observations focusing on the developmental onset of tool-using behavior revealed that children over 18 months of age were capable of engaging in instrumental behavior that observers could agree was mediated by cognitive processes. Since the approach was basically inductive and we were not certain how detailed our observations should be, vast amounts of detailed information on problem episodes were collected.

Sample Findings. It was possible to train observers and coders of observers' narratives to reach agreement of 80% or more in the identification and description of the various PROBA elements. A scheme was progressively developed over the 2-year period for classifying blocks and responses, interpreting narratives, and in general, for working out a methodology to deal with the complexity of observed behavioral events. During the first year, the four children collectively experienced 271 blocks (ca. 2.3 per hour), as defined by the first version of the scheme. In the second year, using the second version of the scheme, observers reported that the children encountered 1,069 blocks (ca. 17.8 per hour). This 2-year difference was not due only to the difference in recording schemes. During the first year, 37% of the blocks were social, compared to 60% in the second year; and during the first year less than 2% were informational, compared to 17% in the second year. Being asked questions and asking questions constituted the vast majority of informational problems. Very few instances were observed, suggesting complex or multistep cognitive processing. Responses to blocks included complying with or ignoring social impositions, crying, manipulating objects, seeking help, and verbalizing. Approximately 14% of the blocks were removed by the child during the first year, compared with 33% during the second year; the remaining blocks were removed by parents, parents and child together, sibs, or someone else. The findings revealed individual differences in the frequency and nature of problems encountered and responses employed to deal with them. From a methodological standpoint, the project demonstrated that it was feasible to study problem episodes in the field and that a comprehensive picture of the episodes required a complex and painstaking process of re-cording, identifying, and classifying elements. This process has still to be sim-plified and streamlined to practical proportions without risking obtaining an incomplete or unrepresentative sample of the individual's problems and behavior.

Project II

An observational study (Spiker, Note 3) was made of problem solving behavior in response to problems encountered by six preschoolers (3½ to 4½ years old) in the preschool setting. Total observation time was 45 hours.

This study was carried out in order to describe the preschooler's problems and problem solving behavior during ordinary school activities by using a simplified version of the method used in Project I.

Sample Findings. The six children exhibited variability in the problems they encountered and in the ways they dealt with them; individual differences were stable across the observational period. On the average, approximately 6% of the 3-hour preschool day involved problems. Problems ranged in frequency between 47 and 67 across children during 450 minutes of observation. Problem solving time on the average was less than 30 seconds and problems occurred most frequently during playtime or in social groups involving peers or peers and adults. On the average, 63% of the blocks encountered were social, approximately 28% were physical, and the remaining 8% were informational. The children were generally more successful than nonsuccessful in removing the blocks to ongoing behavior—57% of the blocks were removed by the child alone or with the help of the teacher or another child. Social blocks were removed 44% of the time, physical blocks 78% of the time, and informational blocks 77%. Social problems consisted mostly of object or territory disputes, verbal requests or commands, and being ignored or physically interrupted by another person; physical problems consisted mostly of objects' being unavailable, difficulty in getting dressed, accidents, and general gross and small motor difficulty in doing things; informational problems consisted mostly of not being able to remember something or simply lacking information. Response to social problems consisted of the pulling, lifting, manipulation, and the like of objects, and of using tools. Informational responses consisted of overtly searching for something, asking information from another, or providing another with requested information.

Project III

Observational study, with video and audio records (Charlesworth et al. Note 2), of informational problem episodes consisting of questions (impositions) and answers (needs) encountered by 21 preschoolers (4½ to 5½ years old) and 2 teachers was conducted during 69 science lessons in the preschool classroom. Total observation time was 15 hours.

This study was carried out in order to document all questions asked during the science lessons, whether they were answered or not, and in what manner. Size of the groups in which the lessons took place was also studied. There were three group sizes—large (18-21 children and 2 teachers), medium (5-7 children and 1 teacher), and individual (1 child and 1 teacher). It was hoped that precise objective descriptions of questions and answers as indicators of cognitive demand and functioning would be helpful in operationalizing the procedures for cognitive enrichment provided by preschool curricula.

Sample Findings. During the 69 lessons, the children asked a total of 930 questions, each child averaging 7 questions per hour. The two teachers together asked 1,673 questions, each averaging 55 per hour. Of the children's questions, 66% were requests for information; 93% of these were lesson related, most being in the form of a request for specification or confirmation of something that occurred during the lesson (unrelated questions dealt with content outside of the lesson). Thirty-four percent of the children's questions were social and mostly involved requests for permission or bids for attention. Of the teachers' questions, 84% were requests for information; of these, 95% were lesson related and consisted of requests for elaboration, specification, and confirmation. Sixteen percent of the teachers' questions were social and most involved requests for action and permission. Whether questions were answered or not depended on who posed the question to whom and in what size group. Approximately half of the children's questions, when asked in groups, were answered by the teachers, whereas over 70% were answered when the children were in individual sessions. About three-quarters of the teachers' questions were answered, regardless of group size. The most significant finding was the relationship between group size and questioning and answering: Children asked significantly more information-seeking questions when in the individual session than when in any of the group sessions. Also, more of the children's questions were answered during the individual session than during the group session.

Project IV

An observational study (Charlesworth et al., Note 1) was made of one Down's syndrome (DS) girl and one normal (N) child (both 22 months old) in their homes. Total observation time was 32 hours.

This study was carried out with the express purpose of comparing the two children (separated by 57 points on the Bayley Infant Scale) in terms of the problems they experienced during an "average" day and how they dealt with the problems.

Sample Findings. The two children experienced different frequencies of problems—the DS child encountered 328 problems (or 814 blocks—a problem can consist of a number of blocks) compared to the N child who encountered 535 problems (or 1,350 blocks). Of the 16 observation hours, the DS child spent 77 minutes on problems, or 8% of the total time, compared to 155 minutes or 16% spent by the N child. Social blocks consisted of 96% of the total for the DS child compared on problems, or 8% of the total time, compared to 155 minutes or 16% spent by the N child. Social blocks consisted of 86% of the total for the DS child compared to 89% for the N child. Two percent of the former's blocks were physical, compared to 6% of the latter's. Informational blocks constituted 11% of the DS child's problems, compared with 4% of the N child's, because the former's mother spent considerable time drilling her child on picture identification problems. The DS child asked no questions, whereas the N child asked three. Problem solving success, as measured by percentage of blocks removed, did not differ significantly between the two children; the DS child removed 36% of all blocks, compared with 41% removed by the normal child. After the block was removed, both children resumed the ongoing behavior disrupted by the block to roughly the same degree—the DS resumed 31% of her ongoing behavior as compared to 28% for the normal child. In general, in some respects the children did not differ from each other. Neither child encountered very complex problems, although the N child had more complex problems involving more blocks than the DS child and spent more time with them. A cursory examination of the DS child's problems revealed that they were more elementary than the normal child's problems. For example, the former was frequently asked to eat, bite, chew, talk to someone, and play patty-cake, whereas the N child was asked to eat with a fork, drink from a cup, say "Thank you," call Daddy to come from the other room, and turn the light on. Such problems and behaviors are considered forerunners of more complex and cognitive demanding episodes to come at a later age.

Project V

An observational study (Raison, 1982) was done of 23 physically handicapped and 23 physically normal children (6 to 14 years of age) in a mainstream and special school setting during typical classroom activities. Total observation time was 105 hours.

This project was undertaken as part of a larger project intended to assess the classroom activities of physically handicapped children and to relate such assessments to individual achievement, curricular features, social climate, and other factors with the ultimate aim of improving education for the handicapped.

Sample Findings. On the average, the handicapped children encountered 7.2 blocks per 5-minute observation period, compared with 5.9 encountered by normal control children. This difference, which was significant, was due (1) to the greater number of informational demands made on the handicapped children than on the normals (the demands were usually in the form of the teacher's asking the child to, say, read, identify, or write something), and (2) to the significantly greater physical needs experienced by the handicapped, such as the need for pencils, paper, and the like, and to accidents caused by the inability to move around objects, hold materials, and so on. The handicapped also received significantly more unsolicited help than the normals did in solving their problems. Responses to the blocks by the handicapped and normals were remarkably similar, the former complying significantly less frequently to requests to perform certain physical acts. Success at block removal was similar for the handicapped and normal children, except that the handicapped had significantly more physical needs removed than the normals. Ongoing behavior of the handicapped consisted of significantly more interactions with the teachers than was the case with normals, who engaged in significantly more peer interaction.

Project VI

Self-observation (in daily records) was done of problems encountered by 12 undergraduate honors students during 2 to 5 days of typical everyday activities. Total observation time was approximately 30 days.

This project was undertaken to test the feasibility of expanding PROBA to include self-observation and self-report on the part of trained adults whose activities could not be observed or monitored in any other fashion.

Sample Findings. Problem episodes included not being able to decide what to wear in cold weather, running out of eggs for breakfast, being told to be quiet, being curious about a course grade, having to answer tough test questions, worrying about a future job, having to write a difficult term paper, not knowing what is wrong with a sick pet cat, being asked by a friend for advice, difficulty finding library materials, getting a sore throat, getting lost driving across town, forgetting how to make garlic bread, difficulty keeping up with others on the basketball court, being asked to move the family car, not knowing if everyone is at home before locking up, and having difficulty reading an Old English assignment. Most of the problems could be classified as needs or impositions and as social, physical, or informational, although some students had difficulty doing so. Frequency of problems ranged approximately from 20 to 60 per day. Informational problems constituted a substantial percentage of the total and were related to schoolwork, carrying out daily chores, or meeting social obligations.

Comments on the Projects

The forgoing findings give an account of the kinds and numbers of problems various groups of individuals faced in their everyday settings and the responses they made to such problems. In the first five projects, an attempt was made to sample exhaustively and objectively problem episodes during prescribed observational periods. Such sampling made it possible to establish qualitative descriptions and quantitative estimates of the cognitive demands that faced the individuals and of the responses they made to them during the normal course of the day. The most surprising finding was that a great preponderance of problems was social and only a relatively few were similar to those used in standard test and experimental settings. For example, problems requiring tool-using solutions were exceedingly rare. What was less surprising was that individuals varied greatly as regards the number and kind of problems they encountered and how they solved them. Such variation, we expect, would be related to variation in standard assessments of developmental progress as well as in indices of early adaptation, such as school performance, interpersonal relations, and general mental health.

In the undergraduate project, there is no way of knowing how valid and exhaustive the self-observations and reports are. Given the relative simplicity of the PROBA scheme and lack of expectations of what would occur, one would think that much of what was reported was true. Underreporting, however, could have occurred because of lack of attention or failure to record fast enough. Also, the actual fre-quency of blocks could have declined over time as a consequence of being aware of them. A number of students reported that becoming aware of blocks and their responses to them motivated them to take a better look at themselves and to work hard in order to reduce their problems. One advantage of the self-report method is that it is possible for investigators to get some idea of problems that are anticipated and solved, so to speak, before they occur behaviorally. For exam-ple, a frequently reported block consisted of remembering that something had to be done at a later date and then making an appropriate effort to ensure that it was. That self-reports varied across individuals in frequency and detail was expected. Terse reports such as those noting in a few words that test questions had to be answered, or that it was difficult to read an assignment, obviously do not reveal anything of the cognitive processes that are involved in dealing with them, but the knowledge that such problems occurred and an estimate of how frequently they occurred is worth having. Such knowledge takes on special significance when related to external indices of success and failure on cognitively demanding life tasks.

While the developmental aspect of problems and problem solving has not yet been adequately investigated, it is clear that successive observations over an individual's life will help shed light on the environmental factors involved in cognitive change and adaptational success. One would expect that, in general, many simple problems decline in frequency over time and are replaced by a smaller number of more complex ones. Using PROBA terms, problems would give way to bit problems, which in turn would disappear as a result of changes in the individual's ability to anticipate them.

Conclusion

As already suggested, the ethological approach, at least as it is expressed in PROBA, has its disadvantages. The process of acquiring compilations of problems and problem solving behavior and of their contexts and consequences is generally tedious, at times very inconvenient, and often not possible with segments of the population who view it as intrusive and unethical. However, systematic exploration of the everyday process of human adaptation is necessary if we wish to understand the occasions and functions of cognitive behavior and how such behavior develops over time. Asking the question "What is going on in the everyday cognitive domain of individuals?" is no less important than asking "Is what is going on consonant with current views of cognitive functioning?" The latter question implies some grounding in a theory that already specifies what is important to study and how to study it, whereas the former question assumes that no theory exists and none can exist until there is some empirical basis upon which to formulate it. PROBA is loosely theoretical in that it posits problems and cognitively mediated responses to problems as important dimensions of cognition in general and of cognitive development in particular. PROBA is atheoretical in the sense that it operates with commonsense definitions of terms and provides no hints as to the connections between problems and problem solving behavior and external indices of adaptation. An illustration of the implications of remaining atheoretical in this sense can be derived from some comments made by Lorenz.

Lorenz (1981) notes that theologists can make a special contribution to the behavioral sciences by demonstrating that a broad survey of the phenomenon under study is necessary before any scientifically worthwhile hypotheses can be generated for more rigorous test. Without such a survey, misleading inferences about the nature, origin, and function of a behavioral trait can easily be made. A recent example illustrates this point very well. For decades, tool using has been viewed as a critical, if not decisive, factor in hominid brain evolution. However, as Lovejoy (1981) points out, this view is seriously being challenged by data on primate reproductive behavior which strongly suggest that the unique reproductive (and hence social) behavior of humans appears more important than tool using in initiating and sustaining significant evolutionary changes. Humphrey (1976) comes to a similar conclusion as a result of observing monkeys in social groups. Whether this new hypothesis will become more attractive remains to be seen, but this is not the point. The point is that the division between the disciplines of cognition and social behavior has been bridged by taking a broad view of adaptation which requires observing all aspects of animal behavior, especially those outside of standard test and/or experimental conditions. In PROBA terms, much significant problem solving may well take place in response to social blocks, and the only way this can be demonstrated as worth pursuing further is by observing the full range of cognitively mediated events in everyday life.

In a discussion of historical movements in the philosophy of science and its current condition, Toulmin (1972) argues that philosophers of science should shift their concerns from the "acceptability" of scientific propositions to their "applicability." By *acceptability* Toulmin means that empirical propositions are conventionally evaluated and judged as acceptable or unacceptable in terms of a priori definitions and logical position within the paradigms that cultivated them; by *applicability* he means that such propositions are evaluated in terms of the standards and requirements of human undertakings and scientific disciplines outside of their paradigms. Toulmin's argument is also appropriate for cognitive psychology today. The acceptability of current definitions of cognitive processes in terms of our standard conceptions of them, or of their empirical existence as demonstrated by laboratory manipulations, characterizes only part of the quest for understanding them. The other part of the quest, the part that emphasizes the adaptive (or maladaptive) role that cognitive processes play in mediating everyday behavior and contributing to developmental changes in adaptation, still has to be undertaken. This undertaking requires extensive and systematic field research as well as a conscious openness to other disciplines, pure and applied, that have as their main objective the understanding of human adaptation and the educational and therapeutic efforts that flow from such understanding. The vacuum alluded to above within evolutionary theory, the particular propensities characterizing the efforts of psychologists during the first century of their science, and the needs of those working in therapy and education for better understanding of the role of cognitive mechanisms in the everyday process of human adaptation can be filled by assiduous, systematic field research. The particular conceptual framework and methodological commitment of modern ethology, with its special emphasis on the context, frequency, function, and long-term adaptive value of cognitively mediated behavior, can contribute to this quest.

Acknowledgments. Preparation of this chapter was made possible by support from Program Project Grant 1 PO1HD 05027 from the National Institute of Child Health and Human Development. Special thanks go to the PROBA workers—the first wave of pioneers, Andrea Bie, Kathy Binger, Sheri Daniels, Debbie Fausch, Susan Frey, Lana Kjergaard, Nancy Sonstegard, and Donna Spiker; and the second wave, Peter Clark, Peter LaFreniere, Diana Morgan, Don Nemcek, Jean Nimmo, and Susan Raison. Final thanks go to Paul Callagy for the last-minute assistance.

Reference Notes

1. Charlesworth, W. R., Kjergaard, L., Fausch, D., Daniels, S., Binger, K., & Spiker, D. A method for studying adaptive behavior in life situations: A study of everyday problem solving in a normal and Down's syndrome child. *Bureau of Education for the Handicapped Report #6*, October 1976.
2. Charlesworth, W. R., LaFreniere, P., Nemcek, D., & Clark, P. Asking and answering questions: Observations of preschoolers and their teachers in various size lesson groups. Unpublished manuscript, 1982.
3. Spiker, D. *An observational study of problem solving behavior in six preschoolers.* Unpublished manuscript, University of Minnesota, 1976.

References

Barker, R. G. *Ecological psychology: Concepts and methods for studying the environment of human behavior.* Stanford, Calif.: Stanford University Press, 1968.
Barker, R. G., & Wright, H. F. *Midwest and its children.* New York: Harper & Row, 1955.
Bindra, D. *A theory of intelligent behavior.* New York: Wiley, 1976.
Bindra, D. Comments on papers by Charlesworth and Trevarthen. In M. von Cranach, K. Foppa, W. Lepenies, & D. Ploog (Eds.), *Human ethology: Claims and limits of a new discipline.* New York and London: Cambridge University Press, 1979.
Bitterman, M. E. The evolution of intelligence. *Scientific American*, 1965, *212*(1), 92-100.
Bonner, J. T. *The evolution of culture in animals.* Princeton, N.J.: Princeton University Press, 1980.
Brainerd, C. J. A review of *Beyond universals in cognitive development* by David H. Feldman. *Developmental Review*, 1981, *1*, 63-81.
Bronfenbrenner, U. *The ecology of human development.* Cambridge, Mass.: Harvard University Press, 1979.
Brunswick, E. *Perception and the representative design of psychological experiments.* Berkeley, Calif.: University of California Press, 1956.

Charlesworth, W. R. Human intelligence as adaptation: An ethological approach. In L. Resnick (Ed.), *The nature of intelligence*. Hillsdale, N.J.: Erlbaum, 1976.

Charlesworth, W. R. Ethology: Understanding the other half of intelligence. *Social Science Information*, 1978, *7*(2), 231-277.

Charlesworth, W. R. Ethology and sociobiology: Contributions to the study of mental retardation. In P. H. Brooks, D. McCauley, & R. Sperber (Eds.), *Learning and cognition in the mentally retarded*. Baltimore: University Park Press, in press.

Charlesworth, W. R., & Bart, W. Some contributions of ethology for education. *Educational Studies*, 1976, *7*(3), 258-272.

Charlesworth, W. R. & Spiker, D. An ethological approach to observation in learning settings. In R. Weinberg & F. Wood (Eds.), *Observation of pupils and teachers in mainstream and special education settings: Alternative strategies*. Minneapolis: University of Minnesota, Leadership Training Institute/Special Education, 1975.

Griffin, D. R. *The question of animal awareness: Evolutionary continuity of mental experience*. New York: Rockefeller University Press, 1976.

Griffin, D. R. Prospects for a cognitive ethology. *The Behavioral and Brain Sciences*, 1978, *4*, 527-538.

Heider, F. *The psychology of interpersonal relations*. New York: Wiley, 1958.

Higgins, J. V., Reed, E. W., & Reed, S. C. Intelligence and family size: A paradox resolved. *Eugenics Quarterly*, 1962, *9*, 84-90.

Humphrey, N. K. The social function of intellect. In P. Bateson & R. Hinde (Eds.), *Growing points in ethology*. Cambridge, Mass.: Cambridge University Press, 1976.

James, W. *Principles of psychology*. New York: Holt, Rinehart & Winston, 1910.

Jerison, H. J. *Evolution of the brain and intelligence*. New York: Academic Press, 1973.

Johnston, T. D. Contrasting approaches to a theory of learning. *The Behavioral and Brain Sciences*, 1981, *1*, 125-173.

Klein, R. G. *Ice-age hunters of the Ukraine*. Chicago: University of Chicago Press, 1973.

Lockhard, R. B. Reflections on the fall of comparative psychology: Is there a message for us all? *American Psychologist*, 1971, *26*(2), 168-179.

Lorenz, K. *Studies in animal and human behavior*. Cambridge, Mass.: Harvard University Press, 1971.

Lorenz, K. *The foundations of ethology*. New York: Springer-Verlag, 1981.

Lovejoy, C. O. The origin of man. *Science*, 1981, *211*(23), 341-350.

Lumsden, C. J., & Wilson, E. O. *Genes, mind, and culture: The co-evolutionary process*. Cambridge, Mass.: Harvard University Press, 1981.

Maier, N. R. F., & Schneirla, T. C. *Principles of animal psychology*. New York: McGraw-Hill, 1935.

Mason, O. T. *The origins of invention*. Cambridge, Mass.: M.I.T. Press, 1966. (Originally published, 1895).

Mason, W. A. Windows on other minds. (Review of *The question of animal awareness* by D. Griffin). *Science*, 1976, *194*, 930-931.

Mills, W. *The nature and development of animal intelligence*. London: Fisher Unwin, 1898.

Patterson, G. R., & Cobb, J. A. A dyadic analysis of aggressive behaviors. In J. Hill (Ed.), *Minnesota Symposia on Child Psychology* (Vol. 5). Minneapolis: University of Minnesota Press, 1971.

Patterson, G. R., Littman, R. A., & Bricker, W. Assertive behavior in children: Toward a theory of aggression. *Monographs of the Society for Research in Child Development*, 1967, *32*(5-6, Serial No. 113).

Piaget, J. *The origins of intelligence in children.* New York: International Universities Press, 1952.

Piaget, J. *The construction of reality in the child.* New York: Basic Books, 1954.

Piaget, J. *Behavior and evolution.* New York: Pantheon Books, 1978.

Ragle, D. D. M. *Problems and problem-solving behavior of children in an American town.* Unpublished doctoral dissertation, University of Kansas, 1957.

Raison, S. *Coping behavior of mainstreamed physically handicapped students.* Unpublished doctoral dissertation, University of Minnesota, 1982.

Razran, G. *Mind in evolution: An east-west synthesis of learned behavior and cognition.* Boston: Houghton-Mifflin, 1971.

Reed, S. C. The evolution of human intelligence. *American Scientist*, 1965, *53*, 317-326.

Romanes, G. J. *Mental evolution in animals.* New York: AMS Press, 1884.

Romanes, G. J. *Mental evolution in man: Origin of human faculty.* New York: Appleton, 1889.

Sackett, G. P. (Ed.). *Observing behavior* (Vol. 1). Baltimore: University Park Press, 1978.

Sears, R. R., Maccoby, E. E., & Levin, H. *Patterns of child rearing.* Evanston, Ill.: Row, Peterson, 1957.

Stern, W. *Die Intelligenz der Kinder und Jugendlichen.* Leipzig: Johann Ambrosios Barth, 1920.

Thorndike, E. L. Animal intelligence: An experimental study of the associative processes in animals. *Psychology Monographs*, 1898, *2*(4).

Thorpe, W. H. *Origins and rise of ethology.* New York: Praeger, 1979.

Tinbergen, N. On aims and methods of ethology. *Z. Tierpsychol.*, 1963, *20*, 410-433.

Tinbergen, N. Ethology and stress diseases. *Science*, 1974, *185*, 20-27.

Tolman, E. C. *Purposive behavior in animals and men.* New York: Appleton-Century-Crofts, 1932.

Toulmin, S. *Human understanding.* Princeton: Princeton University Press, 1972.

Weinberg, R., & Wood, F. (Eds.). *Observation of pupils and teachers in mainstream and special education settings: Alternative strategies.* Minneapolis: University of Minnesota, Leadership Training Institute/Special Education, 1975.

White, N. F. (Ed.). *Ethology and psychiatry.* Toronto: University of Toronto Press, 1974.

Willems, E. P., & Rausch, H. L. (Eds.). *Naturalistic viewpoints in psychological research.* New York: Holt, Rinehart & Winston, 1969.

Wilson, P. J. *Man the promising primate.* New Haven: Yale University Press, 1980.

Wright, H. F. Observational child study. In P. Mussen (Ed.), *Handbook of research methods in child development.* New York: Wiley, 1960.

Author Index

Subject Index

C